An Archive of Skin, An Archive of Kin

AMERICAN CROSSROADS

Edited by Earl Lewis, George Lipsitz, George Sánchez, Dana Takagi, Laura Briggs, and Nikhil Pal Singh

An Archive of Skin, An Archive of Kin

DISABILITY AND LIFE-MAKING DURING
MEDICAL INCARCERATION

Adria L. Imada

UNIVERSITY OF CALIFORNIA PRESS

University of California Press
Oakland, California

© 2022 by Adria L. Imada

Portions of chapter 2 were published previously as "Promiscuous Signification:
    Leprosy Suspects in a Photographic Archive of Skin," in *Representations*
    138, no. 1 (2017). DOI: https://doi.org/10.1525/rep.2017.138.1.1.
Portions of chapter 4 were published previously as "Lonely Together:
    Subaltern Family Albums and Kinship during Medical Incarceration," in
    Photography and Culture 11, no. 3 (2018). DOI: https://doi.org/10.1080/175
    14517.2018.1465651.

Library of Congress Cataloging-in-Publication Data

Names: Imada, Adria L. (Adria Lyn), author.
Title: An archive of skin, an archive of kin : disability and life-making
    during medical incarceration / Adria L. Imada.
Other titles: American crossroads ; 62.
Description: Oakland, California : University of California Press, [2022] |
    Series: American crossroads | Includes bibliographical references and index.
Identifiers: LCCN 2021038202 (print) | LCCN 2021038203 (ebook) |
    ISBN 9780520343849 (hardcover) | ISBN 9780520343856 (paperback) |
    ISBN 9780520975200 (ebook)
Subjects: LCSH: Leprosy—Patients—Social conditions. | Leprosy—
    Hawaii—History. | BISAC: HISTORY / United States / State &
    Local / West (AK, CA, CO, HI, ID, MT, NV, UT, WY) | HEALTH & FITNESS /
    Diseases / Skin
Classification: LCC RC154.5.H3 I43 2022 (print) | LCC RC154.5.H3 (ebook) |
    DDC 616.99/8—dc23
LC record available at https://lccn.loc.gov/2021038202
LC ebook record available at https://lccn.loc.gov/2021038203

30 29 28 27 26 25 24 23 22
10 9 8 7 6 5 4 3 2 1

CONTENTS

PREFACE: ENCOUNTERING
THE PHOTOGRAPHS

Readers opening this book may be surprised, disturbed, angered, or elated to encounter clinical photographs of people taken at leprosy institutions in Hawaiʻi beginning in the 1890s, so I begin with a pause. If you have ancestral ties to ka pae ʻāina o Hawaiʻi (the Hawaiian archipelago), you may be distressed seeing how the process of medical incarceration filed people away and consigned them to social death. Perhaps, however, a photograph brings the face of a relation into focus for the first time. Or you may take comfort in witnessing how patients bestowed care and attention on one another. I cannot anticipate your response. These photographs open up encounters for viewers that I cannot predict, as I could not for myself.

Each leprosy surveillance photograph, now housed at the Hawaiʻi State Archives, is placed in a separate file. Mounted on thick cardboard, the photograph retains a heft and particular smell. Over a period of about five years, I held and touched each of the approximately 1,400 clinical photographs one at a time. Tina Campt has suggested photographs are more than seen; they may resonate with a sonic frequency.[1] My encounters with these images also went beyond the visual to the haptic. Touching each photograph was an encounter with a person. It is hard not to feel moved by the collective weight of these images and the experiences of the people within.

Seeing people in the leprosy detention hospital adorned with fragrant lei ʻawapuhi (ginger blossom garlands) or the face of Cecelia, a young girl who was removed from the district where I grew up, I have cried sloppily in the air-conditioned archives. I know now to stash tissues in my pockets. I also have chuckled at the insolent, sideways, or even flirtatious glances made in front of the medical camera. Other images required much more pause and contemplation—people whose skin revealed open ulcers and who likely were in states of pain, distress, or confusion.

At the risk of offending certain viewers, I have chosen to publish a selection of clinical photographs in this book. These photographs were essential to medical and political processes that transformed people into racialized pathogens and removed them from civil society. I integrate these photographs into my analysis, including as much contextualizing and biographical information as possible to situate a person in broader relationships with kin, communities, land, and water.

A fuller elaboration of the ethics of viewing medical photographs, as well an explanation of the speculative guides, protocols, and consultation upon which I relied, is in the introduction. In conversations with people, some reacted as if the photographic archive were a mortuary unearthing sacred bones. "Hawaiians do not show iwi [bones]," a Kanaka ʻŌiwi (Native Hawaiian) scholar and friend took care to remind me.[2] Other friends with ties to the current Kalaupapa, Molokai, settlement advised me on selecting photographs that would balance analysis with regard for personhood.

Clinical images from what I call an archive of skin reveal bodies in vulnerable states. However, I deliberately excise nudity from photographs and crop images to discourage voyeuristic staring at disfigurements associated with leprosy (Hansen's disease). I indicate where these alterations have been made. Some readers may wish to bypass the clinical images altogether (particularly in chapters 1 and 2) and move directly to patient-centered kinship practices in chapters 3 and 4, and the epilogue.

These photographs are also much more than representations of death, however. While the colonial-medical state violated people in the creation of this carceral archive, the photographs live on as performances by those imaged within. They resonate with violence, grief, and care, signaling the life-making that persisted after medical exile. If you forge past the more difficult medical surveillance photographs, you will see incarcerated people bestowing care upon one another and taking their own sorrowful and funny photographs. They posed with pets, friends, and lovers with wit and humor. One man who was exiled for decades joked about his condition, calling leprosy "leperoses," or the "handsome disease." Like him, people survived exile by laughing and crying.

As much as this book offers interpretations of skin and its significant consequences, I hope to move us to other ways people recognized and claimed each other beyond the surface of the skin. Kimo Armitage, in his novella *The*

Healers, offers one such way of apprehension. The character Laka is a contemporary practitioner of Hawaiian medicine who was born without arms and legs in the Kalaupapa leprosy settlement. Laka's mother had been exiled there after contracting leprosy. Returned to his extended family outside, Laka was raised as their most treasured and brilliant child. He became a celebrated healer. When his nephew Keola comes to seek training as a healer, Laka asks, "Does my appearance scare you?" Keola replies, "No . . . it inspires me that even though you have no arms or legs you have become one of the most renowned healers of Hawaii." From the unspeakable loss of Laka's mother to the leprosy prison emerged Laka, the "wondrous child" of life and healing.[3]

NOTE ON LANGUAGE

In this book, I refer to the Indigenous people of the Hawaiian archipelago as Kānaka 'Ōiwi, Kānaka Maoli, Kānaka, Native Hawaiian, or Hawaiian. Kānaka 'Ōiwi are people whose iwi (bones) are the land. Signifying indigeneity, "Hawaiian" does not reference Hawai'i as a place of residence, but signals a genealogical relationship to 'āina (land).

Following modern Hawaiian orthography, I use diacritical marks—the 'okina (marking a glottal stop) and the kahakō (a macron indicating a long vowel)—for Hawaiian-language terms. I do not italicize words in 'ōlelo Hawai'i (Hawaiian language), in order to avoid marking an Indigenous language as foreign. Words such as "Hawaiian" are English words and therefore do not require diacritical marks. Since nineteenth-century and early twentieth-century sources written in 'ōlelo Hawai'i did not employ diacritical marks, I have preserved the original spelling of names and words in these sources, with the exception of prominent names and places that follow contemporary spelling conventions.

Makanalua, the northern peninsula of Molokai island, was the site of two leprosy settlements: the original Kalawao settlement on the eastern side of the peninsula from 1866, and Kalaupapa, on the western side, where patients began moving in the early 1900s for its more hospitable climate. As this book spans a period when one or both locations were operative, my term "Molokai settlement" is inclusive of Kalawao and Kalaupapa sites.

While colonial biomedicine, incarceration, and stigmatized illness are not transhistorical concepts, I have sought to calibrate descriptions of these experiences in specific historical contexts with the political and cultural preferences of contemporary people.

In 1873, the Norwegian microbiologist Gerhard Henrik Armauer Hansen identified the bacterium that causes leprosy, a minimally communicable bacterial disease. Nearly a century later, in the 1960s, "Hansen's disease" became the term adopted by leprosy patients, their advocates, and some doctors to refer to leprosy. Many patients began to repudiate the stigmatizing and pejorative term "leper." I choose to use "leprosy" when situating Hansen's disease in any historical period prior to this shift. I also avoid using "leper" except when quoting directly from sources. While some might object to the latter term under any circumstance today, other patients adopted a looser, pragmatic vocabulary. John Kaona, interviewed at Kalaupapa settlement in 1987, said, "The doctors gave it the name Hansen's Disease, 'eh? . . . Now, people ask you, 'What is Hansen's Disease?' . . . Me, I just tell them, 'I am a leper.'"[1]

I utilize a range of terms for people who were imprisoned in Hawaiʻi's leprosy institutions, but generally prefer "incarcerated person," which imparts personhood that is retained during incarceration. However, I make use of "inmate" and "prisoner" when emphasizing the carceral aspects of people's capture by colonial biomedicine.

The use of "patient" is not generally in favor today, as it tends to authorize physicians and biomedicine to diagnose, pathologize, and cure over people defining their own experiences of illness and health. However, "patient" is the preferred colloquial term in the present-day Kalaupapa, Molokai, community, referring to someone who was exiled under the Hansen's disease policy prior to 1969. "Patient" is not patronizing as it may have been previously in leprosy management, but denotes a person deserving of elevated regard and respect by the settlement community and beyond. It does not mean this person is a medical patient or is disabled, but incorporates the phenomemology of having suffered because of one's previous medical and legal status, as well as belonging to a shared culture of survival.

CHRONOLOGY OF SIGNIFICANT EVENTS

1820s–1840s   Appearances of illness in Hawai'i that may have been leprosy

1863   Papa Ola (Board of Health) of Kingdom of Hawai'i discusses rapid spread of leprosy

1865   "An Act to Prevent the Spread of Leprosy" passed by Kingdom of Hawai'i legislature

1866   First group of exiled patients arrive at Molokai

1878   Arrival of first resident physician to Molokai settlement

1893   Overthrow of Kingdom of Hawai'i

1898   Annexation of Hawai'i by United States

1900   Organic Act passes; Hawai'i made an incorporated territory of United States

1905   U.S. Congress passes appropriations bill funding leprosy investigation station in Hawai'i

1909   U.S. Leprosy Investigation Station at Kalawao, Molokai, opens

1913   U.S. Leprosy Investigation Station at Kalawao, Molokai, closes

1921   National Leprosarium established at Carville, Louisiana, by U.S. Public Health Service

1941   Clinical trials of promin (sulfone drug) begin at Carville; established as a cure by 1947

1946   Sulfone drug treatment introduced to Hawai'i

1959   Hawai'i becomes fiftieth state of union

1969   Termination of Hawai'i leprosy isolation policy

1980   Kalaupapa established as national historical park by U.S. Congress

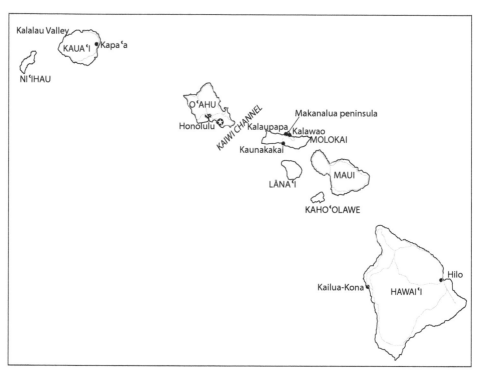

Main islands of Hawaiʻi. Molokai lies less than thirty miles southeast of the most populous island of Oʻahu. The leprosy settlements of Kalawao and Kalaupapa were established on Makanalua, the northern peninsula of Molokai.

Introduction

AN ARCHIVE OF SKIN, AN ARCHIVE OF KIN

I BEGIN WITH THE PHOTOGRAPH of a young boy named Keliiahonui, who was born around 1897 in the Hawaiian Islands (figure 1). His clinical photograph, taken at the Kalihi Hospital and Detention Station in Honolulu on September 11, 1903, marks his official appearance as a leprous person in the Hawai'i Board of Health archive when he was six years old. Keliiahonui was one of approximately eight thousand people with who were sentenced to lifelong incarceration at a remote settlement on the island of Molokai.[1] Photographs like his were foundational to modern medical knowledge and a criminal system of medical segregation.

When Keliiahonui was captured as a leprous suspect by the colonial state, he was also "captured" by the medical photograph. Although there were diverse photographic conventions of patient imaging, Keliiahonui was photographed against a plain background with most of his clothes removed to reveal his somatic stigmata. This photograph marked his transformation from a person to a prisoner-patient; he entered the realm of civil and legal death. His photograph resides today in a file at the Hawai'i State Archives in Honolulu, where I was able to handle the yellowing albumen print. Filed by a single case number, the photograph is organized by the year of his medical examination, 1903. This photograph is a material trace of Keliiahonui's once living presence. Decades after his death in 1914 in the Molokai settlement, his exact grave is unknown.[2] Each photograph represents a person and a life interrupted by medical surveillance and incarceration.

Outbreaks of leprosy in Hawai'i began to cause alarm in the early 1860s, following waves of devastating smallpox and measles epidemics that decimated the population.[3] According to the law passed in 1865 by the Kingdom of Hawai'i legislature, people believed to have leprosy were

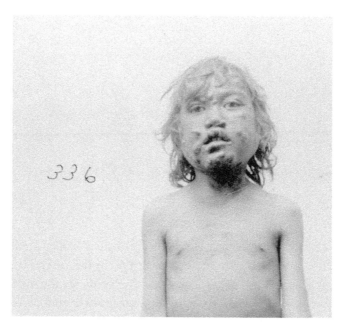

FIGURE 1. Clinical photograph of Keliiahonui, cropped from original full-length. Kalihi Hospital case 336, September 11, 1903, six years. Hawaiʻi State Archives.

removed from their homes and medically inspected. If confirmed as leprous and incurable, they were to be exiled to a "place of isolation" within the Hawaiian archipelago.[4] The kingdom's Board of Health selected Makanalua, the northern peninsula of the island of Molokai, for this purpose. Although Molokai is the island closest to the main island of Oʻahu, they are separated by the rough Kaiwi Channel (map 1). The forbidding cliffs and limited landing shores of Makanalua created a natural prison and discouraged escape (figure 2).[5]

Among the numerous names given by Hawaiians to this place of exile were "luakupapaʻu kanu ola" (grave where the living are buried), "luahi o ka make mau loa" (fiery pit of endless death), and "lahui i hoehaeha" (nation of great agony).[6] Incarcerated patients became subject to the full authority of the Board of Health and its agents. If a person was married, a diagnosis of incurable leprosy gave a non-leprous spouse legal grounds for uncontested divorce.[7] Parents with leprosy had to leave their non-leprous children behind. The settlement was a place where people were left to die of a disease that was then incurable.

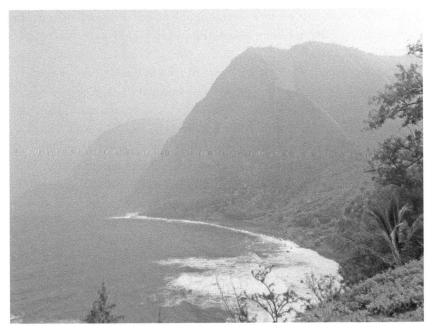

FIGURE 2. Shoreline of Makanalua peninsula, Molokai, near original Kalawao leprosy settlement. Photograph by author.

Leprosy afflicted Natives, settlers, and immigrants of all economic and social backgrounds, but the majority of exiled men, women, and children were Kānaka ʻŌiwi (Native Hawaiians), the Indigenous people of the Hawaiian archipelago.[8] Hawaiians referred to this new illness as "mai Pake" (Chinese sickness), possibly because the first Chinese contract laborers arriving in the 1850s recognized its symptoms or because a Chinese person had this illness.[9] The alarming spread of this so-called Chinese leprosy among Native people was first discussed in the kingdom's Board of Health proceedings in 1863. Less than three years later, the first group of people was exiled, all twelve of them Kānaka ʻŌiwi.

Although referring to "Chinese leprosy," the kingdom's leprosy laws originally focused on Kānaka ʻŌiwi, not Chinese.[10] Immigrant laborers from Asia and Portugal became ensnared in these sanitizing logics as global migration to Hawaiʻi increased in subsequent decades. Thus Chinese, Japanese, Portuguese, Korean, and Filipino settlers and their descendants also were exiled, as well as people of mixed racial backgrounds. European and American settlers constituted the smallest number of incarcerated people. Responses to leprosy in Hawaiʻi shifted over several decades from a disease believed to primarily afflict Natives to one found disproportionately in its "native and oriental" populations.[11]

The Hawaiʻi segregation policy began in 1866 and ended over a century later in 1969, making this the longest and most severe practice of medical incarceration in modern history. The Molokai leprosy settlement incarcerated over six thousand people in its first forty years, from 1866 to 1906, becoming an influential global site for the compulsory removal and lifelong detention of leprosy patients.[12] The outbreak and management of leprosy in Hawaiʻi was closely watched, reanimating global concern about this ancient disease.[13] Other nations turned to Hawaiʻi as a medical-carceral model. Legislation establishing compulsory leprosy segregation was passed in Norway in 1885, the British colonies of New South Wales in 1890, Cape Colony in 1891, Ceylon in 1901, the Philippines in 1901, Canada in 1906, and Japan in 1907.[14]

A disease known but little understood for millennia, leprosy is understood by scientists today as communicable through slow-growing bacteria in respiratory droplets. Leprosy is now known as Hansen's disease, named for the Norwegian bacteriologist Gerhard Henrik Armauer Hansen, who discovered the bacilli in 1873. Leprosy is not highly infectious; transmission requires long-term exposure to untreated patients. It may take decades to manifest.[15] It is also difficult to diagnose, with symptoms confused with eczema, vitiligo, psoriasis, and other skin conditions. However, because *Mycobacterium leprae* affects the peripheral nervous system, the disease can cause nerve damage in the coolest parts of the body—the hands, feet, skin, and eyes—sometimes with disfiguring effects. It can cause deformation of nostrils and facial tissue, loss of fingers and extremities, paralysis of eyelids, blindness, and chronic pain.[16]

Perhaps because leprosy can dramatically deform the face, as Susan Sontag has suggested, the illness became associated with the loss of personhood and bodily integrity in a Western context. A "dreaded" disease like leprosy instills different responses of shame and revulsion than a "lethal" disease.[17] For Western observers in the nineteenth century, leprosy instilled far more dread than tuberculosis, although the latter killed far more people.[18]

The interpretation of leprous bodies as non-human, perverse pollutants became powerfully animated and attached to racial-sexual difference during Western colonial expansion. Represented via disabled raced bodies from the colonies, leprosy provoked stigma and panic in the West in the high age of empire. Leprosy was resignified as an "imperial danger" and "tropical disease" spread by colonized people to white Europeans in the nineteenth century, although it had been endemic in parts of Western Europe and reappeared in England in the 1840s.[19] This linkage between leprosy and racial contamination prompted compulsory forms of removal and segregation.[20]

Whereas people with leprosy in medieval Europe were often relocated in leprosaria outside of towns, this exclusion was adapted and codified as a system of permanent and compulsory segregation in colonial regimes.[21] Leprosy institutions in the age of empire, rather than providing shelter or relief for the sick, shifted to establishing a cordon sanitaire that isolated the infected from the well.[22] In Hawai'i, a legal-medical code institutionalized the radical and racialized exclusion of all those determined to have leprosy. How was this removal of thousands of Native Hawaiians from their natal homes made possible?

For decades prior to annexation by the United States in 1898, settler occupation and colonial pressure subordinated Hawai'i law, health, trade, and land tenure to the West.[23] The Hawaiian Kingdom, in an attempt to appear respectable and civilized in the "family" of modern Western nations, adopted a legal system modeled on the West that transformed its governance and society.[24] This transition to Western law privileged white foreigners, who were familiar with these systems of governance. By the 1840s, these foreigners occupied powerful leadership positions in the Hawaiian government.[25] Some of these prominent settlers later participated in the U.S.-backed overthrow of Hawai'i's monarchy in 1893 and supported American annexation of the quasi-colony in 1898.

This transfer of authority from Hawaiian chiefs to Euro-American settlers was starkly apparent in Papa Ola, the kingdom bureaucracy known in English as the Board of Health (BOH).[26] Missionary descendants and non-missionary settlers dominated the ranks of the Papa Ola leadership. Only physicians trained in Western medicine received licenses to practice medicine in the kingdom, effectively displacing and delegitimizing kāhuna lapa'au (traditional Hawaiian medicine practitioners) and their expertise.[27]

Established in 1851 by the Hawai'i legislature as Native Hawaiians were beset by deadly epidemics, the Papa Ola acted as a key biopolitical instrument of the state to protect and ensure life. Biopower, as analyzed by Michel Foucault, is the power of "making live and letting die." It operates by "optimizing the capacities of a population through interest in health, fecundity, illness and longevity."[28] The exercise of biopower in Hawai'i prioritized the economic investments of the white settler oligarchy and preservation of law and order. Fearing damage to the mercantile and sugar plantation economy, white settlers urged the strict containment of leprous people.[29]

Viewing the hefty budgets, voluminous reports, and files dedicated to eliminating the leprosy problem in the kingdom, one might conclude reasonably that leprosy killed more people than any other disease. No other public health problem received as much sustained attention and infrastructure as leprosy within the kingdom, the quasi-U.S. colony, and (as of 1900) the territory of Hawaiʻi. Yet relative to contemporaneous diseases, leprosy was far less lethal. It was not a significant enough public health threat to warrant the systematic carceral response I discuss in this book.

Outbreaks of mumps, smallpox, venereal disease, measles, and influenza since Western contact in 1778 had led to the decimation of the Native Hawaiian population.[30] By 1915, pneumonia and tuberculosis were the top two causes of death in Hawaiʻi, while leprosy ranked a distant tenth.[31] In comparison with the long simmer of leprosy infections, bubonic plague and smallpox outbreaks in Hawaiʻi were relatively short-lived and episodic. Public health and quarantine efforts directed toward the latter in Hawaiʻi do not exhibit the frenetic attention paid to leprosy. In the broader context of fin de siècle United States, influenza and tuberculosis were far greater public health threats than leprosy, each killing nearly two hundred thousand people, while there were only 278 confirmed cases of leprosy.[32] So why did health agents and settlers in Hawaiʻi mount such a bulwark against leprosy? Anxieties about leprosy encompassed concerns far beyond health, disease, and economics.

COLONIAL EXCHANGES AND OBSESSIONS

Leprosy took on geographic and racialized associations as a tropical disease emanating from the Pacific region in the late nineteenth century.[33] From the vantage point of Europeans and Americans living in metropolitan and colonial zones of contact, leprosy was a highly contagious, incurable, and racially contaminating disease prevalent among a range of non-white peoples: Indigenous Pacific Islanders, Asians, "Negroes," and inhabitants of the Indian subcontinent.[34] The disease's very ambiguity was perturbing: the more knowledge produced about leprosy, the less seemed to be certain.

Disturbing the boundaries between the visible/invisible, clean/dirty, colonized/colonizer, able/disabled, settler/Native, leprosy became a colonial obsession. Physicians could peer at leprosy bacilli under a microscope as early as 1873, but the transmission of the microbe was frustratingly elusive. Health agents in Hawaiʻi and contemporaneous sites in the British Empire debated whether the disease was hereditary or spread by sexual contact, food, soil, or blood. Visible under the microscope, but hidden beneath the skin and in the body, leprosy bacteria could emerge as infections years later, confounding scientists. With leprosy's unpredictable incubation period, a person could appear "clean" or uninfected while potentially harboring and spreading these germs.

Leprosy thus became an apt metaphor for the duplicitous colonial subject. The German microbiologist Eduard Arning unwittingly conflated the uncontrollable leprous body and the unruly Hawaiian body in 1884 when he wrote, "[W]e must look upon every single leper as a hot-bed of disease . . . He, at any rate, breeds and multiplies a poisonous germ; and is, on this account, dangerous."[35]

Nathaniel B. Emerson, a son of American missionaries and the Molokai leprosy settlement's first resident physician, expressed similar bewilderment peering at people's skin, behavior, and moral character. In his clinical notebook, Emerson assessed a thirteen-year-old Hawaiian boy in 1880: "This boy's skin is perfectly clean and free from speck or flaw. And it hardly seems possible that this handsome, healthy and clean boy is a leper." Emerson could not bring himself to trust his own sight: those who appeared "clean" and beautiful could be polluted where the eye could not reach.[36] This boy passed Emerson's inspection and never became sick. However, twenty-five years later, the now-grown boy would see his only daughter sentenced to the Molokai settlement and die there.

Leprosy also became intertwined visually and discursively with promiscuity and immoral sexuality in Hawaiʻi's intimate, porous zones of contact. In this colonial imaginary, leprosy was a dangerous racial-sexual invasion crossing the threshold from soiled to "clean" bodies, a contention that I explore in chapter 3. Hawaiians and immigrants were culpable agents, spreading leprous germs through wanton sexual contact and non-conjugal domestic intimacy. George Fitch, an American-born government physician posted at the Molokai settlement, and his colleagues insisted that leprosy and Native sexual deviance must be related. "The disorder has been allowed to run on unchecked and uncontrolled," Fitch asserted, because of the "uncontrolled licentiousness" of Hawaiians.[37]

While principally represented as a germ spread by contaminated Native bodies, leprosy also remained a visible reminder and symptom of the fallibility and erotic excesses of nineteenth-century colonial society, a society that would not be fortified easily by a cordon sanitaire. Leprosy was a libidinal haunting, a symptom of white civilization's erotic weaknesses. White (male) settlers willfully transgressed by having sex with, living in intimate proximity to, and marrying Native women. Although emerging from putatively repulsive and immoral Native bodies, leprosy contaminated white bodies because white men could not control their own bodies and desires. Concluded Martin Hagan, an Ohio-born physician who had joined the ranks of Hawai'i's government physicians, "Emigrated Americans and Europeans having intimate intercourse with the lepers, sooner or later take the disease."[38]

CARCERAL MEDICINE

The U.S. Supreme Court ruled in Jacobson v. Massachusetts (1905) that vaccinations could be mandated by the state, citing smallpox epidemics and the greater public welfare. This decision confirmed the legal authority of police power in matters of public health. Yet Hawai'i had already severely curtailed individual liberties and criminalized contagion on a wide scale four decades prior to this case. The 1865 Act to Prevent the Spread of Leprosy granted "full power" to health agents to confine and exile all leprous people. The euphemistic terms "conveyance," "isolation," and "seclusion" in this legislation fail to convey the forced removal, containment, and natal alienation experienced in Hawai'i. I rely on *incarceration* to designate the widespread, overlapping practices and institutions of colonial carcerality in which leprosy control was enmeshed, including insane asylums and juvenile reform schools.[39]

Medicine practiced in a colonial society, as Frantz Fanon cogently argued, cannot be separated from the colonialism that enabled it. The colonial condition enabled physicians to gain access to the bodies and culture of colonized subjects.[40] More specifically, I delineate Western biomedicine's role in these carceral practices. Hawai'i's leprosy regime conjoined medicine and law in a carceral system.[41] This system produced and depended on what I am calling *carceral medicine*—a juridical-medical system that worked to incarcerate particular bodies and produce knowledge about those bodies. Carceral medicine worked within and alongside the service of Hawai'i's settler-colonial state to control, subordinate, and sanitize threatening and non-normative bodies, the majority of whom were Native Hawaiians and non-white immigrants.

Disparate personnel—physicians, health agents, bacteriologists, nurses, and missionaries from North America, Britain, Germany, France, Japan, and Spain—lent their expertise and labor in this medical regime as formal and informal state actors. Some were chief architects and administrators of leprosy institutions, mapping influential policies for detention, incarceration, and parole. Others labored for many years on the ground.

A methodical surveillance and detention system was made possible by a grid of government physicians and district sheriffs. Government physicians, all Westerners licensed in Western medicine, were posted in twenty-six different island districts.[42] These physicians had private practices, but also were appointed by the Board of Health. They were responsible for reporting suspicious cases of leprosy to the board and providing monthly reports.[43] "On the constant, vigilant outlook," doctors and district sheriffs dispatched "suspects" to Honolulu, where they were admitted and examined at the city's receiving station and hospital.[44]

Physicians then consigned people to one of three medical-juridical categories that determined a person's freedom and un-freedom: "Not a Leper," "Leper," and "Suspect," as I detail in chapter 2. A "leper" was someone who was "incurable or capable of spreading the disease of leprosy." Those in this category were exiled to the Molokai settlement for the rest of their lives. A "suspect" was someone who was a "doubtful" case or "not in sufficiently advanced stages" to spread the disease. Suspects could be detained or recalled for future inspection. Despite their projected rigidity and authority, these categories could be porous and ambiguous, as I discuss in chapter 2.

In addition to government physicians, still others benefited from the carceral regime as short-term medical tourists who gained unfettered access to leprosy prisoners for experiments, visual curiosity, and private ethnographic research. As historian Regina Kunzel has analyzed, the twentieth-century American prison became a "laboratory of sexual deviance."[45] Leprosy institutions were productive carceral laboratories for foreigners to scrutinize disease, race, indigeneity, and sexuality in a captive, colonized population. An exemplar I deliberate in chapter 1, the German dermatologist and bacteriologist Eduard Arning, experimented on prisoners, photographed Hawaiians, and collected material culture in the early 1880s in an ambitious bid to salvage medical and cultural data from disabled Hawaiians. His access to a range of Hawaiian subjects, he admitted, was afforded because he was a physician. Arning wrote, "This role of physician brought me trust and sympathy, which I could put to good use."[46]

In total, these diverse practices of carceral medicine were similar to and contemporaneous with other Western state technologies that catalogued, organized, and studied criminal or non-normative raced bodies, such as late nineteenth-century German anthropological photographs of races of men; nascent criminal "mug shot" photographs; and the French criminologist Alphonse Bertillon's detailed descriptions of criminal bodies placed in a vast filing cabinet at Paris police headquarters.[47] The Italian physician Cesare Lombroso's studies of "criminal man" and "criminal woman," which included galleries of inmate photographs, tied bodily non-normativity to moral depravity.[48]

People with leprosy were treated and imaged as patients, inmates, and deviant criminals in Hawai'i, as I analyze via overlapping visual and textual representations. The mundane accounting of the Kaka'ako Branch Hospital in the 1880s lists its "inmates present," with a Dr. Clifford B. Wood serving as physician and quasi-warden. The succeeding Kalihi Hospital was surrounded by a fence, but detained men and women climbed through it to fraternize with friends, lovers, and family in Honolulu. Instead of erecting a higher fence, the Board of Health resolved to discipline recalcitrant patients by sending them to Molokai.[49] After the United States incorporated Hawai'i as a territory in 1900, people residing in the settlement were enumerated as "institutional inmates" in the U.S. census.[50] Mirroring and intensifying the language and practices of imprisonment, patients released in the twentieth century were not merely discharged; they were released on "parole" and photographed as parolees.[51]

AN ARCHIVE OF SKIN

These carceral practices lead us back to the child Keliiahonui's clinical photograph. While his clinical photograph first entered him into a criminal registry of leprosy suspects in 1903, a year later this same photograph surfaced far beyond Hawai'i in the influential *Journal of the American Medical Association* (figure 3). Even later, the photograph was repurposed for a public health lecture by the pathologist who led the National Institute of Health.[52] After Keliiahonui's exile to Molokai in 1903, he was also photographed in the settlement, probably by a French-born Catholic priest serving as a medical missionary. This latter image later appeared in early to mid-twentieth-cen-

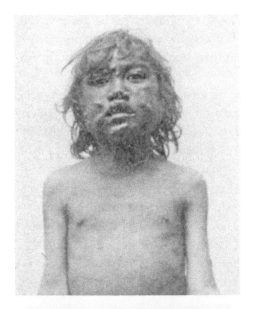

FIGURE 3. Keliiahonui, captioned as "Tubercular Leprosy in a Young Native Girl," in Senn, "Leprosy in the Hawaiian Islands," *Journal of the American Medical Association,* August 13, 1904. Cropped from original.

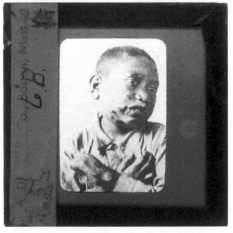

FIGURE 4. Keliiahonui, Catholic lantern slide, ca. 1910. Slide LS8-48, Congregation of the Sacred Hearts of Jesus and Mary U.S.A. Province.

tury Catholic lantern slides and a French-language biography of the Belgian priest Damien de Veuster (figure 4).[53]

Photographs of Keliiahonui taken during incarceration thus circulated to diverse locales and publics far outside of the Hawai'i leprosy archive during and after his short life. Clinical photographs remained indefinitely in the archive, taking on a life of their own even after the people they indexed had died. The dispersed photographs provide us a sense of how far and wide images of incarcerated patients moved through time and space. Keliiahonui is but one person, but he represents thousands of other Hawaiʻi patients who were photographed and archived by the state and then seen and interpreted by transnational medical, religious, and lay publics through the twentieth century.

What distinguished this modern regime of medical incarceration from previous ones was its intense investment in visual technologies. The camera was adapted and put to effective use for carceral medicine, and a vast, prolific archive of leprous bodies emerged from the colonial-carceral state, as I detail in chapter 2. This book begins in a visual culture of leprosy that I call an *archive of skin,* an archive that exposed and organized raced-sexed bodies into intelligible and visible entities. What was this archive of skin? More than any other colonial or "tropical" location, Hawaiʻi produced spectacular images of leprosy patients that were collected, archived, and displayed. Despite this broad circulation, we know remarkably little about the production and institutional contexts of these visual archives of skin and even less of their meanings.

Every leprous suspect captured in Hawaiʻi from at least 1898 was photographed individually during medical examinations at a Honolulu detention facility and entered into the Board of Health's leprosy files. This visual cataloguing of Indigenous and Asian bodies constitutes one of the most extensive in America's Pacific empire. Approximately 1,400 of these images survive from a fifteen-year period between 1895 and 1909, but there were likely thousands more shot as the practice continued at least until the 1950s.

These are portraits of criminality and disability—repressive portraits, to borrow Allan Sekula's phrasing.[54] Photographs established important medical and legal evidence for lifelong incarceration and exile, confirming a clinical diagnosis of leprosy and documenting a suspect's somatic condition upon capture. Above all, the photograph dominated the clinical record. The photograph was the central part of the leprosy case file in Hawaiʻi, traveling with a patient's clinical file, sometimes for decades. Unlike contemporaneous identification systems that relied on textual descriptions, the case files were less "commitments to paper" than commitments to *images.*[55]

The Hawaiʻi Board of Health archive of skin is distinct as a genre of medical photography because it was instituted and financed by the colonial state. American physicians made and collected photographs of unusual clinical cases as early as the 1840s for diagnosis and documentation.[56] However, the Hawaiʻi archive was far more extensive and deliberate than an assembly of pathological images taken by individual physicians. Analyzed in chapter 2, this archival practice required funding, preprinted forms, equipment, time, and storage of the proliferating image-documents: a state apparatus.

Why such an investment in photographs? Photographs, as a particular kind of "archival form" and power, are distinct from bureaucratic paperwork.[57] Photographs offered the seductive promise of iconicity and indexicality for settler-colonial officials and lay observers. As Susan Sontag and Christopher Pinney have discussed, the photograph is iconic in that its images resemble its referents. But the photograph is also *indexical,* meaning that the image bears a "physical trace of the material world."[58] Sontag describes a photograph's indexicality as "a trace, something directly stenciled off the real; like a footprint or a death mask."[59] The camera, when put to use on patients, was believed to communicate medical truths and capture tracings of the real body. Photographs would extend the omniscient eye of the doctor—the "clinical gaze" opening up the "tangible space of the body," as analyzed by Michel Foucault.[60] The intimate interface between the photographic grain and a patient's epidermis ostensibly would produce scientific objectivity and juridical self-evidence.

In clinical medicine, physicians observe the body and interpret somatic signs for diagnosis, prognosis, and therapy. Mediated representations of the body, such as the visual case study rendered through illustrations, engravings, or three-dimensional models, have been an integral part of Western medical training since at least the medieval period. But in the late nineteenth century, the medical camera became a favored technology for physicians: it was "the scientist's true retina."[61] With its mimetic qualities, photography was put to use in Hawai'i for communicating putatively objective clinical symptoms like lesions, tissue loss, and nerve damage associated with leprosy, though photographs yielded conflicting, ambiguous evidence in practice.[62]

Leprosy appears to be the only disease and disability systematically photographed by the Hawai'i Board of Health and with sustained attention to individual bodies. In contrast to its approach to leprosy, the board documented the contemporaneous 1899–1900 bubonic plague in Honolulu's Chinatown through the geographic space of infection: wide shots of buildings, groups of residents and onlookers, and quarantine camps. Individual sufferers and decedents were not photographed.[63] Once people died of plague, they disappeared, while leprous people, dead or alive, lingered in the archive through narrative records, family histories, and photographs.

The imaging of leprous bodies also took place outside of and parallel to the official state archive. The production and proliferation of images was radically promiscuous, as many non-state actors like visiting researchers and religious caregivers photographed, collected, and distributed images of incarcerated patients for their own diverse purposes. During approximately the same time frame in China, a transnational "circuit community" of Western physicians residing in China collected and exchanged information about Chinese medical subjects, as Ari Heinrich has analyzed.[64] A circuit community in Hawai'i disseminated enough tantalizing visual and ethnographic information about people with leprosy that physicians were inspired to come in person to visually inspect and photograph them in the islands.

Visitors clamored to enter the leprosy settlement. As the British physician Arthur A. Mouritz wrote during his post as resident physician of the Molokai settlement, over forty applicants were turned down and refused permission to enter the settlement, "the chief desire of these people being to see the lepers and take photographs."[65] Although these particular applicants were refused permits, many others did obtain visual access to the bodies of incarcerated people, as Keliiahonui's own imaging reveals. At the Kalihi Receiving Station in Honolulu, which functioned as a medical detention facility, physicians visiting from places like California requested visual access to prisoners. The BOH president granted permission to a doctor in July 1906, writing to the warden, "This will introduce Dr. E.J. Caldwell, of Rio Vista, Calif, who desires to see a leper. Kindly take him about the station."[66]

In its broadest strokes, we might say the visual economy of leprosy encompassed four major, overlapping representational modes at the turn of the century: 1) archiving by the state for medico-juridical and criminal surveillance; 2) ethnographic and biomedical mapping of Hawaiian bodies and disease; 3) tourist and political media and exhibitions;[67] and 4) Catholic religious media. Why is this visual culture important, and how might paying attention to these visual economies shift our understanding of leprosy and disability?

While much has been written about leprosy in world history and in Hawai'i in particular, photographs of incarcerated people seldom are considered. If they do appear, they serve as illustrations of disease, somatic changes, or medical and social conditions, with little contextualization or accompanying analysis.[68] Patient photographs have been largely treated as incidental, rather than constitutive, elements of biomedical knowledge production, medical surveillance, and incarceration. Yet the extraordinary visual culture of leprosy was vital to the ideological conjoining of contagion, race, and disability.[69] It attached disease and disability to the bodyminds of Indigenous and colonized people. In turn, these people's caregiving practices became visible, knowable, and maligned in the United States and places far away.

The archive of skin was an enduring way of seeing and interpreting race, sex, and disability in the Pacific. Taking a careful look at this archive of skin enables us to understand how subordinated colonial subjects and racialized immigrants were imaged, organized, and categorized as criminals, sexual deviants, and piteous wards over a period of about six decades from the late nineteenth to mid-twentieth century. Photographs were valuable state and biomedical resources girding epistemologies of racial-sexual pathology, disability, and alterity. Influential beyond Hawaiʻi's internal leprosy management system, this visual culture populated diverse transnational media, fascinating viewers and resignifying leprosy as a broader racial-sexual contagion emerging from the Hawaiian Islands. These images, more than representing a generic "tropical pathology," mapped leprosy onto Native Hawaiian and Asian immigrant bodies.[70] Thus photographs taught spectators to interpret racial-sexual difference as attached to disease, disability, and bodily non-normativity.

As I seek to illuminate, images of people with leprosy found avid viewers and voyeuristic consumers in diverse locales. These photographs provoked erotic fascination, disgust, fear, pity, and empathy. They *arrested* the viewer far more than textual representations of leprosy: photographs horrified, shocked, and stirred. Images function differently from narrative, as Laura Mulvey has analyzed in the context of cinema. A screen image arrests through visual spectacle, evoking pleasure and horror for the spectator, whereas narrative struggles against powerful visuals to mount a meaningful story and character development. In the archive of skin, patients were visual spectacles defined by their "to-be-looked-at-ness."[71] They suggested and evoked more than was possible in narrative. Well into the twentieth century, the iconography of the raced-sexed leprous body has been as durable as the scientific and religious knowledge it was intended to bolster. This knowledge flooded outward to other trans-local sites, informing policies and practices of medical incarceration and ethnographic interpretations of race, sex, and disability.

AN ARCHIVE OF KIN

These images, however, are multivalent and far from fixed. The archive of skin was also what we might call an *archive of kin*. Put another way, two competing knowledge systems and epistemological frames of the body, ability, personhood, health, and caregiving are at work in these images. If the archive of skin disaggregated communities into discrete individual case files that exposed the body in the pursuit of pathological disease and behavior, images visualizing kinship, interdependence, and collectivity operated within, against, and alongside the alienating archive of skin. The archive of kin is a *counter-archive,* then, that reveals affective approaches to personhood and interdependence, pursuing connection over alienation. Most fundamentally, this counter-archive of kin allows us to apprehend continuities of kinship and collectivity during exile.

As a boy of about seven or eight years, Ponepake (also written as Boniface) Lapilio was exiled as a leprosy patient to the Molokai settlement in 1889, along with his older sister Mele Lapilio. They were from Kamō'ili'ili (now known as Mō'ili'ili), Honolulu. Ponepake Lapilio married another patient, a Hawaiian woman named Louisa Lui, in 1902, and they had several children.[72] When his portrait was taken by a Catholic priest in the Molokai settlement about 1906, Lapilio chose to pose with another patient, a man named Bernard Palikapu (sometimes recorded in BOH records as Polikapu). Palikapu had arrived in 1897; he was almost twenty years senior to Lapilio and came from a different island. Palikapu had been divorced from his wife upon his exile to Molokai.[73]

These two men likely had not known each other before their separate arrivals in the settlement, but they grew close, as revealed in this photographic sitting (figure 5). Both men had lived in the male dormitory, Baldwin Home. On this occasion, the twenty-five-year-old Lapilio sits in a chair holding his infant child, while Bernard Palikapu stands above him. Palikapu's hand rests on the younger man's shoulder, suggesting familiarity. Encouraged by the convention of the intergenerational studio portrait, a viewer today perhaps would apprehend these subjects as three generations of the same family, but they were not related by blood or marriage.

The baby in the portrait was either Lapilio's first or second child. Lapilio and his wife Louisa named their second child Bernardo (Benenato) Palikapu Lapilio, that is, the namesake of the elder Bernard Palikapu. Names were chosen with great care and consultation, for they were Hawaiians' most personal and "precious" possession, shaping a child's character and influencing health and happiness.[74] In this act of honorific naming, Ponepake and Louisa Lui Lapilio tied their child's future to the elder man. The portrait further sealed the three subjects as kin.

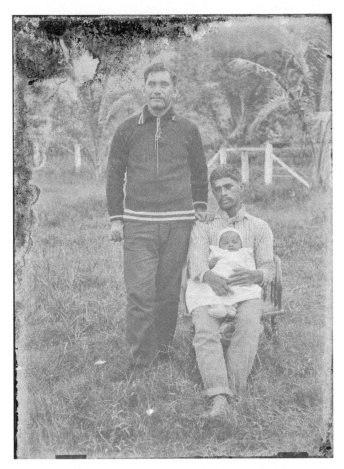

FIGURE 5. Left: Bernard Palikapu. Right: Ponepake Lapilio holding his infant child. Kalaupapa, Molokai settlement, ca. 1906. SG 105, Congregation of the Sacred Hearts of Jesus and Mary U.S.A. Province.

Yet only a few years later, in 1908, the namesake Bernardo Palikapu Lapilio and his brother Joseph William Lapilio were removed from this family and placed in the Kalihi Boys' Home for non-leprous children in Honolulu. Four other Lapilio children born later in the settlement were also removed to Honolulu institutions.[75] Leprosy was experienced as violent disruption as authorities medically, legally, and socially parsed the "clean" from the "unclean." Doctors and social reformers instituted the removal and out-adoption of "clean" children from leprous relations, as well as the sterilization of patients in various time periods to limit reproductive bodies. Catholic missionaries also remade kinship in leprosy institutions through orphanages and surrogate parenting and by encouraging gender segregation and heteronormative domesticity. Children born in the settlement were removed, but also could return to the settlement as inmates if they were later diagnosed with leprosy.

Hawaiian descriptions of leprosy tended not to focus on disgust or revulsion, but interpreted leprosy as a performative condition—that is, as an affliction that performed great suffering and transformations on one's social relationships. Hawaiians referred to leprosy as "mai hookaawale ohana" (illness that separates families), "mai hookae a ka lehelehu" (illness despised by the public), and "mai aloha ole" (illness without mercy), among other names, because a person would be cut off from natal communities and exiled. The archive of skin merged the pathology of the disease with the person, but Hawaiians still perceived the person while the body changed.

Although patient-centered kinship like that of Ponepake Lapilio can be approached as a significant kind of counter-knowledge, the archive of kin also is a fraught and ambivalent site. I hesitate to treat it as a celebratory repository of patient "agency" apart from the colonial state or biomedical regimes.[76] The desires and subjectivities of those within this archive remain elusive and partial; these "counter-colonial" desires were neither clearly oppositional nor accommodating to the colonial state, as I have theorized previously.[77] Following Laura Wexler's analysis of the state's investment in making certain kinds of families visible, I resist romanticizing the archive of kin as an archive of recovery, dignity, and agency, for the "family" or Indigenous kinship was not autonomous from state practices of regulation and violence.[78]

Leprosy surveillance and incarceration put immense pressure on the unit of the family. In the minds of Western physicians, health agents, and bureaucrats, it was Hawaiians' social and cultural practices of kinship that made them culpable for the spread of disease. They interpreted the proliferation of leprosy among Hawaiians as an *excess* of aloha (love), kinship, and sexuality: a communal people loving and living together too liberally and refusing to shun sick relations. A Canadian American physician who served as a Hawai'i Kingdom physician wrote in 1886: "The habits and customs of these people disclose the causes of the wide and rapid spread of leprosy among them. The Hawaiians are the most amiable, good natured, social people on earth ... They are always visiting from island to island and congregating together, never excluding any on account of disease, however contagious or loathsome.

They surround smallpox sufferers and kiss, embrace and sleep with lepers without any suspicion of results."[79]

The family thus became a focal point of biopolitical regulation and visual surveillance, with doctors and health agents producing "genealogical grids" such as elaborate family trees, kinship charts, sketches, and photographs of Hawaiian people and families to trace leprosy contagion and sexual practices.[80] Nathaniel B. Emerson, a missionary son and resident physician at the Molokai settlement in 1879, produced prolific ethnographic case notes that splayed open family relationships, conjugality, reproduction, and sexuality. Among the chief questions Emerson deliberated in his leprosy case histories were, "Married? To leper? Children? Are they lepers?"[81]

As this scientific spotlight on prolific forms of kinship suggests, people did not simply die after exile. While leprosy institutions reduced patients to "bare life" or "life unworthy of being lived," to use Giorgio Agamben's formulation, these institutions were far more than mortuaries.[82] They were active and productive sites of *life-making* where babies were born, children and animals were adopted, and new partnerships and relations were shaped and forged. In a Foucauldian sense, power operates through the proliferation of, rather than a repression of, knowledge, and in these carceral institutions, new knowledge, life, affective ties, and kinship emerged.

In my attention to kinship, I turn toward practices of relationality, intimacy, belonging, caregiving, and interdependence, or what Elizabeth Povinelli describes as "intimate forms of recognition."[83] These practices were often illegible or discredited within grids of biological reproduction, disease etiology, consanguineal ties, and lineal descent mapped by state and medical authorities.[84] What did these forms of kinship recognition look, sound, or feel like? Persistent forms of life-making and kin recognition can be apprehended through "visual kinship" and non-visual sensory registers encompassing tactile, haptic, sonic, material, and embodied relations.[85] If kinship was rigidly defined in biomedical and legal contexts as biological descent, affinal ties, and consanguinity, incarcerated people reconceived relatedness through homosocial, a-filial, and lateral networks. They forged conjugal and non-conjugal intimacies, and performed caregiving to adoptive, collateral, and non-human companions. Acts of naming, provisioning, feeding, laundry, leisure, and nursing emerging from the archive of kin can tell us much about non-lineal, non-reproductive relations and approaches to disability.

The multi-sensory archive of kin thus reveals how interdependence flourished outside of biological kinship. As families became sites of violent disruption, displaced and incarcerated people developed life-sustaining forms of kinship and interdependence, however provisionally. Family and friends chose to accompany patients to the settlement as mea kōkua (unpaid helpers), effectively giving up their own civil rights and property to become quasi-wards of the Board of Health, as described in chapter 3. Ponepake Lapilio, after being released as non-leprous, petitioned to become a mea kōkua for his wife in 1909. Patients became caregivers for one another in the absence of cures, adequate nursing, and reliable medical treatments. Gendered acts of laundry, caregiving, and cohabitation have left traces in this archive of kin.

While sited in the Molokai settlement and Kalihi Hospital, this book does not offer a comprehensive history of leprosy institutions in Hawai'i, nor of the lived experiences of people within them. There is a robust literature that reconstructs the social and political lives of people with leprosy in Hawai'i in the nineteenth and twentieth centuries.[86] Although intriguing continuities link Hawai'i to leprosaria in colonial zones across time, those relational claims are beyond the scope of this book. Instead, this book is concerned with kinship and disability culture—visual, material, and affective—forged in the everyday of empire. People were sorted, surveilled, and confined, but they contested these imperial impositions in ordinary and extraordinary ways, producing their own life-making affinities beyond the totalizing effects of carceral institutions.

DISABILITY OR DISEASE?

Disability is another important epistemic framework that accounts for the incommensurability between the carceral management of leprosy and people's kin-based caregiving. In this book I am marking a critical difference between leprosy as a *disease* and leprosy as a *disability*. Far more than a disease, leprosy terrified because it signified a racialized and sexualized disability. As a disability, it imperiled the able-bodiedness and wholeness of a range of differently valued bodies—settler, Native, and immigrant—in settler society and broader publics. Disability was by no means an accidental rubric, but a distinct form of settler-colonial biopolitical management. Douglas Baynton has usefully and explicitly connected race, disease, and disability, arguing that disease and disability often were attached to people racialized as nonwhite.[87] However, the significant relationship between disability and colonialism has not always been made concrete or explicit, although raced-gendered disability and colonialism were often co-constitutive processes.[88]

The construction of leprosy as a disability was valuable indeed in the context of U.S. empire-building. Far from being a twentieth-century Western metropolitan phenomenon, disability was mobilized productively for overlapping legal and medical arguments controlling incompetent and unruly bodies in the U.S. imperial archipelago. The reverend Sereno Bishop, a prominent American missionary son in Hawai'i, for example, pointedly relied on "disability" as an analytical paradigm in 1888 to mark Hawaiians' failure to thrive. Bishop named leprosy as one key component of their disability.[89]

Leprosy commanded attention and fear not only as a disease or medical condition, but also as a *disability* in the context of settler-colonial society and broader publics. That is, by the late 1800s, leprosy was recognized as a stigmatized, raced-sexed social condition identified with the offensive, incompetent, and non-compliant bodies and behaviors of Hawaiians and Asian immigrants. As Baynton has observed, "[T]he *concept* of disability has been used to justify inequality against other groups by attributing disability to them."[90] Susan Schweik also has provided a most useful demarcation of disability as an "intolerable bodily variety and vulnerability," and a form of ugliness in public that requires policing.[91] Leprous bodies were sequestered not as much for their risk to public health, but because their bodily and social differences were perceived as intolerable forms of disability.

Eugenics and the sorting of human bodies based on race/sex/ability/competency intensified the vexed epistemological and ontological problem lying at the core of colonial practices—who was "clean" and who was "dirty"? Who was diseased and who was able-bodied? Who deserved to reproduce and raise children and who did not? Eugenics was forged not only in white supremacy projects that subordinated African Americans, American Indians, and non-European immigrants, but also during fraught encounters and struggles over Native bodyminds and lands. Settler colonialism relied on the representation of disability, incapacity, and incompetency in order to socially and legally exclude putatively weak, irrational, deficient Hawaiians (and in a later period, immigrants) in favor of stronger, able-bodied, reasonable, morally and physically superior Euro-American settlers.

Leprosy incarceration was a particular response to visible forms of disability that disturbed race-sexed boundaries and hierarchies. Note the urgent tone in a 1886 letter written by an American physician informing the Board of Health of a Hawaiian leprosy suspect on O'ahu: "I have just given Pilipo

. . . a thorough examination and find him unquestionably a Leper! He must have been so for a considerable time, his body is covered with tubercles, and it will be but a short time when he will not be *presentable on the street!*"[92] The threshold for Pilipo's apprehension as a leprosy patient was his aesthetic unpresentability in public, not whether he was a public health risk or capable of spreading the infection.[93]

The Molokai resident superintendent and physician George Fitch made similar assertions in the 1880s. Fitch did not believe leprosy was contagious, but still advocated for the strict legal incarceration of patients based on their deformities and "repulsiveness" to people of "ordinary sensibility." He wrote, "[A]s a measure of *public decency,* the community must put the leper away from others by process of law" (my emphasis)."[94] Segregation laws were necessary not because disabled Natives were a medical danger, but because they did not see themselves as loathsome, as Fitch emphasized: "For these people seems [*sic*] utterly incapable of understanding, or feeling, why they should not exhibit themselves in all their repulsiveness anywhere and everywhere." If not for these laws of segregation, they would be seen "on every street and highway."[95] Fitch informed the board he would leave Hawai'i if segregation were abolished.

The Supreme Court of the Hawaiian Kingdom similarly relied on visual metaphors of wholesomeness, beauty, and ability when it ruled the incarceration of leprosy patients was constitutional in 1884. Considering the 1865 Act to Prevent the Spread of Leprosy authorizing the forced removal and isolation of leprous people, the court ruled that the law was "a wholesome law." The court explained that although leprosy was not a crime, without such a law, ". . . these fair islands would become a *pest-house to be avoided by the whole civilized world.*"[96] Thus the BOH retained its exercise of "police power" to protect the able-bodied majority from the unsightly, diseased, and disabled.

People with leprosy threatened because they indexed disturbing values and attachments at odds with those of Euro-American settlers. As living examples of uncontrollable and grotesque forms of disability, these people could spread myriad forms of disablement and unfit behavior to respectable settler citizenry. From this vantage point, Hawaiians afflicted with leprosy did not seem to suffer from embarrassment or shame, and their infections suggested the proliferation of promiscuous and non-conjugal sexual practices. Furthermore, able-bodied people who performed acts of love and care for leprous people were themselves interpreted as disabled, suffering from *blindness,* or a kind of critical misperception.[97]

If we approach disability as a non-compliant way of being in the world, as Disability Studies scholar Karen Nakamura has productively proposed,[98] then we might better understand how Native people and immigrants were poised as susceptible to disability and transgressive behavior in the eyes of Western settlers. Yet many with unconventional bodyminds deployed *non-compliance* as a tactic and creative response to medical incarceration. People refused these assessments of incompetence, failure, and disease. The musician Mekia Kealakai exalted his wife, Akiu Haupu, who had passed away at the Kalaupapa, Molokai, settlement in August 1894 with a kanikau (poetic lament). Kealakai's remembrance, published in a Hawaiian-language newspaper later that month, likened his beloved to a lei (garland) and "an 'ō'ō bird (*Moho nobilis*) with a joyful voice."[99] Apprehended in the archive of kin through remembrances, caregiving, and the claiming of vulnerable bodies, this disability culture defied conventional, state-oriented views of ability, ugliness, and social death.

IMAGINED INTIMACIES

During the same period when leprosy incarceration removed Indigenous people and immigrants with disabilities from public view, another visual economy dominated the Euro-American imaginary of Hawai'i—that of hula and Hawaiian women's bodies. How and why might hula and leprosy be linked? While researching my first book on hula performance in the U.S. empire, I slowly became aware of leprosy appearing in American narrative and visual accounts of Hawai'i at the turn of the century.[100] I began to notice a parallel and sometimes overlapping imaginary of leprosy and hula in illustrated travelogues from the time of the U.S.-backed overthrow of the Hawaiian Kingdom in 1893.

One notable travel guide published in 1897, for instance, spectacularized the bodies of Native Hawaiian women and hula dancers and introduced them as debauched pleasures to Americans (figure 6). In this volume, the American travel writer also warned of leprosy lurking in Hawai'i: "The Hawaiian Islands have been termed by some of their enthusiastic admirers 'The Paradise of the Pacific.' . . . But the Hawaiian Islands are not Paradise. . . . One of the most dreadful diseases known to man haunts that land of beauty."[101] This prose was set next to a photographic montage of Hawaiian women or nonbinary people with leprosy: three clinical portraits of people who show

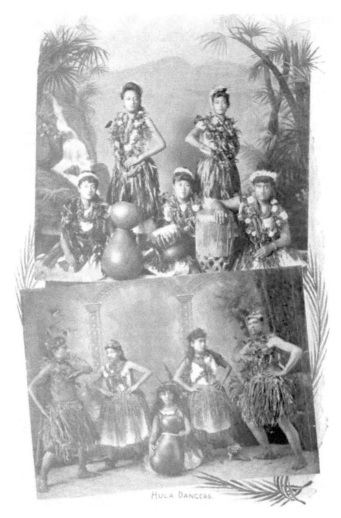

FIGURE 6. "Hula Dancers." Published in John R. Musick, *Hawaii: Our New Possessions* (1898).

advanced disfigurements, and a more ambiguous domestic setting of women holding babies in a non-conjugal household. The infants signified the inexorable reproductive capacity of leprous women. I suspected hula and leprosy were competing visual economies: both hula and leprosy visualized Hawaiians as fascinating subjects capable of intimate relations with outsiders.

However, leprous bodies were imagined as repugnant, while feminized hula bodies were largely desirable. As the United States incorporated the territory of Hawai'i into its political body, the bodies of hula performers mitigated dreaded images of leprous people. Leprosy and hula, then, may be considered entwined parts of what I have termed an "imagined intimacy": hula as an imagined intimacy producing the benevolent integration of Hawai'i and the United States; and leprosy as the nightmare outcome of those intimate and eroticized encounters—what happens if and when leprosy and leprous bodies infect white American bodies.[102]

Another American travel writer amplified this theme of a beauteous, yet risky, paradise, describing Hawai'i as a "Garden of Eden" with a serpent, a shadow, and a "skeleton" in its closet. He concluded, "Hawaii's skeleton is the leper; its closet grim Molokai."[103] We see leprosy represented as the shadow in Hawai'i's closet in the early twentieth century: for a white oligarchy trying to attract economic investment, tourists, and settlers, leprosy was a shameful, stigmatized illness leaving a black mark on the islands' economic development and political future.[104] For those incarcerated and their families, it was often experienced over many decades as a trauma causing great suffering and silences.

Ellipses in the life histories of hula performers began to make better sense when I brought medical incarceration into the same frame. One of the dancers whom I interviewed left Hawai'i in the 1940s to join her cousins in New York City.[105] I only had a vague sense of this woman's motivations for leaving Hawai'i. She had intimated that she had joined the hula circuit as a way for her to connect with her family. While on the road, this young woman called an older Hawaiian dancer her surrogate "mother." As I learned much later, this girl had been separated from her birth mother. Her mother had been diagnosed with leprosy and removed to the Molokai settlement, dying there in 1936.[106]

The characterization of leprosy as a trauma that cannot be easily named or must be hidden away in a closet shares something of a kinship with queerness historically. Like same-sex desire or non-heteronormative forms of sexuality and kinship, leprosy was often treated and experienced as bodily and sexual perversity—a "disqualified" identity, in the formulation of queer studies scholar Heather Love.[107] In carceral-medical practices and a range of literary, visual, and historical media, leprosy became conflated with non-normativity, bodily aberration, and perverse sexuality and kinship. These associations between sexuality and disease indeed did much to lay the interpretative groundwork for the criminalization of HIV over a century later, when gay men and homosexuality became culpable for the spread of HIV, the so-called "gay plague."[108]

In expressions of shame, secrecy, stigma, loss, self-loathing, rejection, invisibility, and melancholy, incarcerated people with leprosy have shared an affective relationship with queerness, even as some actively opposed the illness' associations with perversity and aberration.[109] Hansen's disease (HD) patients in Hawai'i insisted on visibility while agitating for autonomy, better health care, housing, state accountability, and rights in the 1960s and 1970s. Settlement patients had made similar demands from administrators since the late 1800s, but they became impossible for the State of Hawai'i to ignore in relation to a broader Native Hawaiian self-determination movement.[110]

During a dramatic patient-led protest that persisted from 1978 to 1983, for example, HD patients occupied Hale Mōhalu, the Pearl City, O'ahu, facility where some received medical care and lived privately. The state intended to move them to a different hospital. The standoff between HD patients and the state government culminated in the arrest and removal of two disabled patients and sixteen supporters in 1983. Hale Mōhalu was bulldozed, and the patients removed to the new hospital, but this grassroots opposition brought significant publicity and moral and political authority to patients during negotiations over housing, medical care, and the preservation of the Molokai settlement.[111]

In the wake of these struggles, the public scholarship and memorialization of Hansen's disease patients has embraced survival, pride, and the persistence of dignity among patients and their caregivers.[112] This victory over the shame of leprosy echoes "gay pride" activism of the late twentieth century, which disavowed stigma and suffering in the queer historical experience. In "pride" and "coming out" accounts, shame and trauma are conquered through narratives of redemption, recuperation, and sacrifice.[113]

However, I am attempting to relay unresolvable conflicts and a complex range of experiences that do not easily fit into Manichaean terms of victory or defeat, pride or shame. When thirty-eight-year-old patient Richard Marks declared, "I am a leper," on the cover of *Beacon Magazine of Hawaii* in February 1968, he claimed a disqualified identity.[114] Yet this "coming out" narrative was far from triumphant, as Marks expressed rage and frustration at the hypocritical and humiliating treatment of himself and his wife.

Taking a cue from queer and disability studies scholars and the creative labor of HD patients, I historicize these struggles by accommodating anger, violence, humor, trauma, suffering, disability, and forms of persistent survival without offering dignified victories over pain and shame. These approaches may allow us to see people "living with injury," as Love delineates, without having to repair or rehabilitate these injuries or to produce heroes that stamp out shame. I recognize that these are two divergent approaches to history: one that is honorific and restorative, while the one I am offering is multivalent, ambivalent, and necessarily incomplete.

AN ETHICS OF RESTRAINT

If these subjects have been injured and already hypervisible in an archive of skin, can and should they be named and imaged within? How might they be ethically and responsibly included and discussed? Feminist, anti-racist, Indigenous, and decolonizing politics and scholarship insist on ethical orientations: that researchers make their investments, privileges, and blind spots transparent.[115] These questions of accountability and ongoing obligations have animated and unsettled my research process and choices.

As a non-Native descendant of plantation laborers who were settler immigrants to Hawai'i, I often enjoy privileged access as an interpreter of knowledge through entangled webs of immigration and imperialism. If I am to care for the relationships that give Hawai'i life now and in the future, I recognize abiding obligations to not cause harm to the subjects within, their ancestors, collateral kin, and future relations. For although these people may no longer be living in human form, they are far more than biomedical objects or inert sets of data, but persist as cherished relations.

But how might this best be accomplished? To whom might I seek guidance about the protection of people's privacy and whether my research may be beneficial or harmful? Indigenous methodologies have outlined collaboration and engagement with Indigenous communities as decolonial praxis: asking subjects whether your research is beneficial and to produce research for and with subjects.[116] As useful as a starting point these decolonizing principles are, I remain less satisfied with a collaborative methodology centered around living subjects. I have mindfully opted out of active collaborative research, but rather, have drawn upon what I call an *ethics of restraint*. This ethics and praxis of restraint is a deliberate step away from authorizing strategies, that is, the seeking of approval, absolution, or authorization from living subjects.

Specifically, the living subjects are a small cohort of former Hansen's disease patients residing at Kalaupapa settlement. I discuss the transformation of this settlement into a national historical park in the epilogue; formerly incarcerated patients chose to remain in the community after the leprosy segregation law was rescinded in 1969. Today fewer than ten patients reside there. I began this research on Hansen's disease and visual culture assuming I should consult with them, imagining that they would be best positioned to guide my research and tell me which materials they might be comfortable or uncomfortable having discussed.

However, the youngest former patients are now in their late seventies. One of the first and best pieces of advice shared by a non-patient resident when I visited the Kalaupapa settlement in 2013 was that the patients are "talked out." They have been interviewed, documented, photographed, and filmed, and they are aging and fatigued. Some are in fragile health and wish to be left alone in peace.[117] The resident shared this story: a filmmaker came to Kalaupapa settlement and wanted to interview an elderly former patient, whom I'll call Aunty N, on camera. Aunty N initially agreed, but then did not show up at the appointed time and begged off, saying she was sick. The filmmaker then showed up on her doorstep. He kept knocking on the door, but she didn't answer. It was Aunty N's way of refusing the interview.

Informed by this story of refusal and similar ones shared by trusted interlocutors, I did not seek direct interactions or interviews with former patients (a few unexpected encounters are discussed in the epilogue). This is an agential refusal, aligned with Audra Simpson's theorizing of Kahnawake anticolonial "refusal" of anthropological inquiry enacted upon them.[118] My method instead has adopted active forms of distancing and restraint. Whereas the ethnographic research for my first book on hula relied on intimate relationships with older Hawaiian women who shared memories, experiences, and friendship, this research on Hansen's disease is premised on deliberate detachment and deference. I have refused to seek the authorizing presence of "real" patients, a phenomenon echoed in the attraction of dark tourism to sites of tragedy, death, and suffering. Another colleague, an accomplished Kanaka ʻŌiwi historian, drolly calls this phenomenon the "contact high" some non-Hawaiian researchers seek in the presence of Hawaiian subjects, whether dead or alive.

Thus, my form of engagement involves abiding by existing boundaries; my responsibility is not to speak "for" patients or to represent them. However, being aware of boundaries does not mean passive avoidance. During my fieldwork and consultation process, I instead talked to surrogates who work with and have developed deep relationships with patients and people connected to the settlement. They include a settlement resident who is a relative of a patient and has conducted oral histories with patients; the primary care physician who treats people at Kalaupapa settlement; a former state department of health director; a retired Native Hawaiian physician who has worked with patients and staff since the 1970s; and former caregivers—all people who have developed trust with patients past and present. I also have spoken with a range of people about their memories and encounters with Kalaupapa and the Makanalua peninsula: elders who have visited and had pāʻina (informal parties) with patients; kumu hula (hula masters) and cultural practitioners; students who visited the settlement; and people with kinship ties to topside Molokai and Kalaupapa.[119]

I have turned to these surrogates and asked them to weigh in on my choice of materials and photographs. Which stories might be too sensitive for me to narrate? Which photographs do you think might be potentially offensive? Do you agree with my interpretations? While their responses have been invaluable guides, these negotiations and questions are neither straightforward nor settled. Enacting responsibility to one's subjects and interlocutors can become uncertain terrain when people express different or shifting opinions.

SPECULATIONS ON PHOTOGRAPHS

While trying to answer these questions, I remain most uncomfortable and wary about the use and republication of clinical photographs in this study. Over the course of this research, I assembled approximately two thousand extant photographs of leprosy patients in Hawaiʻi from archives based in Hawaiʻi, Germany, Maryland, Philadelphia, and Louisiana. This extensive visual culture was a cornerstone of carceral-medical institutions and a scopophilic visual regime in the nineteenth and twentieth centuries. Who owns or claims photographs taken of people under duress?[120] Does publishing clinical photographs from these archives only serve to reinscribe that epistemic violence? Does the inclusion of images from the archive of skin amplify voyeuristic access to racialized people with disabilities and disfigurements? Would it be better to then withhold all images from readers of this book? I recognize I am caught in a vexing ethical bind with few straightforward answers.

Photographs often are interpreted as more indexical of the body and "speaking" truth more than textual sources, and therefore treated as more problematic, provocative, and ethically suspect. After I placed an order for high-resolution scans of historical clinical photographs in Hawaiʻi, a senior archivist wrote me, asking what I was planning to do with the images. She was concerned about where and how I would use and publish them, and rightly so. Doctors have treated clinical images as captured tracings of a real body. So too, have some patients and their broader relations treated photographs as powerful attachments to material bodies and memories. On the opposite side of the fixed nature of indexicality, however, is speculation. These photographs have produced interpretative speculation and ambiguity from the beginning of their creation and reappearance in multiple contexts.

As another person entering the field of interpretation, I continue to speculate about best ways to analyze images while refraining from the uncritical refiguration of subordinated and disabled people. I have been thinking alongside and conversing with scholars who have adopted diverse, but allied, approaches to what archival studies scholar Michele Caswell calls the "ethics of looking." Disability studies scholar Jay Dolmage has not published any photographs in his book on eugenics and immigration, choosing instead to make some available as a "shadow archive" on the publisher's website. Julie Livingston does not use or publish photographs of Batswana cancer patients in her book, but deliberates narratively on the visual nature of cancer and its treatment. Reflecting on the violent imaging of people of African descent during enslavement, Christina Sharpe includes only a thin band from two famous nude medical daguerreotypes of Delia and Drana taken in 1850. This altered image reveals only the enslaved women's eyes to emphasize "*their looks out and past and across time.*"[121]

I have found my speculations and decisions perhaps most closely aligned with those of Caswell. Referring to an archive of prisoner photographs taken by Khmer Rouge before their subjects were tortured and executed, Caswell includes a few of these standardized mug shots in her book, insisting upon understanding and preserving the context of their creation within bureaucratized state genocide. She concludes viewers "have an ethical imperative to look at these photographs, as long as such looking is properly contextualized."[122] She also usefully positions herself as a "co-witness" shaping historical memory and memorializing genocide.

Most importantly, and specific to the clinical images of people with Hansen's disease that concern the first part of this book, I have discussed the photographs with several patient surrogates and interlocutors. Relying on their suggestions, I have developed a set of tentative and speculative protocols for the photographs included in this book. Selecting particular photographs that allow critical analysis of this history of patient exposure, I avoid publishing the most spectacularized forms of visual stigmata and nude patient photographs, though the colonial archive of skin is replete with these. When it is necessary to analyze how people were imaged without clothing and in vulnerable positions, I crop the original images and explain that I have done so.[123]

I recognize these images may trouble and upset some viewers, but hold to an ethical and political commitment to contextualize and analyze them as best I can. I teach pre-medical students, and I keep them and others in mind as I write. I include some difficult and problematic images in an obscured colonial history of disability and medicine for constituencies like my students, in hopes that we will craft better and more ethical practices of looking at contingent bodies going forward. In order to discourage easy access to the archive of skin, readers will not find photographs inserted in a glossy section in the middle of the book; they are integrated purposefully into the narrative. Each photograph of a person is analyzed, rather than treated as a mere illustration or clinical condition. I also attempt to provide biographical and genealogical information about imaged subjects in order to convey lifeworlds and relationships beyond the experience of illness and incarceration. Family members seeking to learn more about exiled relatives may find these biographies and sources elaborated in the notes.

Moreover, I do not assume there is a single, stable interpretation or valence of medical photographs. These photographic archives of skin are a kind of "encounter with the dead," just as perhaps all photographs are losses in the making.[124] Yet these photographs are far more than a registry of loss. Even during surveillance shots, where people are the most objectified and exposed for the camera, we may see them appropriating the clinical space and enacting performances of care, affection, or indifference. For many, this would be their first time sitting for a photograph, as discussed in chapters 1 and 2. While the medical camera was meant to impart a transition to social death, it is also possible to apprehend intimate relationships and claiming in front of the camera. I attempt to counterbalance such surveillance with photographs of people appropriating photographic technologies for their discrepant purposes. As much as possible, I have traced the images of people across time and space through different archives, so that we may see them acting in multiple social and cultural contexts and in relationship to others.

I also do not wish to overendow the violence and alienation that may be read in the images, for present-day and future viewers may experience a variety of responses that cannot be anticipated. In one mode of contemporary resignification, a clinical image taken at Kalihi Hospital may become an image cherished by a great-grandchild—the only image remaining of a forebear removed from the family. Chamorro scholar Anne Perez Hattori analyzes the reconnection of people from Guam with clinical photographs of Chamorro people removed and incarcerated at the Culion leprosy colony in the Philippines. These descendants perform their own reunification with the people imaged within clinical photographs by imparting names, clans, villages, and relationships to make the photographs speak "anew."[125] This practice of reclaiming connections is also happening in Hawai'i, as I discuss in the epilogue.

All the while, I recognize that the image selection is imperfect, tentative, and may need to be rethought; I am not foreclosing better practices, protocols, considerations, or future discussions. Precepts and principles, however tightly outlined and reasoned, are rarely so neatly executed or received in practice. In committing to ethical research on historical trauma that is unresolved in a community, perhaps the most transparent statement would be to admit that I am unsure and that obligations and responsibilities shift. As in any small community, people have different ideas of best practices; abiding by one person's wishes and values may mean stepping on someone else's toes. I remain grateful, however, to many who shared their 'ike (knowledge), those who told me, "I trust you to make the right decision," and those who gently or not so gently told me to retrace my awkward steps.

ON NAMING, PRIVACY, AND REMEMBRANCE

While photographs pose a significant area of consideration, the use of names is also a concern. Will discussing the experiences of incarcerated people reveal the identities of those who did not wish to be publicly associated with leprosy or inadvertently imperil their descendants? Does a leprosy diagnosis in the nineteenth century count as private medical information that deserves to be protected even if privacy laws in the United States generally do not apply to deceased people?[126] Can the privacy of people, both deceased and living, be balanced responsibly with historical interpretation?[127]

I have sought ethical guideposts and clues to the desires of incarcerated people in early twentieth-century Hawaiian-language newspapers and other forms of public memorialization. Patients exiled in the early 1900s gave their names to writers in the leprosy settlement and allowed them to be published. In 1909, patients in Molokai petitioned the BOH and territorial legislature to be re-examined by physicians in hopes of being declared non-leprous and granted freedom. A fellow patient writing under the names S. K. M.

Nahauowaileia and S. K. Maialoha submitted the petitioners' full names, ages, and towns of origins in letters addressed to several Hawaiian-language newspapers. His detailed, compassionate accounting was printed in these newspapers.[128] While seemingly a medical list, it was not intended to shame people, but to publicize attempts to return to loved ones, friends, and kin.

These reports offer a public record of struggle against being forgotten. The writer himself was an exiled patient who included the total years "in the land of the sick" and the land from which his companions were removed. This practice suggests to contemporary researchers like me that some of those exiled might support their names and genealogical information being disclosed today. Similarly, tributes and poems to those who had been exiled or had died were published in newspapers throughout the twentieth century.[129] Survivors wished for the names and one hanau (birth sands, or genealogically rooted birthplaces) of their loved ones to be recorded and circulated through printed promulgations.

Working from these implications, I have chosen to use the real names of nineteenth- and early twentieth-century patients, rather than pseudonyms, in this book.[130] If people later in the twentieth century disclosed their own Hansen's disease status in formats like newspapers, documentaries, testimonies, and published oral histories, I use their given names. There are some exceptions: if people used a pseudonym during their lifetimes or expressed not wanting to be identified with Hansen's disease, I have abided by that choice.

Pseudonyms are not an ideal way to reconcile confidentiality with people's specific experiences in this study. Naming practices suggest places, time, genealogy, occupation, and context.[131] Yet beyond the immediate work of history, inoa (names) hold deep significance and mana (spiritual power) for Kanaka 'Ōiwi subjects. Shaping a person's personality, fate, fortune, and misfortune, names are neither endowed nor removed lightly, as Mary Kawena Pukui has described.[132] They exceed the life of an individual physical body, signifying ongoing relationships with the past and the future.[133]

I began this book with Keliiahonui, an exiled child who died without his birth parents in the settlement. But his name is important—it tells us he was not alone. He carried an inoa invested with authority and anticipation throughout his life. Keliiahonui is possibly a contraction of Kealiiahonui, which means "chief with many breaths"—a person endowed with perseverance. The child Keliiahonui's homeland was Hilo, Hawai'i, not the island of Kaua'i, but his name may evoke or pay tribute to two Kaua'i ali'i. The high chief Aarona Keliiahonui was the son of the last ruling chief of Kaua'i.

Following Aarona Keliiahonui was Prince Edward Abnel Keliiahonui, Aarona's namesake and grandnephew, who was sent with his brothers to a California boarding school. We may continue to speculate who, what, or where the boy's name references, but using Keliiahonui's actual name enables him to be seen as a person with wider connections, kinship, and expectations beyond the reach of the medical record. There is power in that recognition and remembrance today.

ONE

Ocular Experiments and Unruly Technologies of the Body

As every seed requires its peculiar conditions of soil, atmosphere, etc., to allow it to strike, and, when struck, to grow up to be itself a seed-bearing plant, so does the leprous germ require a certain disposition of the human soil to strike and thrive. What this peculiar disposition may be, we are at present unable to define.

DR. EDUARD ARNING,
Report to the Hawai'i Board of Health, November 14, 1885

NATHANIEL B. EMERSON'S STRUGGLES as an artist began not long after he returned to Hawai'i in 1878. Emerson, the son of American Protestant missionaries in Hawai'i, had been born on the island of O'ahu in 1839. After completing medical training at Harvard and the College of Physicians and Surgeons in New York City, he was asked to assume the post of resident physician at the Kalawao, Molokai, leprosy settlement.[1] Emerson became the first Western-trained physician to treat exiled patients there since the establishment of the settlement in 1866.

Like many of his contemporaries, Emerson was baffled by the spread of leprosy in Hawai'i. He appeared to be focused on two main concerns: determining whether a person had leprosy and how the person might have contracted it. Emerson began compiling detailed case histories of people with ambiguous pathologies inside and outside of leprosy detention facilities. Diagnosis was not always straightforward, as his notes reveal. Leprosy at times presented distinct pathological signs, but could be confused easily with scabies, eczema, fungal infections, and syphilis. Furthermore, Emerson wanted to determine how the disease was communicable and whether particular people were prone to infection. Was leprosy contracted through sexual contact or blood? Was it hereditary? Did poor hygiene, shared food, or bedding spread infection?

Within case histories filled with ethnographic data, sexual histories, and family relationships, Emerson began sketching and painting men, women, and children in pencil, ink, and watercolor. Pasted or drawn directly next to his detailed clinical histories of suspected leprosy cases, these rough sketches reveal a desire to accurately represent somatic symptoms as well his difficulties imaging the human body.

Emerson examined leprosy suspects who were detained at the Kakaʻako Branch Hospital and Receiving Station in Honolulu. In one of his early cases, Emerson described an eleven-year-old Hawaiian girl named Kauapaliloa. He diagnosed her on November 5, 1879, with an "eruptive and anesthetic form of leprosy." When he conducted a physical examination in 1880 following her exile to the Kalawao settlement, he updated his journal with this entry: "This girl is rather a good looking, well formed, well developed girl. Has a delicate pinkish hue in her brown skin as of leprosy, no tubercles. Has on the skin of her body and limbs a considerable number of light colored pohaka [splotches] which are found on her shoulders, chest, abdomen, back, on each rump, on thighs, legs, arms, and forearms and over the right chin, and along the jaw. The following art will show location of the pohaka."[2] Immediately below his handwritten text, Emerson attempted a crude sketch of Kauapaliloa in frontal and rear views (figure 7).[3]

Throughout these journal entries, Emerson attempted to attach observed pathologies to sketches:

—"The following art does not exaggerate the deformity of this hand."[4] (sketch of a hand in ink)

—"This is a fiendish and awful burlesque of a hand, something like an abortion. Finger nails of the left hand are wrinkled and distorted."[5] (sketch of a hand in ink)

A competent speaker of Hawaiian, the missionary son Emerson collected family and sexual histories that might help him understand how leprosy was connected to practices he considered transgressive. His probing questions of patients included, "Married? To leper? Children? Are they lepers? Where did he take L[eprosy]?" For a twenty-one-year-old man, Emerson recorded the following in July 1880: his clinical symptoms, a sketch of the "hideous deformity" of the man's face, and a detailed sexual history. Emerson wrote, "He says that before he took this disease he lived with a married woman who,

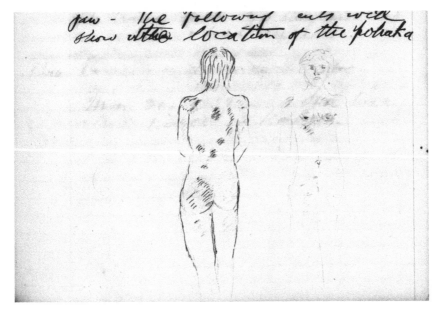

FIGURE 7. Ink and pencil sketches of Kauapaliloa, 1880. Nathaniel B. Emerson, Leprosy Cases 1–184, EMR 1314, p. 355. The Huntington Library.

as it proved has this disease. Slept in the same bed with her. Her name Kaui, she died a leper here at Kalawao."[6]

How would Emerson organize this chaotic discursive and visual data about Indigenous practices, sex, disability, and disease? And how would he arrive at a method of imaging, diagnosing, and tracking bodies and their behavior? Despite the frequent inclusion of uncooperative drawings, Emerson's notes betray a certain anxiety. Emerson was caught between an excess of visual evidence of leprosy and a paucity of stable signifiers to represent them. In his reach for a visual system, he vacillated between confident proffering of his illustrations and apologies for his meager renderings. On one page next to a sketch of a woman, he confessed, "The accompanying is not a very successful drawing of her face and chest."[7]

When the bacteriologist and pioneering leprosy researcher Eduard Arning arrived in Hawai'i from Hamburg, Germany, in 1883, Emerson found part of his answer. Arning had been recruited by the Hawaiian Kingdom's foreign minister and Board of Health president, the colorful American-born Walter Murray Gibson, to investigate the origins and spread of leprosy in Hawai'i.[8] A German physician not yet thirty years old, Arning readily welcomed this

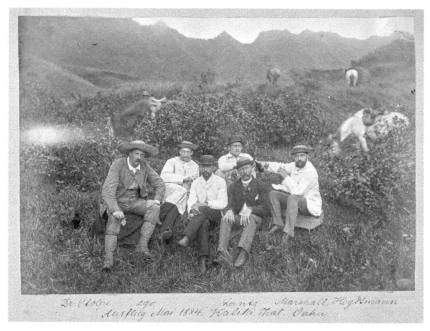

FIGURE 8. Eduard Arning on ethnographic excursion at Kalihi Valley, Oʻahu, May 1884. Arning is second from the left. Arning's caption translates to "Dr. Stolpe, me, Lantz, Marshall, Heydtmann." Arning Ethnographic Album, p. 33. Arnsteiner Patres, Germany.

opportunity because he was guaranteed unique access to more than seven hundred leprosy patients.[9]

During a nearly three-year residence in Honolulu between 1884 and 1886, Arning conducted bacteriological research on people in Hawaiʻi. At the same time, Arning photographed hundreds of Hawaiians, Pacific Islanders, Japanese immigrants, and white settlers, concentrating his tireless ethnographic collecting and photography on Hawaiian people, practices, and material culture (figure 8).[10] He photographed approximately twenty-six individual leprosy patients at the same Kakaʻako Branch Hospital where Emerson had conducted exams and patient interviews a few years prior. One of these patients was a Hawaiian girl whom Arning identified as Ester Kanepuu. He included her as an example of "lepra anesthetic," or anesthetic leprosy, in his photograph albums (figure 9).[11] Arning went on to refine his techniques and bring these photographs back to Germany.

Grappling with empirical visual evidence that could do justice to his textual descriptions, Emerson may have been relieved, if not delighted, to meet Arning in Honolulu and learn of his methodical photographic approach.

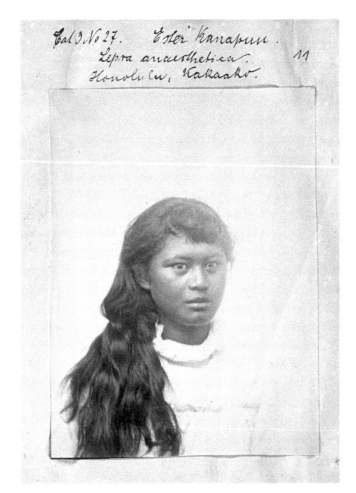

FIGURE 9. "Ester Kanapuu, Lepra Anesthetica, Honolulu, Kakaako." Arning Leprosy Album, p. 12, Negative Catalogue 3.27. The girl Arning identified as "Ester Kanapuu" was known as Ekekela Kanepuu, from Iwilei, Oʻahu. Ekekela and another family member named Halakii Kanepuu were admitted to Kakaʻako Branch Hospital on May 16, 1884. Arnsteiner Patres, Germany.

Emerson admired and supported Arning's leprosy research, although they do not seem to have collaborated directly in Hawaiʻi. The men's correspondence continued even after Arning returned to Germany in 1886. Both men were physicians who pursued anthropology and Hawaiian artifact collecting as avocations, as I will discuss; both could contend for the title of first non-Native ethnographer of Hawaiʻi. Arning, however, was about fifteen years younger than Emerson. He trained in dermatology and the bold new field of microbiology, which was hunting the bacterial scourges of syphilis, tuberculosis, gonorrhea, and leprosy. Inspired by German physician-ethnographers, he also learned glass plate photography in Germany.

Arning's forays into photography may have been encouraged by dermatology and ethnography, for both fields experimented with new photographic materials and technologies to document and illustrate somatic differences. Dermatologists sought to capture pathological conditions emerging on the skin, while anthropologists sought to preserve the practices of Naturvölker (natural people) firsthand, that is, representatives of the non-Western world whom they believed were disappearing rapidly.[12]

Arning's photographs of approximately fifty patients during his investigations of leprosy at his Kaka'ako laboratory and the Molokai settlement managed to produce what Emerson could not with his meager sketches: the photographs offered prolific types of leprous bodies for diagnosis, visual comparison, and ethnographic speculation. This chapter considers the early idiosyncratic imaging of leprosy patients in Hawai'i by Arning and other Euro-American scientists as they developed methods of merging ethnographic, visual, and medical data in the late nineteenth century. These visual representations—ranging from functional clinical photographs to self-consciously artistic compositions—brought disease, disability, and racial-sexual alterity into the same interpretive frame.

In what I call ocular experiments, scientists attempted to capture and image a diverse range of healthy, sick, and ambiguous people and their cultural artifacts in a broad study of disability and extinction. While lesser known than biomedical experiments performed by physicians on incarcerated people, these ocular experiments constituted significant knowledge production about the bodies, cultural practices, and dispositions of Indigenous men, women, and children. Ultimately these explorations could not answer how leprosy was transmitted or who would become infected, but nevertheless accrued into forceful claims about the civilizational "weakness" of Hawaiians. In turn, these unruly empirical approaches would be adapted into Hawai'i's carceral-medical apparatus over the next century.

ETHNOGRAPHIC AND BIOMEDICAL ALBUMS

Two albums of photographs reside today in a Catholic archive in Werne, Germany. Eduard Arning lent them to the Arnsteiner Patres, the German branch of a Catholic congregation, in 1936.[13] Arning took hundreds of photographs of Hawaiʻi during his residency from 1884 to 1886, and brought the negatives back to Germany with him.[14] Arning lent these albums to this Catholic congregation not due to a particular religious devotion, but because of the group's longstanding connection to Hawaiʻi and its leprosy mission.[15] Arning might not have intended the photographs to reside here permanently, but he died later that year and was unable to reclaim them.

During his Hawaiʻi residence, Arning photographed scenery, clinical patients, various residents and visitors, and material culture of ethnographic interest. We do not know what kind of camera Arning used in Hawaiʻi, but he likely had learned glass plate photography in Germany. Invented in the 1870s, glass plate photography preceded celluloid film as a medium. Dry glass plates greatly simplified the process and geographic range of photographers, as they no longer had to prepare glass plates with wet chemicals right before exposure or develop them immediately after in the field. Arning's laboratory at Kakaʻako Hospital likely contained a darkroom, where he developed his negatives and printed photographs.[16]

Arning organized and catalogued these glass plate negatives, perhaps even upon his return to Hamburg. The two albums in the Arnsteiner Patres archive suggest two distinct approaches to Arning's imaging of Hawaiian people and artifacts: the ethnographic and the biomedical.[17] Arning labeled the first album in his own handwriting, "wichtige ethnographische und landschaftliche Aufnahmen" (important ethnographic and scenic photographs). The album includes scenes of material culture, sacred religious objects, and people in situ and in arranged settings between 1883 and 1886. Arning described Hawaiian women lying on their stomachs as "Charakteristische Bauchlage" (typical prone position) (figure 10). He captioned the adjacent photograph "Group of Hawaiians in Kalihi Valley," where he had taken an ethnographic excursion with a visiting Swedish anthropologist in 1884 (figure 11).

The second album is one of leprosy and pathological skin conditions—primarily photographs of incarcerated leprosy patients taken by Arning during these same years in Hawaiʻi (figure 9).[18] Arning photographed men, women, and children in makeshift laboratories and clinics as examples of the leprosy cases he was categorizing and studying.

In these parallel albums, Arning appears to present two separate and distinct approaches to visualizing Hawaiian life in the late nineteenth century: first, the living, in situ "cultural" activities of Hawaiians, and second, individual pathological bodies representing types of leprosy. However, we know

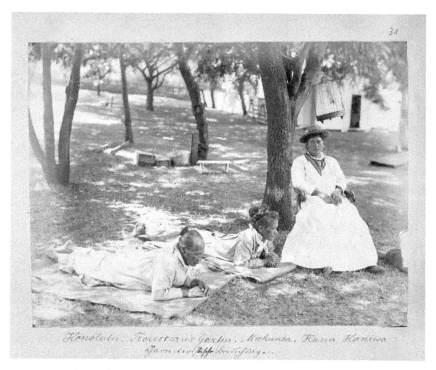

FIGURE 10. "Honolulu, Trousseau's Garden. Makanea, Hana, Honiwa. Charakteristische Bauchlage" (typical prone position). Eduard Arning Ethnographic Album, p. 31, undated, ca. 1884. Arnsteiner Patres, Germany.

that he was photographing these subjects at the same time. As part of his fastidious research method, Arning recorded many specific locations, dates, and descriptions of his photographs. When we bring the ethnographic and leprosy photographs into the same frame of reference, we begin to see them as part of an intertwined process of knowledge production about proclivity to disability and death. What was he trying to see and make intelligible?

Upon his return to Germany, Arning began writing an ethnography to accompany his photographs and material culture collection. At a lecture given at the unveiling of his vast Hawaiian collection at the Berlin Ethnological Museum (Museum für Völkerkunde) in February 1887, Arning asserted, "[O]ne could view Old Hawaii as vanished forever." He stressed, "The speed with which Old Hawaii perished cannot be attributed only to the sudden flooding by Anglo-Saxon culture; no, ancient Hawaiian culture carried in itself the germ of its demise."[19] Relying on the bacteriological metaphor of the germ taking root in fertile soil, Arning maintained that some

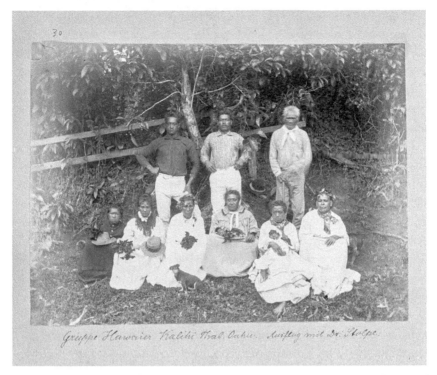

FIGURE 11. "Gruppe Hawaier Kalihi Thal., Oahu. Ausflug mit Dr. Stolpe" (Group of Hawaiians in Kalihi Valley. Excursion with Dr. Stolpe), ca. May 1884. Eduard Arning Ethnographic Album, p. 30. Arnsteiner Patres, Germany.

element in Hawaiian lifeways made their extinction inevitable. How did this cultural "germ" take form and where could he detect it in Hawaiian bodies, culture, and people?

DISABILITY AND THE SALVAGE PARADIGM

An a priori principle for Arning was the extinction of Hawaiians: he was not interested in verifying whether Hawaiians were going to die, only *how* and *why* they would. Arning had been influenced and mentored by prominent German anthropologists who similarly straddled the professions of medicine and anthropology. German anthropology, also known as ethnology in the 1870s, divided the world into two groups: cultural people ("Kulturvölker") and natural people ("Naturvölker"). In this view, Europeans possessed written history and therefore belonged in the former category. Anthropologists like Adolf Bastian, a trained physician and founder of the Berlin Ethnological Museum, believed natural people (e.g., Indigenous people) were perishing due to the inexorable advancement of civilization.[20] Arning would echo these views when he presented his Hawai'i collection at the Berlin Ethnological Museum in 1887: "[D]espite all assurances by the government that better hygienic conditions are curbing further extinction, the demise of the full-blooded Hawaiian race is probably only a matter of decades."[21]

In the settler-colonial milieu of Hawai'i, Euro-American missionary descendants and businessmen had gained significant political and economic influence, destabilizing the authority of the Hawaiian mo'ī (ruling chief or sovereign) Kalākaua.[22] Members of this oligarchy actively worked to depose chiefly sovereigns, using Hawaiian extinction and racial inferiority as rationales.[23] The reverend Sereno Bishop specifically drew upon the paradigm of disability to characterize Hawaiians as a dying people in an 1888 address to the Honolulu Social Science Association. Asking, "Why are the Hawaiians dying out?" Bishop linked disability to racial incompetence and sexual excess. He proceeded to itemize the "elements of disability" of Hawaiian people, including unchastity, drunkenness, oppression by chiefs, infectious and epidemic diseases like leprosy, and idolatry.[24] In Bishop's blunt rhetoric, Hawaiians were disabled and had failed to thrive. Their disability was a collective racial-sexual inferiority that would extinguish them. As a newspaper editor and vociferous advocate of Hawai'i's annexation to the United States, Bishop supported the overthrow of the Hawaiian Kingdom by white settlers in 1893 and annexation in 1898.

American physician George Fitch, who worked as medical officer at the Molokai settlement in the 1880s, similarly yoked Hawaiian civilizational collapse to disability. Fitch assessed Hawaiians as improvident, frivolous, and promiscuous, and thus bound for extinction. His 1892 article "The Etiology of Leprosy" relied on a floridly discursive anthropology of medicine to explain what he interpreted as Hawaiian susceptibility to disease. Fitch expounded, "Like all other uncivilized races, they are extremely improvident—when food abounds they gorge themselves; when it is scarce they go hungry." Speaking bluntly about their perceived sexual deviance, Fitch declared, "There is no word meaning chastity in the [Hawaiian] language."[25]

Arning remained distinct from the likes of Sereno Bishop and the pro-American oligarchy in Hawai'i—he was neither zealous Christian nor landowner with stakes in the islands' industry or political-economic purse strings. A dispassionate bacteriologist, Arning contributed a particularly ingenious twist to these settler views of Hawaiian incompetence: Hawaiians had no value in living, yes, but their value was in disability and dying. He would take advantage of their ostensible disability by studying them and making use of their bodies while they were dying.[26] His expropriation of imprisoned patients for scientific experimentation was emblematic of this approach to carceral medicine—Hawaiians will soon be dead, so take and learn as much as possible.

German ethnologists rushed to collect in the late nineteenth century, before non-Europeans disappeared.[27] Caught within this urgent paradigm, Indigenous people were treated as already dead. If salvage ethnography was an effort to save, collect, retain, and preserve the material culture of a "dying" and disappearing people, Arning was what we might call a salvage clinician.[28] As a salvage clinician, Arning aimed to leverage disability into valuable data, scraping and extracting as much as he could from Indigenous bodies before they disappeared.

The rapid mortality of Hawaiian patients produced what Arning described as favorable "experimental conditions" in Hawai'i. He described Hawai'i as an ideal site to experiment on living leprosy patients because they had a much shorter life than Europeans. Hawai'i's patients lived for about three to five years with leprosy, compared to fifteen to twenty years in European countries.[29] Indeed, as a special investigator for the Hawaiian government, Arning enjoyed liberal access to incarcerated people at leprosy institutions and the O'ahu prison. Arning could use leprosy patients as clinical material because of carceral-medical conditions and colonial subordination.

The Kaka'ako Branch Hospital grounds consisted of series of a dozen wooden buildings on a muddy, low-lying waterfront in Honolulu (figure 12).[30] This is where Arning set up his laboratory, conducted clinical experiments, and photographed the majority of his leprosy subjects. His letters to the Board of Health reveal his ability to requisition particular patients for his laboratory. He wrote directly to BOH president Walter Murray Gibson on December 20, 1884, requesting seven "males" and four "females" by name.[31] While Arning did not detail what he meant by "placed under my special care," it likely included photography and other experiments, as he discussed in subsequent reports to the board. A photograph of one of these four girls remains in his leprosy album, that of Ester (Ekekela) Kanepuu (figure 9). Between 1883 and 1885, he conducted an inoculation experiment on at least three people with leprosy to test whether "new centres" of leprosy could develop in the body after vaccination with non-sterile lancets.[32]

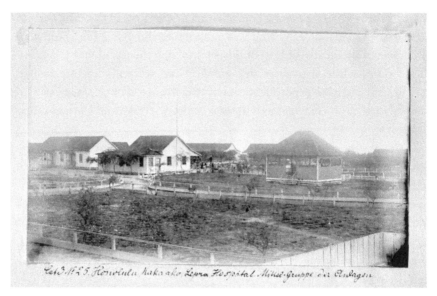

FIGURE 12. "Honolulu. Kakaako. Leprosy Hospital, Middle Group of the Grounds." ca. 1884. Eduard Arning Leprosy Album, p. 5, Negative Catalogue 3.25. Arnsteiner Patres, Germany.

Like his continental contemporaries, Arning participated in what historian Andrew Zimmerman has called the "skin trade" to secure his empirical data. Nineteenth-century German natural scientists accessed prisons, graveyards, and colonies to source human bodies and body parts for anthropological and medical science. Several decades prior to the rise of National Socialism and biomedical experimentation on prisoners in Nazi concentration camps, Arning gained access to hundreds of leprosy suspects incarcerated at Kaka'ako Hospital and the Molokai settlement.[33]

Historian Susan Lederer has argued American physicians in the nineteenth century would have been shunned if they had engaged in human experimentation.[34] While this may have been generally true on the U.S. continent, Hawai'i was an important exception to this code of conduct, even prior to its formal status as a U.S. colony. Far from exerting self-regulation over human experimentation, German, American, and British carceral physicians drew captive bodies from Hawai'i's leprosy institutions for experiments and documentation, practices that continued throughout the twentieth century. These physicians contributed to the ideological and material infrastructure of the leprosy regime, while benefiting from privileged access to inmates.[35]

In the 1880s, British physician Arthur A. Mouritz inoculated non-leprous caregivers living in the settlement, while American physician George Fitch inoculated six detained leprosy patients, all girls under the age of twelve, with syphilis to test his hypothesis that syphilis and leprosy were related diseases (see chapter 3).[36] And, as I discuss below, Arning was to carry out the most infamous of these experiments on an imprisoned Hawaiian man named Keanu in 1884.

"A CERTAIN WEAKNESS"

In his laboratory, Arning's objective was to determine how leprosy was transmitted by artificially cultivating and inoculating the microbe, using contemporary principles of germ theory.[37] The field of bacteriology encouraged experimentation on humans and animals. To prove that a microbe caused a disease and had a particular mode of transmission, physicians hunted the bacillus. First, they needed to identify the germ under the microscope, then produce the disease in a healthy organism. The organism was a living animal, and if possible, a human subject.[38] The scientist Gerhard Armauer Hansen had identified the leprosy bacillus under a microscope in 1873 in Norway, but the specific mode of leprosy's transmission remained unknown.

Trained under German bacteriologist Albert Neisser, who had discovered the bacteria *gonococcus,* responsible for gonorrhea, Arning took an exacting approach to bacterial research.[39] He fashioned a laboratory at Kaka'ako Hospital in Honolulu, where patients were held before being sent to Molokai. He experimented with growing *M. leprae* (the leprosy bacilli) outside of the human body in all matter of living and non-living organic material and "artificial soils." These soils included guinea pigs, rats, rabbits, pigeons, meat gelatins, vegetables, sterilized sheep's blood, and the manufactured food cultures of Hawaiians: seaweed gelatins, fish gelatins, and the Hawaiian staple, poi.[40]

In his first report to the BOH and its president, written on April 10, 1884, Arning discussed five months of research and future proposed microscopic work. He was able to find the bacilli in the tissue of dead and living patients in Hawai'i, but not in the blood or in the spots and sores of anesthetic leprosy patients. In hopes of learning more about the "paths the germ follows in the organism," he proposed spending future months attempting to grow leprosy bacilli outside the human body on various media, including in a monkey.[41] He predicted that these would be associated with "many discouraging failures."

Indeed, after eighteen months of trying to get the bacilli to grow in air, water, gelatins, bouillon, vegetables, and having inoculated all manner of living subjects, Arning was left to report in November 1885, "I have not once succeeded in obtaining an independent and pure growth of the bacillus leprae."[42]

Although microbiology appeared a stable field of investigation—counting bacilli in excised tissue in a laboratory—it still could not reveal why particular people developed leprosy. It was slow and frustrating research yielding no method of incubation. Arning hypothesized about the "peculiar conditions" in people that led the leprous germ to "strike and thrive": "It is evidently a disposition which may coexist with apparent good health, as many examples of strong robust men, developing leprosy, show us . . . I do believe that a certain weakness to resist its attack may be transmitted."[43] The microbial causes for this "certain weakness" remained elusive, so where could he turn?

Arning turned to a visual laboratory outside of the hospital proper: the entire island habitus. Using Hawai'i as his laboratory, Arning imaged diverse bodies and ethnographic objects as data. Clues to these conditions might be revealed in photographs and by peering at raced-sexed bodies in their habitus. Arning's experiments on living clinical subjects were one such productive interface between microbiology—germ hunting—and photography.

Arning's biomedical research in Hawai'i has been discussed in relation to notorious, canonized experiments he conducted on a Hawaiian man named Keanu, while his photographic efforts are far less known and have been treated as "ethnographic." Bruno Latour's method of studying science suggests entering through "the back door of science in the making."[44] By examining the late nineteenth-century science and hermeneutics of leprosy, we may locate Arning's ocular experiments in the porous spaces between laboratory and field, as he framed Indigenous disability and civilizational decline.

CREATING TYPES

In August 1884, a man named Keanu was sentenced to death by hanging. Keanu had been convicted of murdering the Japanese husband of his lover Kamaka in Kohala, Hawai'i. Called the "Kohala murderer" by the English-language press, Keanu was a forty-eight-year-old man with genealogical ties to Kohala and Makapala on Hawai'i island.[45] Not long after the sentencing, Arning and the Board of Health requested permission from the kingdom's privy council to have Keanu's death sentence commuted, which it granted in late September 1884.[46] In exchange for commutation of the sentence, Keanu signed a written agreement to be infected with leprous tissue. Arning inoculated Keanu on September 30, 1884. Arning had found an ideal human subject to test a theory of leprosy transmission: a robust Hawaiian man in apparent good physical health with no family history of leprosy.[47]

At the first Congress of the Society of German Dermatology in 1889, Arning delivered a detailed account of the medical procedure he had performed on Keanu; this was later published in the conference proceedings.[48] He created a blister on Keanu's arm and rubbed fluid from a leprosy ulcer into it. He also removed a nodule from a nine-year-old girl at Kaka'ako Hospital, whom he described as an "exquisite" case of tubercular leprosy. He implanted this girl's tissue into an incision on Keanu's right arm.[49] Arning's objective was to establish whether leprosy could be transmitted between people via inoculation.

Within three years of the implantation, Keanu had developed distinct symptoms of leprosy. He was still imprisoned in O'ahu jail and his condition was perceived as a menace to the other prisoners; Keanu was then shipped to the Molokai settlement in 1888. He died there on November 12, 1892, eight years after Arning's original experiment and after Arning had returned to Hamburg, Germany.[50] Arning claimed that his experiment proved that inoculation could produce leprosy infection; physicians and leprologists in German, American, and British medical journals debated the evidence and claims. Some took the "convict" experiment as proof of the "contagious" and communicable nature of leprosy.[51] By today's bioethical standards, using a death row inmate in a painful experiment in lieu of state execution would be verboten. At the time, some medical peers expressed nervousness about the ethics of the experiment, while others only questioned its putative claims.[52]

While Arning's experiment has become well known in the history of leprosy and microbiology, what was little known now and then is that Arning photographed Keanu at the commencement of his experiment. His photographic studies of Keanu and other human subjects have been treated as ethnographic instead of clinical, perhaps because of Arning's own insistent taxonomic division.[53] The photographs are interpreted as records of Hawaiian lifeways and cultural practices, rather than documentation of clinical symptoms and diseases. Yet the relationships between these two categories are far more entangled, as portraits of Keanu and other subjects reveal.

On September 28, 1884, the same day Arning examined Keanu and recorded his detailed clinical history, and two days prior to the suturing

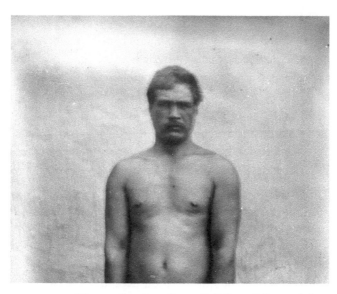

FIGURE 13. "Keanu. Hawaiian. Front. Full figure." Cropped from original full-length nude photograph by Eduard Arning, September 28, 1884. Eduard Arning Ethnographic Catalogue, Negative Catalogue 2.13. Hawaiian Historical Society.

procedure, Arning photographed Keanu at the Oʻahu jail. One of these photographs survives today, revealing Keanu in a frontal, full-length nude shot (figure 13). It is reproduced here in a cropped format. Arning took at least three other photographs of Keanu: in full-body profile, half-length frontal view, and half-length profile view, although the location of the latter three images is not known.[54]

For having assumed such a celebrated part of Arning's medical career, Keanu is curiously absent in his leprosy album. Nor did Arning list photographs of Keanu in his "Lepra" (Leprosy) catalogue of negatives, which he carefully organized and annotated. Instead, he deliberately filed them in his "Anthropologie" photograph series. Arning annotated the subject of photograph 2.13 simply as "Keanu. Hawaiian. Front. Full figure" in the catalogue.[55] Arning made no reference to Keanu as a prisoner or special medical subject.

Arning later suggested a particular reason for filing Keanu in his anthropological series. He wrote that Keanu's general state of strength was very good the day of the exam, so much so that "Keanu's photograph appears in my anthropological collection as *a type of the powerful Hawaiian*" (my emphasis).[56] Arning thus filed Keanu as a *type*—a typical Hawaiian man, an example of Hawaiian masculinity. Arning visualized Keanu as an ideal prototype of a healthy and strong Hawaiian, an individual standing in for a larger group of Hawaiian men. He needed Keanu to be a healthy subject in order to transform him into something else: Arning, in fact, had struck an explicit agreement with the Hawaiian government that the sourced prisoner be absolutely free of leprosy symptoms.

My point is not that Keanu was misfiled and actually belonged in Arning's leprosy catalogue; rather that the placement of Keanu in the ethnographic section highlights the fungibility of Arning's categories. Arning could have inserted ethnographic subjects into his leprosy catalogue, and leprosy patients in his ethnographic catalogue. Despite these distinct labels, his methods of sourcing and imaging people and objects were remarkably similar. His taxonomies were artificial constructs, part of a larger disorderly system in the making—that is, the science of human extinction. These subjects, regardless of final placement and cataloguing, were visualized as part of an investigation of racialized disability and human extinction.

TAXIDERMIC VISIONS

Including Keanu, Arning photographed at least fifty incarcerated leprosy patients in total, although the location of some of these negatives and prints is currently unknown. At Kaka'ako Hospital, he photographed approximately twenty-six individuals with leprosy and a few formal groups of Hawaiian patients, according to his catalogue. On other occasions, he visited the Kalawao, Molokai, leprosy settlement, where he photographed at least eight individuals. The majority of these subjects were Kānaka 'Ōiwi (Native Hawaiians), while two were Chinese immigrants and two others were white Europeans or Americans.

Though Arning later parsed his photographic collection into separate areas of knowledge—medicine and ethnography—we can begin to understand the simultaneity of his collecting habits by merging his clinical notes with his photographic annotations. After implanting the leprosy tissue into Keanu, Arning examined him daily for the first month, then about once a week for several months.[57] Arning's clinical notes, translated from his original German, read:

January 5, 1885. The injection site completely healed on the left arm. K. [Keanu] again complains of pain in his left shoulder and left wrist. The latter is also a bit painful to exercise. General health undisturbed.

January 26, 1885. The site of the inoculation wound is marked by a two-centimeter-long, four-millimeter-wide, keloid-like red strip and a pale zone surrounding this strip on all sides, not a diminution of sensibility within this area. [. . .] Pressure on the ulnar nerve is not particularly painful.[58]

Arning conducted such inspections of Keanu, hoping to detect the possible spread of leprosy infection from the original inoculation site. As his experiment on Keanu unfolded, however, Arning photographed other Hawaiians, patients and non-patients alike, as racialized ethnographic subjects. Arning would file these portraits in his "Anthropologie" and "Lepra" negative catalogues. On January 12, 1885, a week after Keanu's injection site had healed, Arning photographed a fourteen-year-old girl named Kina Keahi for an ethnographic portrait. He described Kina as a "half Chinese girl. Father—Chinese, Mother—full-blooded Hawaiian." In the next few weeks, he photographed at least two more subjects described as "ethnographic": a Hawaiian named Kahalelau, presumably a man, wearing a loincloth of "pure kapa" (bark cloth), on January 18, 1885, and M.C., a twenty-two-year old woman, on February 2, 1885. Arning annotated M.C. as "Half white. Father, English, mother pure Native."[59]

During the same month, Arning transformed the spare leprosy hospital in Kakaʻako into an ethnographic studio setting. He posed this girl in a checked dress for a portrait. With a lei (garland) on her crown, she holds flowers stiffly with more blossoms at her feet (figure 14). The use of flowers was a purposeful prop deployed by Arning; by the late nineteenth century, flowers had become familiar signifiers of Hawaiian female sexuality in tourist and ethnographic print media. While the girl remained nameless, Arning labeled her with a diagnostic term: "lepra nervorum" (leprosy of the nervous system). Arning drew liberally and idiosyncratically from a repertoire of visual conventions available to him as a European scientist and tourist, as this framing of disease and racialized sexuality reveals.

How and why did Arning's various subjects participate in these scenes of exposure? Arning's subjects did not necessarily need to sit still in front of the camera for a long time; the exposure time for dry plate photographs required less than a second. However, Arning still needed to pose and position Kina, Kahalelau, and others in front of his camera as he created the mise-en-scène. Arning did not say how he was able to achieve such compliance, nor are there

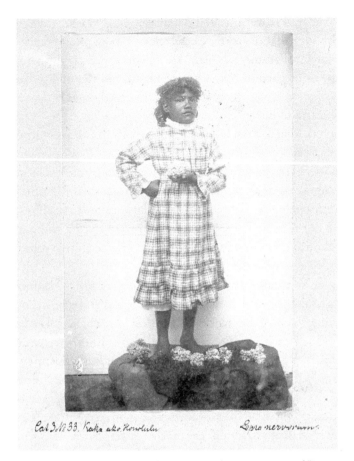

FIGURE 14. Girl in checked dress, name unknown. Captioned "Lepra Nervorum." Eduard Arning Leprosy Album, p. 26, Negative Catalogue 3.33. Arnsteiner Patres, Germany.

records of his subjects' experiences. However, leprosy patients were already intimately familiar with the inexorable institutional power of the Board of Health, Western medicine, and law.

Keanu had little choice; he had "consented" to Arning's full experimentation in exchange for the commutation of his death sentence. Detainees at Kaka'ako Hospital may have sat for photographs because they wanted to remain in Honolulu, rather than exiled to Kalawao settlement, where they would not be able to see their families. In 1883, a Hawaiian-language newspaper announced the German doctor's arrival in Honolulu with anticipation of new leprosy treatments. Hawaiians also may have viewed Arning as a gateway to medical treatments and potential cures.[60] Others who were not under health surveillance may have been curious about photography and this particular foreigner's camera, as many Hawaiians approached studio photography at the time. Even in rural areas of Hawai'i in the mid-to late 1800s, Hawaiians of maka'āinana (non-chiefly) status eagerly sought the services of Euro-American and European studio photographers.[61]

Although Arning had not been trained formally in cultural anthropology in Germany, he adopted early anthropology's primary mode of photography for the majority of his leprosy portraits: photographing a nude subject against a plain background, with clear lighting, and in front and profile views.[62] German anthropologists favored these standards in order to allow physical comparison of the subjects within. A standardized setting without clothes and props limited extraneous data that might have permitted more distinct personhood to emerge in the frame.

In addition to creating anthropological types, Arning documented his subjects with language that merged anthropological and medical detail. Of Keanu, Arning wrote, "The coloring of the skin is a rich chocolate brown, as is generally the case with the Polynesians as a sign of health."[63] Arning's skin color schema thus became a type shared by a much larger group of healthy "Polynesians." This method of combining individual case history with anthropological typicality carried over into his ethnographic research. For Pualokelani, a girl, Arning inscribed: "11½ years from Moiliili, Oahu, allegedly of pure Hawaiian extraction. The mother guarantees a Hawaiian genealogy of 4 generations. Skin color appears to be noticeably dark in accordance with the Pacific color scale no. 43. Eyes no. 2, hair kinky, very shiny, strong hair growth hanging down in front of the ears."[64]

Arning's strong reliance on physical anthropology's visual conventions carried over into portraits of three divergent subjects. In June 1885, Arning photographed a thirteen-year-old Hawaiian girl named Kealoha, a leprosy patient detained at Kaka'ako Hospital (figure 15). He posed Kealoha according to contemporary conventions of physical anthropology, unclothed with a light sheet for a background. The full-length frontal and rear views were meant to reveal lighter patches of skin, a possible symptom of leprosy. He filed Kealoha in his leprosy catalogue.[65]

Arning's photographs of the Hawaiian girl named Pualokelani were composed in a style strikingly similar to that of Kealoha (figure 16), unclothed in full-length frontal and side profile views. However, Pualokelani was not a Kaka'ako Hospital leprosy patient; she was one of his ethnographic subjects.

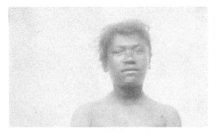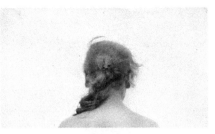

FIGURE 15. "Kealoha, 16 years old. Lepra papul. circinata. Kakaako, Honolulu." Cropped from original full-length nude photograph by Eduard Arning, June 1885. Eduard Arning Leprosy Album, p. 31, Negative Catalogue 3.39a and 3.39b. Arnsteiner Patres, Germany. Kealoha was closer to thirteen years old when Arning took these photographs.

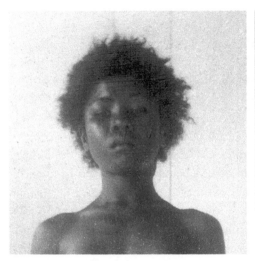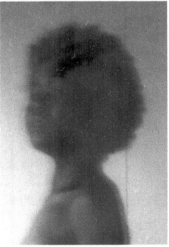

FIGURE 16. "Pualokelani (heavenly rosebud) ... Frontal full figure. Profile full figure." Cropped from original full-length nude photographs by Eduard Arning. Eduard Arning Ethnographic Catalogue, negatives 2.18b and 2.18c. Hawaiian Historical Society.

Pualokelani, age 11 ½, as Arning indicated in his ethnographic notes, was meant to represent a girl of "pure Hawaiian extraction."

A third photograph suggests how Arning's eye for Hawaiian material culture conformed to these photographic and ethnographic standards. Here in 1885, he captured a guardian deity in side profile and frontal views before a plain background in full length (figure 17). Arning identified this wooden figure unearthed from a Kaua'i taro field as "Luaalii." According to a Hawaiian informant, the wooden sculpture represented the guardian god Luaalii. It was 37.5 cm high, a god "to whom the Hawaiians prayed before

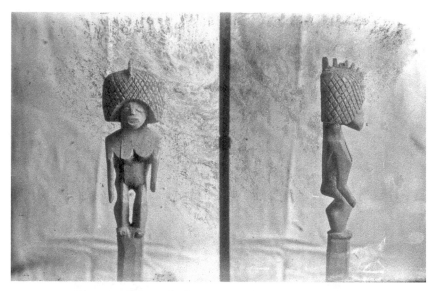

FIGURE 17. "Wooden idol Luaalii from Kauai." Photographs by Eduard Arning, 1885. Eduard Arning Ethnographic Catalogue, negatives 1.56a and 1.56.b. Hawaiian Historical Society.

going on a journey by sea or by land and before going to war."[66] Like their living human counterparts, sacred objects could be unearthed from their functional contexts, assessed, measured, imaged, and described.

Perhaps Arning himself did not know exactly why and what he was collecting and documenting fastidiously as he gazed into the folds of the skin and standardized the poses of human and non-human beings. What or whom might he be hoping to see? Arning pondered whether leprosy could be more than microbial, relying on botanical metaphors of seed and soil to speculate about how a subject's "disposition" made him/her prone to the disease. There was a "certain disposition of the human soil" that made the leprous germ take root, he reflected.[67] Photography enabled Arning to begin organizing a Hawaiian predisposition to disease and disability in the *absence* of outward somatic differences or clinical symptoms. His camera might aid in capturing an individual or collective disposition to disability—an "affective profile," to borrow Ann Stoler's term for criteria silently indexing moral character and sentiments.[68] Photography offered an avenue of discovery—a way of exposing Hawaiian bodies and translating their ambiguous interiority beyond what his Hawaiian informants were willing to narrate.

The consistent aesthetic production between his ethnographic and leprosy photograph series suggested *all* Hawaiians were prone to disease, whether or not showing leprous symptoms. The almost rhythmic positioning of their bodies in front and profile views served to arrest them. Pualokelani and Kealoha manage to appear both living and dead at the same time, preserved in the frame as specimens. Arning photographed the living with a taxidermist's eye, as if they were already dead. Hewing to anthropology's salvage paradigm, Arning presented a timeless version of the ethnographic present, suspending his subjects in time and space.[69]

Arning relied on this method of visual and ethnographic inspection and data collection because he found Hawaiians dishonest and unreliable. He claimed they dissembled and could not be objective observers. He wrote to the BOH in 1886, "I . . . am afraid I have wasted time and patience in trying to derive reliable information from the Hawaiians. Lack of observation of their personal health and willful deceit are so mingled with truth in their statements, that I defy anybody to collect reliable statistics such on which it might be possible to base proofs for hereditary or congenital transmission of Leprosy on these Islands."[70] More specifically, when notating Keanu's family history, Arning added, "I note that, as is the case with all case histories, it is only cum grano salis [a grain of salt] to be taken with the Hawaiians, who are very inclined to falsehoods."[71]

Yet, while Arning disparaged Hawaiians for their supposed duplicity, he also relied on them as key informants for ethnographic research. He extracted information about kapa making, fishing practices, hula, healing, adornments, and much more, which he summarized in an ethnography that accompanied his extensive collection. Arning described, "Right from the beginning, when my collection had only a few pieces, I had the habit of showing it to the old Hawaiians who came to me as patients or out of curiosity. In this way I could learn things about the pieces and also about ethnographic pieces still with friends or relatives; this often led to the acquisition of those pieces."[72]

If Hawaiians were untrustworthy, Arning turned to their bodies for evidence. Their bodies could be photographed, measured, weighed, scraped, and examined under a microscope. Bodies laid bare before Arning's camera would not lie, he believed. Keanu was a case in point—Arning spoke and wrote English well, but it is very possible Keanu did not. Beyond the issue of language, Arning mentioned briefly in his case history that Keanu had lost hearing in both ears after an accident herding wild livestock. Arning later referred to him as a "deaf and dumb convict," suggesting Keanu was hearing impaired and could not speak.[73] At the time of his clinical exam, Keanu may not have been able to understand Arning at all. However, Arning was not dissuaded; communication aside, he would glean as much data from Keanu's body. Keanu's body would speak, even if he himself could not.

In an allied vein, Arning's dependence on the human body for data extended to the raiding of remains and Hawaiian burials. On a trip to the Kalawao, Molokai, settlement, he convinced the resident Catholic priest to allow him to dig up a "body of a tubercular [leprosy] case." As Arning described, the body "had been buried for nearly 3 months, and was in the most active state of putrefaction . . ."[74] Arning tested the decaying tissue to see if leprosy bacilli remained.[75] The bodies Arning exhumed from Kalawao included cheeks, eyes, ears, and chins.[76]

On other field excursions, Arning looted sealed burial caves for intertwined ethnographic and medical research. On Oʻahu, he entered a cave and took a piece of kapa that had been wrapped around a bundle of iwi (bones). In Moanalua Valley, he pried open a cave sealed with stones and took a skeleton and other iwi with him. He inspected the bones for signs of leprosy and syphilis. At another cave on the same cliff, he removed eight skulls for the Berlin Ethnological Museum and took these back to Germany with him.[77] German and American anthropologists built their ethnological collections from such looted bones. Skulls were the most prized booty for Western institutions. Other body parts, like hair, salted skin, and dried hands, could be sourced effectively from colonial hospitals and prisons.[78] As Arning demonstrated in his salvage practices, all bodies, whether dead or alive, were for the taking.

Symbolizing a person's relationship to land and ancestors, iwi are sacred to Hawaiians. The retinue of aliʻi (chiefs) washed the flesh from iwi and secreted the bones away in caves to prevent them from being violated by enemies. Believed to retain a person's individuality after death, iwi link people to their aumakua (ancestral gods) and birth lands. Removals of iwi were and continue to be regarded as desecrations that bring lasting shame and humiliation to living descendants.[79] Using the Native American Graves and Repatriation Act (NAGPRA) of 1990 and international law, Kānaka ʻŌiwi have repatriated and reburied thousands of iwi kūpuna (ancestral bones) from universities and museums in the United States, the United Kingdom, and Germany over the past thirty years.

Although Arning was one of the earliest scientists to utilize leprosy patients for visual and ethnographic experiments, many others would flock to Molokai with cameras. These men found a productive carceral laboratory to investigate racialized pathology, sexuality, and disease. Among these medical tourists and bone collectors was Benjamin Sharp Jr., a professor of invertebrate zoology at the University of Pennsylvania and the Academy of Natural Sciences in Philadelphia. Like Arning, Sharp was an amateur photographer who photographed people, material culture, and ethnographic scenes in the Hawaiian Islands, while unearthing and removing human skulls and remains for scientific study.[80] During his 1893 Hawai'i expedition, Sharp traveled to the Molokai leprosy settlement and staged at least twelve photographs of inmates with leprosy. He later cropped and matted glass lantern slides to isolate his subjects and place their somatic differences in relief. Sharp presented these images to American physicians on at least one occasion: a lecture on "Sandwich Islands" leprosy at the Pennsylvania Medical Society.[81]

The American syphilologist (syphilis specialist) and health reformer Prince A. Morrow relied on photographs to support a more obstreperous position on the necessary containment of leprous people. In 1889, Morrow gained access to nearly 1,100 people incarcerated at the settlement. He asked white American settler and ethnologist William T. Brigham to take photographs of pathological cases there. Morrow used this "Hawaiian collection" of photographs for illustrated lectures and medical writings.[82] He crowed, "The Hawaiian or Sandwich Islands afford to-day, perhaps, the best field for the observation and study of leprosy of any leprous center in the world." The people imprisoned at the settlement provided "abundant opportunities for the clinical study of every possible form and phase of the disease."[83]

Indeed, a few months after his tour of the settlement, Morrow delivered a lecture at a meeting of the New York Academy of Medicine. His lecture was elaborately illustrated with fifty lantern slides of "typical forms of leprosy" that conflated leprosy and Hawaiian bodies.[84] They were "typical" not just of the forms of the disease, but by implied association, of "typical" Hawaiian patients (figure 18). Brigham and Morrow's photographs staged Molokai prisoners as clinical types, as Arning had framed his as anthropological and clinical specimens.

PLATE XVIII.

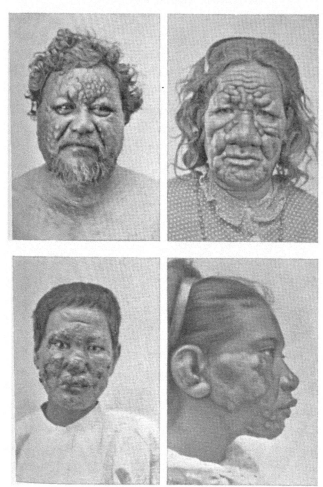

TYPICAL FACIES OF TUBERCULAR LEPROSY.
(From the author's Hawaiian collection.)

FIGURE 18. "Typical Facies of Tubercular Leprosy. From the author's Hawaiian collection." Photographs taken by William T. Brigham at Molokai settlement, 1889. Published in Morrow, *A System of Genito-Urinary Diseases, Syphilology and Dermatology* (1894), p. 570. The names of these people are unknown.

Relying on statistics and his alarming visual archive of non-normative and disabled bodies, Morrow fanned popular fears of leprosy spreading from people in the Pacific to Euro-Americans when he argued vigorously against U.S. annexation of Hawai'i. Were the United States to incorporate Hawai'i, a "gigantic evil" threatened to disseminate the "seeds of leprosy" to Americans.[85] Morrow attributed this disease and disfigurement to Hawaiians' wanton promiscuity. The photographs focused on the most advanced cases of leprosy—hands missing fingers, faces with nodules and thickened tissue— to provide seemingly indexical evidence of Hawaiians as culpable and fearful "bearers of deadly contagion." As photography became a less expensive and more accessible technology incorporated into print culture in the twentieth century, Hawai'i's leprosy inmates would continue to populate photographs that reinforced this discursive and visual field.

INCOMPLETE TYPICALITY

Three years after his return to Germany, Arning unveiled his collection of Hawai'i artifacts at the Berlin Ethnological Museum (Museum für Völkerkunde) in 1889. Publicly endorsed as an ethnographer on this occasion, Arning asserted his objects would provide "as accurate a view as possible of the Hawaiian culture that is gone forever."[86] As wooden calabashes were polished and placed behind iron and glass displays in a museum, so, too, were his human specimens preserved in photographs and glass tubes (figure 19).

Arning donated bones, sacred deities, baskets, tools, calabashes, and woven lauhala (pandanus) mats to the Berlin Ethnological Museum; this still constitutes one of the most significant and extensive Hawaiian collections in Europe. The gypsum casts he made of heads of Hawai'i's leprosy patients were destroyed during World War II.[87] His photographs, however, survived the war and are held in at least two repositories in Germany.

There is at least one documented instance of Arning showing his leprosy photographs during his lifetime. At the first German dermatological society conference, which convened in Prague in 1889, Arning informed his medical peers that his casts and photographs would demonstrate "typical forms of leprosy" and stages in the development of leprosy.[88] His photographs did not attempt to track a specific person's disease through time; rather, each photograph represented a type of leprosy: anesthetic leprosy, tubercular leprosy,

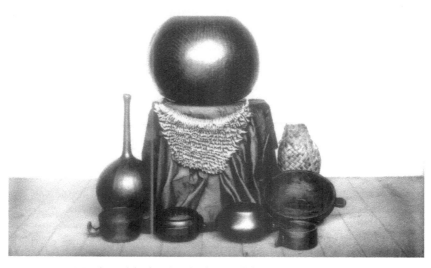

FIGURE 19. Wooden calabashes, bowls, dog tooth leg ornament, and lauhala basket collected and displayed by Arning. Photograph by Eduard Arning, October 1884. Eduard Arning Ethnographic Catalogue, negative 1.66. Hawaiian Historical Society.

and so forth. It was a synchronic, not diachronic, approach to imaging disease.

Ultimately, Arning's photographs attempted to offer objective types, models, and visual standards of pathological bodies against which other bodies could be compared and measured for diagnosis. He was interested in establishing typicality, not particularity. Rosemarie Garland Thomson has analyzed medicine's role in exhibiting the disabled body in clinical settings "in order to pathologize the exceptional and to normalize the ordinary."[89] While Arning's photographs rendered disability visible, they more specifically conjoined disability and Indigenous alterity. Arning's "medical gaze" offered a refinement of the clinical view of the body—his photographs integrated the pathological body and racial-sexual difference.[90]

Viewers of Arning's leprosy album were encouraged to see bodies transformed by disability and disease as manifestly tied to Hawaiian racial-sexual alterity. Captions indicating that these subjects were Hawaiian were unnecessary, for the album presented a series of pathological cases from Hawai'i. The photographs allowed inspection of unclothed Hawaiian men, women, girls, and boys close-up and in exquisite, fine-grained detail. These were Indigenous bodies to be stared at—a series of partial and full bodies lined up within uniform boxes. Visual access to genitalia—breasts, buttocks, penises—

further opened the possibility of anatomical and sexual comparison between Hawaiian men, women, and children and their European counterparts.

Arning had labored to refine his glass plate technique in the clinical space since he shot an early blurry full-length portrait of Keanu in November 1884. In his clinic the following year, Arning was able to better control for lighting and background, so that light-colored patches, deep wrinkles on the face, and fine details on the surface of the skin came into relief. He worked assiduously to make these bodies visually and aesthetically interesting.

In total, Arning's visual system established a knowledge system in which colonized people and non-European Others were condensed into a series of distilled bodies. Historian Andrew Zimmerman has referred to this as the human rendered as "pure body" in nineteenth-century German anthropology. Within this "heightened state of corporeality," colonized people were denied full subjectivity and sovereignty.[91] Yet these photographs left Arning with visual types meshed with a dizzying and inconclusive array of empirical data. Ultimately these photographic types did not allow him to draw clear conclusions about who would become leprous and who would not. He developed a relatively uniform system of imaging peculiar and unusual bodies, at least those appearing as such to Western viewers, but not a stable way of predicting in which of these leprosy would take hold. Arning's ambitious experiments left a broad imprint, however.

EXPERIMENTAL LEGACIES

After reviewing Arning's leprosy research for two years, the irascible Board of Health president Walter Murray Gibson accused Arning of not delivering tangible results quickly enough. A public disagreement over the value and cost of his scientific experiments ensued, and Arning was informed that his services would not be renewed by the Hawaiian government in December 1885. Gibson's secretary requested Arning leave duplicate photographs and casts of leprosy patients with the board. Arning declined, saying he had paid for these out of his salary for his own private use. He expected to use them in future publications.[92] Arning took all of his clinical photographs and casts back to Germany, much to the dismay of a cohort of prominent Honolulu business leaders and physicians who admired Arning's efforts. They petitioned the board to retain Arning so that his scientific experiments could continue, even offering to pay his salary for two years.[93]

Nathaniel B. Emerson was one of these ardent supporters. Emerson later wrote to Arning and tried to induce him to return to Hawai'i to continue this research.[94] Arning would not step foot in the Hawaiian Islands again, but for decades after his 1886 departure from Honolulu, his photographic method of investigating the body was taken up in manifold ways.

Emerson became a secretary of the BOH Committee on Treatment of Leprosy and enthusiastically spearheaded a bacteriological experiment in 1895 at the Kalihi Receiving Station, the facility that replaced the Kaka'ako Branch Hospital. This experiment drew inspiration from Arning's methodical and rational approach to germ chasing, though ultimately it, too, proved inconclusive. Twelve research subjects, mostly young Hawaiian boys and teenagers previously exiled to Molokai, were requisitioned and brought to Kalihi Station. One of the twelve was Ponepake Lapilio, the boy discussed in the introduction; Lapilio later would pose for an intergenerational portrait with his infant son and an older man at the settlement.

Like Arning's earlier experiments, but more grandiose in their aims, these bacteriological experiments in 1895 sought to solve the puzzle of whether leprosy was curable. They aspired to identify the "best means for its relief and eradication from the human system." This was an enigma Emerson had been aiming to solve since he had first examined and sketched leprosy patients almost twenty years prior. Emerson wrote optimistically, "Careful notes have been taken and photographs made of the patients and will be kept up during the different stages of the treatment."[95]

These boys were detained at Kalihi for at least two years, in 1895 and 1896, while their bodies were probed and photographed. According to Kalihi Hospital records, the boys were administered treatments such as zinc, arsenic, cod liver, ointments, ichthammol pills, and medicated baths; their skin ulcers, appetite, and weight were monitored. None of these approaches would amount to a cure. Despite the aspirational tone and embrace of photographic recordkeeping projected by Emerson, the surviving clinical files suggest that the photographs were far more haphazard and taken only occasionally. The photographs appear casually lit and composed. They often were treated as irrelevant to the laboratory work of the bacteriologist or, worse, performed in ways contrary to the needs of the bacteriological staff.[96] As with Emerson's own earlier forays into positivist drawings, the clinical photographs could not provide stable and consistent visual evidence of pathology.

On two of the photographs, the lead bacteriologist handwrote, "Note: arm and forearm not contracted as shown in photo. But hand and fingers shrunken and contracted." The physician needed to intervene narratively and explain these discrepancies between the photograph and his own visual observation. Another bacteriologist on the medical team tolerated but took little interest in the photographs, writing in his report: "The photographs were taken with the assistance of Mr. Bolster [Balster] as my knowledge of that subject is very limited."[97]

Although these particular scientists were indifferent to photographs, Arning and Emerson would be vindicated as champions of photography. Photography of leprosy patients would become official BOH policy and practice just a year later, in 1898. All confirmed leprous people, not just those being subjected to experimental treatment, would be photographed. The board approved a motion at a meeting in May 1898 that "all persons pronounced by the Board of Medical Examiners to be lepers shall be photographed and a record preserved of the name of the patient, number of the case, date of examination, and a description of the symptoms upon which the diagnosis was based."[98]

This visual approach to pathological bodies in Hawai'i was by no means exceptional, as police systems across Europe at the turn of the century ushered in similar methods of cataloguing the "criminal body," as Allan Sekula has analyzed.[99] However, Arning's ocular experiments had produced a local institutional template for the Hawai'i Board of Health's archive of skin to adapt. One scientist had already achieved so much. Arning's medical and ethnographic imaging would be translated into a broader juridical and carceral instrument—one concerned with capturing, sentencing, and entering these bodies into a criminal archival system, as I discuss in the following chapter.

AFTERLIVES

While Arning's experimental subjects lived out their sentences in detention, his art and medical career flourished upon his return to Hamburg, Germany. Equipped with a darkroom in his stately home, Arning continued to hone his skills as an amateur art photographer. He co-founded an amateur photography society in 1895 that mounted increasingly prominent international exhibitions. This turn-of-the-century art photography movement spanned Europe and the United States, exploring artistic expression beyond the realism and mimesis of photography's origins.[100]

Arning primarily adopted a naturalistic approach to his ethnographic and clinical subjects in Hawaiʻi. Yet he already had begun mixing conventions in some of these earlier photographs, experimenting with infusing mood into realist frames. In the portrait of a Hawaiian girl during medical detention, he created a composition of tonal contrast: a white collar framing darker skin, light-colored flowers in her hand and at her feet, and a black and white plaid dress (figure 14). Surrounded by light and space, she is poised as a lonely figure in an ephemeral moment. In Germany, Arning went on to craft tonal, atmospheric scenes of fleeting life, and his photographs were selected for exhibitions, awarded prizes, and printed in photograph journals.[101]

During this time, Arning established a private medical practice for skin and venereal diseases in Hamburg. In 1906, he was appointed senior physician in the country's largest dermatological ward, in St. Georg Hospital.[102] He also taught medical students at the newly founded University of Hamburg, published scientific papers, and organized the 1921 congress of the Deutsche Dermatologische Gesellschaft (German Dermatological Society), retiring with many professional honors. Arning and his wife, Helene Sophie, raised three children. Among their great-grandchildren is a man who has wrestled with the legacy of his ancestor's experiments. It was through Ruthard von Frankenberg, who conducted extensive research on Arning, that I finally located Arning's album of leprosy photographs, after three years of dead-end correspondence with German museum curators.

In 2000, Frankenberg found Arning's photographs and research materials in the archives of the Arnsteiner Patres in Aachen, Germany. After I contacted Frankenberg about my own ongoing research on Arning, he mailed me all of his personal notes, transcriptions, and copies of Arning's albums and documents from the Arnsteiner Patres archives. Frankenberg shared why he chose to give these materials to a scholar from Hawaiʻi whom he had never met: "For me all this is like fulfilling a duty towards my late great-grandfather Eduard Arning. From time to time I pray for Keanu the murderer and for Arning who probably killed him by his shocking in-vivo experiment. A doctor is not an executioner."[103] While Arning's subjects numbered at least fifty and possibly dozens more, how they lived and what they endured under Arning's watch are questions that do not have full answers.

Arning's carceral-medical experiments were not limited to the strictly clinical; they also included the unearthing of iwi kūpuna and ethnographic photography. We know the names of some people via Arning's documentation and clinical notes, but little about their lives before and after his experiments. Ranging from young to old, they included men, women, and children. Some, like the fifteen-year-old boy Kahalemake, died at the Molokai settlement within several years after the experiments concluded. Others survived longer.[104]

We can only speculate about what people felt while standing and sitting in front of Arning's camera. Did they ever get to view their own photographs? How did they experience the process of being exposed as clinical material? As Arning considered his subjects extinct specimens with utility as biomedical and ethnographic resources, he could not envision them living beyond their capture as types. Instead their tissue and photographs were preserved in medical research and natural history museums, serving as surrogates and reminders of their living bodies.

Arning placed one of these subjects, a thirteen-year old girl named Kealoha, in his leprosy album. Photographed unclothed in a physical anthropological framing in June 1885, she was labeled as "Lepra papul. circinata. Full Figure. Frontal" (figure 15). Although Arning had imaged Kealoha as a pathological type in isolation, she had a rich afterlife following this photograph. Far from alone in exile, she posed for at least one other photograph, establishing herself in specific relation to other people.

Two years after Arning photographed her at Kakaʻako Hospital, Kealoha was sent to the settlement on September 27, 1887. There, she married a man named Louis (or Lui) Nailima, who was almost thirty years her senior. By the time she was twenty-eight years old, Kealoha had had five children with Lui Nailima.[105] At least two of her sons survived and resided near her in the settlement—Joseph Hoaeae Nailima, born in 1894, and Louis Kahalewai Nailima, born in 1897; they were also incarcerated patients.

Colonial histories, Ann Stoler has argued, should consider how power was constituted through intrusion into the most intimate zones of the body and mind.[106] Ironically, people may have been less exposed to a culture of inspection after they were exiled to Molokai. Segregated and expected to die there, patients and their daily routines appear to have been less scrutinized by Western clinicians than in Honolulu detention facilities.

Around 1915 a woman and two younger men posed for an informal photograph portrait in the settlement, most likely taken by a Catholic missionary (figure 20).[107] This glass plate negative survives today in the archive of the Congregation of the Sacred Hearts of Jesus and Mary in Hawaiʻi; Catholic brothers and fathers shot hundreds of portraits of Molokai settlement residents in the early twentieth century. There is a strong family resemblance

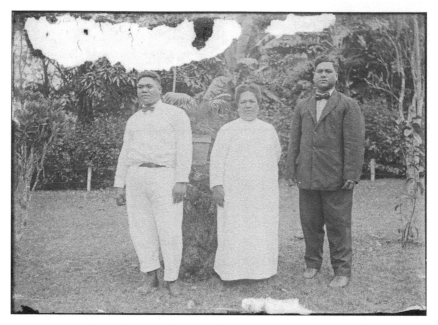

FIGURE 20. Left to right: possibly Joseph Hoaeae Nailima, Kealoha Nailima, and Louis Kahalewai Nailima, Kalaupapa settlement, Molokai, ca. 1915. SG 390, Congregation of the Sacred Hearts of Jesus and Mary U.S.A. Province.

between the three individuals in the portrait; they may be Kealoha Nailima and her sons Joseph Hoaeae Nailima and Louis Kahalewai Nailima.

Within the taxonomy of Arning's leprosy and ethnographic albums, the appearance of this family would be incongruous and unexpected, perhaps even disruptive. The three stand *en plein air,* unmarked by signifiers of illness or incarceration. It is neither a formal nor a tightly composed portrait: Joseph slouches and looks off at an angle, while Louis and his mother are angled toward one another. They are clothed modestly in an informal cotton wardrobe of the day, not exquisite finery. They do not wear clothing or floral adornments that would signify them as "Hawaiian," as did many of Arning's subjects in his ethnographic or leprosy series. They are not holding floral garlands; they do not pose as representatives of Hawaiian racial types. Nor are the Nailimas posed as clinical examples of leprosy, but stand within their own chosen grouping. With their bodies fully clothed and placed outside of the clinical setting, it is hardly possible to tell that they were exiled leprosy patients.

Unlike the anthropological-clinical type meant to sediment legible generic qualities, a portrait is linked to a particular person and allows that individual to be represented and recognized, as Richard Brilliant has theorized.[108] The portrait of the Nailimas is replete with idiosyncratic and individual details—the middle part of Kealoha's hairstyle, the half-visible belt and shirt of Hoaeae, the slightly crumpled shoulders of Kahalewai's jacket. These varied textures come into tension with Arning's photograph of Kealoha as a *typical* case meant to represent a group. The latter removes or diminishes individual characteristics to emphasize uniformity, while portraiture is a mode imparting personhood and particularity. Furthermore, the Nailima family portrait emphasizes lived relationality between specific individuals.

By the estimates of Arning, board physicians, and other Western observers of leprosy, Kealoha and her sons were not expected to live much beyond their moment of capture by the state. However, the Nailimas had personhood and vital kinship that far exceed Arning's photographs of pathologized disability. The sons had many children of their own, some of whom were taken away to institutional homes for non-leprous children by the territorial Board of Health.

A few years prior to posing for this photograph, Joseph Hoaeae, Louis Kahalewai, and a third brother named Kuheleloa signed up to be re-examined by a Board of Health physician, hoping to be declared non-leprous and secure their freedom from incarceration. Patients had petitioned the Hawai'i legislature for re-examination, resulting in bacteriological testing in 1909. Release from the settlement would be granted if the clinical exams and tissue appeared free of leprosy bacilli.[109] Hoaeae and his brothers had been born in the settlement and only knew life there, but they contested the terms of their incarceration nevertheless. The Nailima brothers were not among the group of patients released, but they continued to live in close proximity in the settlement throughout the twentieth century.

When Louis Kahalewai Nailima and Keahi Humphreys Schutte had a son in 1917, they named him Kuheleloa, the same name as Louis's brother. This honorific naming is a reminder of intimate ties fortified in the settlement.[110] Kealoha Nailima survived until 1922, at the age of fifty-one, long enough to welcome the arrival of this moʻopuna (grandchild) and many others. And so the people she cherished lived on in ways Arning would not have been able to imagine.

TWO

A Criminal Archive of Skin

IN 1903, A PHOTOGRAPH OF A HAWAIIAN leprosy patient appeared in the lead article of the *Journal of the American Medical Association* (figure 21). The author, a Philadelphia physician named Judson Daland, identified the male subject only by his clinical symptoms: "Leprosy, showing the characteristic plantar ulceration and changes in the fingers." The photograph, along with those of seven other patients from Hawai'i, dominated the text and drew the viewer's eye to open sores on his feet and fingers. Offering intimate optic encounters with leprous bodies, this image and its companions merged leprosy with specific Hawaiian pathological cases. Daland linked racial difference to this disease, confidently declaring that Hawaiians were subject to a "peculiar susceptibility" to leprosy, while whites were not.[1]

A decade later, another American physician re-used the very same clinical image of this man for a different purpose. This time, the photograph was used to promote a putatively successful surgical cure for leprosy. The caption in the 1913 *New York Medical Journal* read, "Illustrating surgical treatment of hand and foot," although no surgery had been performed.[2] The appearance of this clinical photograph ten years apart suggests how leprosy photographs performed much cultural work. Euro-American scientists relied on images of raced bodies with altered skin and body parts to draw attention to medical and public health narratives. At the same time, these images firmly attached this dreaded disease to people and bodies from the Pacific.

However, what was the specific origin and history of this photograph? How did it come to travel from Hawai'i to American medical journals and generate such flexible meanings? Why was it taken and whom did it represent? Some answers can be found by tracing this photograph back to its original entry in the Hawai'i Board of Health archive in 1902 (figure 22). The

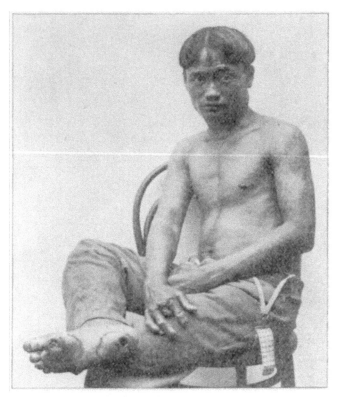

Fig. 7.—Leprosy, showing the characteristic plantar ulceration and changes in the fingers.

FIGURE 21. Photograph published in Daland, "Leprosy in the Hawaiian Islands," *Journal of the American Medical Association* 41 (November 7, 1903).

person imaged was a nineteen-year-old Hawaiian man named John Kapuahi, also known as Keoni Kapuahi.[3] Kapuahi's file was created when he entered the leprosy detention compound, also known as the Kalihi Hospital and Receiving Station, in the port city of Honolulu, on February 3, 1902.[4] A few weeks later, his photograph was taken in the hospital. Determined to have an incurable case of leprosy, John Kapuahi was sent to a settlement on the Makanalua peninsula of Molokai island in March 1902. He died there at the age of twenty-six in 1910.

Hawai'i not only isolated and exiled thousands of leprosy suspects beginning in 1866, but its health bureau began to photograph and archive individual cases in the 1870s. This imaging became more systematic after the United States illegally annexed Hawai'i in 1898. Hawai'i produced spectacular images

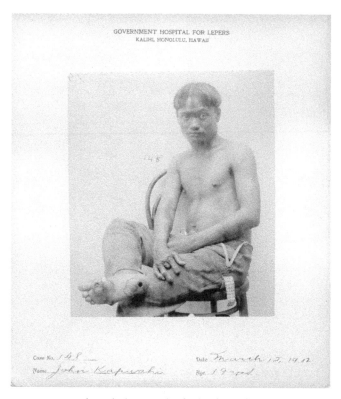

FIGURE 22. Clinical photograph of John (Keoni) Kapuahi. Kalihi Hospital case 148, March 12, 1902, nineteen years. Hawai'i State Archives.

of leprosy patients that were collected, archived, and published in transnational political and medical venues. These images may constitute one of the earliest and largest visual archives of leprosy created and maintained by a colonial government.[5] Yet despite this broad circulation, we know remarkably little about the production and institutional contexts of this visual archive and even less of its meanings.

In this chapter I trace the production and archival force of these leprosy photographs, what I'm calling an archive of skin. I discuss the construction of this archive of skin and the promiscuous signification of its contents, drawing upon approaches to "archiving-as-process rather than archives-as-things" proposed by Ann Stoler and Warwick Anderson in their respective studies of colonial archives and biomedicine.[6] With few exceptions, studies of leprosy and tropical medicine pay only passing attention to photographic technologies and visual culture beyond illustrations of medical and social categories.[7] Yet these leprosy photographs were critical, not incidental, to the foundations of an archival system of medico-juridical segregation and racialized biomedical knowledge.

Internally, photographs established evidence for the legal and medical category of leprosy that consigned a person to lifelong exile. Though public health officials asserted their truth-value, clinical photographs of leprosy were weak signifiers, producing incoherent, ambiguous, and often contradictory data for diagnosis. Photographs could perhaps *illustrate* certain advanced somatic signs of leprosy; these visual stigmata included skin lesions, tissue loss, and contracted fingers. However, photographs could not reliably predict who was a probable contagious carrier or might become a future case.

Yet this weak signification also exerted strong force, enabling promiscuous and flexible applications for colonial administrators. Despite an epistemological unruliness that at times confounded its own adherents, the archive of skin proved valuable as a flexible instrument of juridical and carceral management that embedded criminalized disease into Native Hawaiian and non-European immigrant populations. As Allan Sekula has argued forcefully, a new "criminal body"—and one that was often classed and racialized—was created through photographic archives in the nineteenth century.[8] Contemporaneously the field of psychiatry invented the female hysteric in the photographic "image factory" of the Salpêtrière Hospital, as Georges Didi-Huberman has theorized.[9] Extending Sekula's and Didi-Huberman's analyses into a colonial-biomedical context, I argue that the criminal body merged with the raced-sexed leprous body in this archive of skin. These photographs took on more acute value as a technology of carceral medicine, when enforcement practices such as medical parole were adopted to increase compliance in Hawaiian communities in the twentieth century.

The photographs also remained indefinitely in the archive, taking on a life of their own even after the people they indexed had died. Far outside the Hawaiian Islands, they circulated prolifically, generating political capital and advancing claims of racial-sexual pathology. These images arrested viewers, arousing fear, disgust, pity, and erotic fascination. Bodies altered by leprosy became valuable resources that girded epistemologies of biomedicine, missionary philanthropy, criminality, and colonial alterity. As elaborate ways of knowing, they enacted and revealed settler and imperial anxieties about racial-sexual intimacies and disabilities in Hawai'i. Images from the archive of skin were consumed by wider audiences following the 1898 U.S. annexation of Hawai'i, as the kingdom's Board of Health evolved into a territorial institution and collaborated with federal public health personnel. The territorial Board of Health curated and distributed select archival photographs to American counterparts as an eroticized political resource.

Colonial biomedicine and public health institutions fixed an intense eroticized gaze on Indigenous and immigrant leprosy suspects, who were sometimes captured wholly or partially nude in order to best expose deformities and somatic differences. However, the most spectacularized forms of visual stigmata and nude patient photographs are not reproduced here in full, as a deliberate methodological and ethical consideration that I relay in the introduction. The people represented within were more than biomedical subjects, but persist as kūpuna (elders) whose iwi (bones) and experiences are treasured by people living today.[10] The conclusion of the chapter thus attempts to balance the scopophilic clinical gaze with photographs of people weaving an intricate community of care.

A MEDICO-JURIDICAL ARCHIVE OF SKIN

The archive that remains of a century of leprosy management by the Hawai'i Board of Health (BOH) is both detailed and incomplete.[11] During a fifteen-year period between 1895 and 1909, the BOH archived approximately 900 files and 1,400 individual clinical photographs of patients. These images represent only part of a much longer process of photographing leprosy patients. Known in Hawaiian as Papa Ola, the Board of Health began photographing patients sporadically beginning in 1878.[12] It officially instituted the practice of photographing confirmed leprosy patients in 1898, which continued at least until the 1950s. Collectively, then, these extant images represent an archival practice and investment in photography that spanned more than half a century.[13]

On the one hand, this archive of skin is part of a much longer practice of illustrating dermatological cases. Perhaps the "most visual of all" medical fields, dermatology mapped the surface of the skin with visual evidence and analysis, Katherine Ott has established.[14] Among skin diseases, leprosy has been one of the most visually represented. Illustrations of its sufferers date back to the Middle Ages, and the first colored lithographs of leprosy patients in Norway were published in 1847.[15] Yet this more generic iconography did not strongly tie leprous bodies to race, nationality, place, or cultural practices. Photographs circulating from Hawai'i's leprosy institutions, however, would link illicit sexuality and domesticity with raced-sexed difference and disability.

Furthermore, the archive of skin emerging from Hawai'i is distinct as a genre of medical photography, for it was not produced by individual physicians, but was instituted and financed by the colonial state. While American physicians advocated photography for documenting unusual or spectacular clinical cases in the 1880s, and some photographed their own patients for diagnostic purposes decades earlier,[16] the Hawai'i archive represents a broader scale and functional organization of colonial-medical photography. It may constitute the most extensive visual and biopolitical cataloguing of Indigenous and Asian bodies within America's Pacific empire.

The leprosy suspects who entered Kalihi Hospital and Detention Station were treated as inmates and lost the liberty to come and go. The compound was enclosed by an eight-foot-wide perimeter and eight-foot-high double fence to prevent escape from within and entry from outside.[17] People usually remained at this facility for a short period before they were exiled to the Molokai settlement for life.[18] It was here that photographs were shot after the suspect's medical intake examination.

Photographing each leprosy suspect was likely a costly and time-consuming endeavor. The hospital did not have its own photographer, so this labor was outsourced to a studio photographer in Honolulu.[19] The clinical photograph was a medical and juridical piece of evidence. The board relied on photographs to confirm a clinical diagnosis of leprosy and to document the suspect's somatic condition. Though the earliest clinical photographs in the archive date back to 1895, the BOH made photography an explicit part of medical diagnosis in 1898: "[I]t was ordered that all persons pronounced by the Board of Medical Examiners to be lepers shall be photographed and a record preserved of the name of the patient, number of the case, date of examination, and a description of the symptoms upon which the diagnosis was based."[20]

The 1865 Act to Prevent the Spread of Leprosy gave "full power" to health agents to remove and exile all those it deemed leprous in Hawai'i.[21] The examination process thus entangled medical categories of contagion and infection with carceral practices. Individuals were parsed into three medical and juridical categories during these visual inspections: "Not a Leper," "Leper," and "Suspect." A "leper" was someone who was "incurable or capable of spreading the disease of leprosy." These people were exiled to Molokai for life.[22] A "suspect" was someone who was a "doubtful" case or "not in sufficiently advanced stages" to spread the disease. Suspects were separated from confirmed cases at the detention compound and kept under observation.[23]

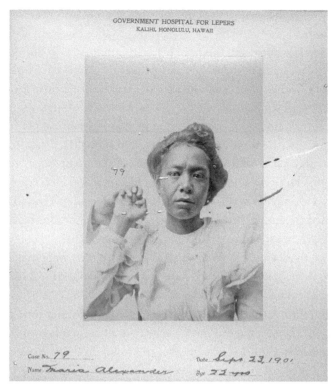

GOVERNMENT HOSPITAL FOR LEPERS
KALIHI, HONOLULU, HAWAII

79

Case No. 79   Date Sept 23, 1901
Name Maria Alexander   Age 22 yrs

FIGURE 23. Clinical photograph of Maria Alexander. Kalihi Hospital
case 79, September 23, 1901, twenty-two years. Hawai'i State Archives.

Of those inspected, the largest number were sentenced as "lepers," followed
by suspects, and a much smaller set of non-leprous people.[24]

Above all, the photograph dominated the clinical record. In Hawai'i, the
photograph was a central part of the leprosy case file, traveling with a patient's
clinical file, sometimes for decades. The photograph, measuring about eight
by ten inches, was printed on albumen paper and mounted on thick cardboard. The photographs are heavy, bored through with insect holes and
occasionally dusted with droppings, as is the photograph of twenty-two-year-
old Maria Alexander, shot in 1901 (figure 23).[25]

The Board of Health published its procedures and publicized legible outcomes that lent the appearance of scientific objectivity, juridical fairness, and
impartiality.[26] Since a positive diagnosis of leprosy led to lifelong detention
and separation from one's natal community, the board sought to document
rational and incontrovertible proof of infection. How would the camera
assist with such evidence?

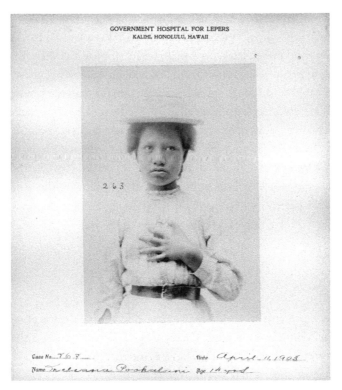

GOVERNMENT HOSPITAL FOR LEPERS
KALIHI, HONOLULU, HAWAII

2 6 3

Case No. 763   Date April 11, 1903
Name Meleana Pookalani   Age 14 yrs

FIGURE 24. Clinical photograph of Meleana Pookalani. Kalihi Hospital case 263, April 11, 1903, fourteen years. Hawai'i State Archives.

Scholars of nineteenth-century medical photography have argued Western physicians readily adopted photographic technologies because they believed the camera extended, and even improved, the objective medical gaze and diagnostic abilities.[27] In Hawai'i, the medical camera came into use after a government physician's initial examination indicated leprosy. Ideally the pathological symptoms first notated by the physician would be visible in the photograph that was shot several days or weeks after the initial intake. Exposing skin and body parts like hands, arms, feet, ears, and face, the photograph was expected to render pathologies visible, confirm the clinical diagnosis noted on the record, and thus provide medical and legal proof.

The 1903 file of a fourteen-year-old Hawaiian girl named Meleana Pookalani reveals the relationship between the physician's eye and the truth claims of the medical photograph. In three consecutive sections printed on Meleana's intake record—"hands: atrophied," "contracted," and "fingers"— the physician filled in the corresponding answers: "yes, left," "yes, left," and "left re[tracted] and contracted" at her physical examination on April 2, 1903. The link between leprosy and her affected hand was affirmed by the photograph taken over a week later, on April 11, 1903 (figure 24).[28] In it, Meleana spreads the fingers of her left hand and holds them against her chest; she was likely instructed to do so in order to expose a hand that the physician had denoted as affected. As with Meleana, the medical camera worked best for indexing advanced signs of leprosy, once they had manifested on the surface of the skin. Thus, the photograph was only taken after a suspicious or positive diagnosis of leprosy, not to aid in diagnosis. If the photograph in Hawai'i leprosy files was not a diagnostic instrument pinpointing the affliction of an individual patient, what was its utility? It served as a carceral tool for biopolitical profiling, analogous to a criminal mug shot.

CRIMINAL PROFILES

The archive represents an effort to gather as much visual data as possible, and an insistent empiricism haunts these files. Whereas nineteenth-century American and European physicians like Eduard Arning assembled medical photographs of spectacular bodies for their personal research collections (discussed in chapter 1), this archive of skin grew within a colonial administrative context as the systematic cataloguing of suspects. It drew its inspirations and aspirations from the intertwined visual genealogies of criminology, physical anthropology, and medicine.

Nineteenth-century criminologists advanced theories that moral degeneracy and criminality could be located visually on a body. Italian physician and criminologist Cesare Lombroso identified somatic signs, including small heads, flat notes, and large ears as "anomalies" and symptoms of degeneracy and dangerousness in the 1870s. Likening criminals to racial savages, Lombroso collected skulls, brains, and photographs of criminals and assembled galleries of these visual and biological materials in a museum of criminal anthropology.[29] Criminals were degenerates who could be identified through visual data, he and his contemporaries asserted.

Working in the Paris police department, Alphonse Bertillon transformed criminal identification by recording physical descriptions, measurements, "peculiar" bodily inscriptions like tattoos, and photographs of prisoners. His system of anthropometric identification was instituted in the United States and Canada in 1887 and spread to other European and colonial penal institutions in the 1890s.[30] Both Lombroso's and Bertillon's systems interpreted visual stigmata to reveal a criminal body prone to recidivism. Francis Galton's composite of criminal types and the eugenicist classification system for identifying "feeble-mindedness" were other visual collections of crime and disability aimed to identify future subjects based on visual profiles.[31]

The Hawai'i archive of skin did not produce a profile of a singular leprous "type" or exemplary "types" against which physicians could compare incoming cases, but it aspired to catalogue and decode bodies visually. Like criminologists mapping the body for criminality and recidivism, doctors hewed to a similar logic and scoured the body for signs of leprous infiltration. White spots, bent toes, thin eyebrows—all were potential clues. The recidivism of born criminals became animated in the promise of capturing the relapsed or "reactivated" leprosy patient. A person determined to be "clean" was still dangerous and could emerge as a leprous body years later.

If trained physicians were thwarted by their own eyes (that is, they failed to "see" leprous germs lurking within these bodies), photographs offered the "capacity of foresight," the possibility of anticipating the future of these bodies.[32] Didi-Huberman characterizes this faith in nineteenth-century photography as "showing what the eye could never perceive."[33] The leprosy archive achieved this prognostic ability not by producing a sensitivity better than that of physicians' retina, but by achieving a kind of oversight. The archive's greatest achievement was in overlooking the proliferation of individual differences to view case histories as a suspicious collectivity. In other words, the archive achieved *foresight through oversight:* skimming over individual differences in skin and symptoms and melding them into a collective of pathogenic criminality. This archive may have stumbled over individual diagnoses and symptoms, but its grandest accomplishment was creating unity out of difference.

By creating a large photographic archive of leprosy suspects, the colonial health bureaucracy captured suspects and created a visual catalogue of those currently under suspicion and likely to become leprous in the future. In essence, the clinical photograph was coextensive with the police photograph, known later as a mug shot: a visual record of the suspect upon capture. The shot ceremoniously entered suspects into the archive and put them on notice that they and their relations were under surveillance. Generally speaking, people determined to have leprosy were not photographed again to track the development of symptoms. Rather, once sentenced as leprous, they were expected to die in exile. This practice appears to have been briefly amended in the early 1920s as select patients were photographed in before and after shots during a short-lived experimental treatment and parole system, as I elaborate later.

As a surveillance mechanism, the clinical photograph did not need to reveal any signs of leprosy. Merely being cast in these poses was an indictment, framing its subjects as suspects. Thus all men, women, and children who were photographed were functionally cast as leprous bodies in the making, whether they had obvious markings, faint markings, or none. More important than determining the clinical outcome of an individual patient was the task of creating an expanding archive of suspects.

Being a suspect in the filing system meant one was in biopolitical purgatory, subject to recall and inspection. As the board stipulated in 1890, the only way to be cleared of suspicion was if "there ceases to be a doubt as to the nature of the disease under which they suffer."[34] Twenty-five-year-old Hannah Paona was ruled a suspect in 1891 when she was first apprehended and assigned case number 76. As a suspect for the next fifteen years, she was under medical observation and subject to sheriffs' seizure and a leprosy examining board at any time. She had to self-report symptoms and submit to examination by a haole (white foreigner) government physician at least once a month on her home island of Maui.[35] When Hannah Paona was reexamined and required to expose her legs in her intake photograph in 1904, she was officially ruled leprous as case number 381. Yet her exile to the leprosy settlement had been prefigured by her suspicious diagnosis fifteen years prior.

RECONCILING OPTICAL EVIDENCE

Despite this apparent confidence in the camera, findings or diagnoses of leprosy could be contradicted by the image itself. Unlike smallpox, plague, and measles, where somatic changes and death took only days, leprosy could take years to surface on the skin and was notoriously difficult to diagnosis. Its external presentation could mimic eczema or syphilis. Some symptoms of leprosy, like erythema (superficial red patches), were difficult for the camera to capture, highlighting the discrepancy between the doctor's expectations and the camera's ambiguous output, as in the case of Mary [Keawe] Akim. An examiner at Kalihi Hospital noted a suspicious "eruption of the face of patches like erythema" on May 9, 1898. He wrote on Akim's record, "She is a leper: the infiltration of the face is characteristic."

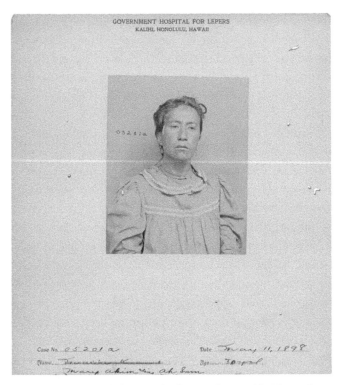

GOVERNMENT HOSPITAL FOR LEPERS
KALIHI, HONOLULU, HAWAII

Case No. 05201a   Date January 11, 1898
Name.   Age   30 years
Mary Akim tin ah Sam

FIGURE 25. Clinical photograph of Mary Akim. Kalihi Hospital case 05201a, May 11, 1898, thirty years. Hawai'i State Archives.

However, these patches are not noticeable in Akim's photograph (figure 25), taken two days later. The medical camera could not faithfully replicate the "characteristic" patches that the doctor saw with his eyes. The examiner reversed his findings and wrote below the original note, "She was declared as a S. [suspect]—for examination. No bacilli found."[36] The notation of "no bacilli" meant that no leprosy bacilli had been observable by microscope in the suspect's scraped tissue. Rather than bestowing self-evident knowledge, the camera revealed itself a "subjective apparatus."[37] These turn-of-the-century records underscore how the photograph and the microscope were brought into the same interpretative field, provoking uncertainty.

Beginning in the 1890s, clinical photographs were increasingly read alongside an analogous form of visual evidence: bacteriological readings.[38] Photographs revealed the surface of the skin, while microscopes purported to expose what lived beneath it. Both visual technologies were ineffective for conclusive leprosy diagnoses and offered conflicting or irreconcilable forms of evidence. Bacteriologists in the 1890s were frustrated by not being able to obtain microscopic confirmation of leprosy bacilli when symptoms like skin lesions seemed to be evident on the body. Tissue samples were taken from the body and slides stained carefully to reveal the presence of bacilli, but even with advanced training, cases of "false-negatives" persisted, as the lead bacteriologist at Kalihi Hospital explained in 1897.[39]

To which kind of visual evidence would physicians give weight? In Mary Akim's particular case, the clinician's eye may have prevailed, as she was subsequently exiled to Molokai. However, clinicians and judges oscillated between these ambiguous forms of evidence in the twentieth century. Hawaiʻi board bacteriologist Jonathan T. McDonald described the difficulty of choosing the right tissue to snip on a body; there was a high likelihood these tissues would yield "negative smears" or a few groups of bacilli under the microscope. McDonald acknowledged the juridical weight of clinical determinations that consigned someone to lifelong exile, writing, "While the microscope is thus first in importance, it is in practice the last agent to be employed; it is only after all the various symptoms have been canvassed that an appeal to it is made as a *court of last resort*" (my emphasis).[40]

These contradictions between forms of optical evidence threatened to undermine the very segregation law on which the Board of Health relied. In 1909, patients and their families petitioned the territorial legislature for re-examination by the Board of Health. Nineteen of these legislative resolutions passed. Eleven people held in leprosy institutions were re-examined. They showed enough visible improvement to be ruled not leprous and were released from BOH custody with clearance certificates. Ranging from ages six to seventy-nine years old, they had been institutionalized from three to twenty years. A Hawaiʻi daily newspaper opined that these people were "victims of a terrible mistake." One of these eleven people was a seventy-nine-year-old Hawaiian man named Naiwi from Pālama, Oʻahu, who had been apprehended and examined in 1906, showing "deformed" hands and "very few" bacilli.[41] Naiwi and the other ten patients may not have been cured, but their bacterial counts had waned as leprosy is now understood to do, presenting as remission.[42]

Hearing news of these releases, over 170 patients requested re-examinations at the settlement. These requests were so numerous that physicians traveled to Molokai in 1909 to conduct exams instead of patients coming to Kalihi Hospital in Honolulu.[43] These well-publicized cases destabilized the authority of the territorial Board of Health. Had doctors misdiagnosed or misperceived leprosy? Should a legal declaration of leprosy require the microscopic presence of bacilli? The Hawai'i attorney general ruled in 1919 that the board did not need to find bacilli in a patient to declare a person leprous. This decision thereby granted maximum discretion to board physicians to adjudicate clinical and microscopic evidence as they saw fit.[44] These tensions between the microscope, the physician's eye, and the camera thus were reconciled through a capacious system that could accommodate diagnostic ambiguity and incommensurability. *Not seeing* could be a form of power itself.

Yet these discrepancies in "optical empiricism," as Allan Sekula has described the phenomena, opened up opportunities for patients to challenge the validity of their medical sentences.[45] The experience of a Hawaiian man named Frank Carr suggests how patients also usurped photography as a form of evidence. Exiled in 1901 to Molokai at age thirteen, Carr had married a fellow patient there, a young woman named Emma Kalanikupaulakea Nakuina in 1907. Kalanikupaulakea Nakuina's mother, Emma Ka'ilikapuolono Metcalf Nakuina, successfully petitioned for her daughter, son-in-law Carr, and niece Manu Beckley to be brought from Molokai to Kalihi Hospital and treated there by a physician at the family's own expense. Carr underwent treatment for over a year. Due to his "wonderful improvement under the treatment," Carr and his attorney requested permission to photograph Carr at the hospital, presumably in order to provide evidence to secure his release. The board approved J. J. Williams, an established Honolulu studio photographer, to take Carr's photograph in June 1909.[46] Carr died about a year later, leaving Emma Kalanikupaulakea Nakuina a distraught twenty-year-old widow in the settlement. While it is unknown whether Carr's photograph was entered into evidence for a re-examination petition, this episode reveals how incarcerated patients, especially savvy and more affluent ones, interpreted photography as leverage for self-advocacy.

INTIMATE RELATIONS AND SKIN

Leprosy affected people of all ages, nationalities, classes, and ethnicities in the United States, Europe, and its possessions, including white settlers. Although leprosy was officially and colloquially called ma'i Pākē (Chinese sickness) or "Chinese leprosy" in Hawai'i, its carceral management became associated with Kānaka 'Ōiwi (Native Hawaiians). By far the largest group of people imaged in this archive of skin was Kānaka. In the twentieth century, as more

Portuguese, Chinese, and Japanese settler immigrants and their descendants were exiled, their images also were taken and circulated. Portuguese recruited to Hawaiʻi as plantation laborers were European, but they were not racialized as "white" or "Anglo-Saxon" in Hawaiʻi settler society.[47]

While white Europeans and Americans may have experienced lower rates of infection, they were neither ensnared in the carceral net with the same intensity nor readily entered into the visual archive. Why was this the case? The Board of Health, which itself was composed largely of wealthy white settlers, only reluctantly detained and exiled whites for having leprosy. These cases seem to have been unreported, underreported, or kept secret by the board to avoid embarrassment to Hawaiʻi and their home countries.[48] Europeans and Americans who had means to do so left Hawaiʻi upon learning they had contracted leprosy. They were known to escape exile by going to the United States, Japan, or Germany for treatment. French-born BOH physician Georges Trousseau encouraged white foreigners to repatriate and even paid the return fare for those lacking the means in the 1880s.[49]

Euro-American scientists and physicians debated whether leprosy was a hereditary condition. Despite this lack of consensus, many treated leprosy as a racial disease.[50] Physicians practicing in Hawaiʻi believed that Hawaiians, and to a lesser degree, Asians, were prone to infection due to purported biological susceptibility and cultural habits. In American medical journals, they characterized what they viewed as Hawaiians' domestic disorder, promiscuity, communal eating, sleeping arrangements, and lack of cleanliness as links to leprosy.

American physician and former Molokai settlement physician George L. Fitch, writing about the etiology of leprosy in 1892, relied on florid prose to describe Hawaiians engaging in illicit relations with one another and white foreigners: "Before the advent of the whites in Hawaii, marriage, as we understand the word, one male and one female consecrating themselves to each other only, was practically unknown."[51] Besides promiscuous intercourse, Fitch alluded to Hawaiian improvidence, drunkenness, and incest as causes of their moral and physical degeneration. By contrast, white settlers lived in legible heteronormative domestic households; these subjects were thought to possess a naturally "high degree of immunity."[52] Hawaiians were explicitly and implicitly blamed as the cause of infection in Euro-Americans.

This habit of discursively scrutinizing the intimate spaces of Hawaiian bodily practices underwrote the ethos and visual practices of colonial medical inspection, the intake form, and the clinical photograph. The BOH physician queried each suspect about a family history of leprosy that corresponded to specific lines on the preprinted form for the condition of the suspect's father, mother, brother, and sister. The question, "Any relative or intimate associate past or present leprous?" demanded either a confession or a disavowal: it required a suspect to admit to associations with kin and friends who had been caught, or to renounce those very same relations.

When fifty-five-year-old Kaulili Kuula was examined as case 382 in March 1904, her response was recorded on her record as: "Had a cousin sent to M. [Molokai] as a leper but have never lived in the same house with a leper and have never associated with lepers." To defend her uninfected status, Kuula was required to assert her domestic space as clean and to keep herself distinct from certain kin. Twenty-one-year-old Makanui Kanehe had to report more relations, including her husband. Kanehe said in December 1902, "I have had 5 cousins sent to Molokai as lepers and more at home under suspicion who have never been before the board. My husband is here with me for examination."[53] Kinship—a sustaining set of genealogical ties, social and political relations for Hawaiian communities—became cause for suspicion and indictment for the adjudicating medical panel.

If the medical form made visible a patient's social relations, the clinical photograph offered doctors intimate encounters with a patient's skin. Suspects entering medical detention were made to expose their bodies and afflicted skin for the medical camera. Non-European men, women, and children were occasionally imaged nude or partially nude. We see this erotic convention structuring two particular images taken of young Hawaiian women in 1903, though I have reproduced only the upper portions of these photographs. Twenty-one-year-old Makanui Kanehe covers her breasts with crossed arms, while her shoulders are bared in the shot (figure 26). Eighteen-year-old Oliwaliilii was captured in a three-quarter length pose that same year, unclothed from the waist up and back turned to the camera, in order to reveal erupted skin on her back (figure 27).[54] Similar to pornographic images of women from this period, Oliwaliilii's clinical pose suggestively reveals the outline of one of her breasts.

These two images represent a more extensive erotic repertoire in which unclothed patients were posed cupping their genitals and breasts with their hands. Male patients, young and old, were also captured nude or in loincloths in several angles that called attention to their genitals and buttocks.[55] Health agents in Hawai'i exhibited a voyeuristic fascination with altered skin and the racial-sexual alterity of their subjects in these photographic portraits.[56]

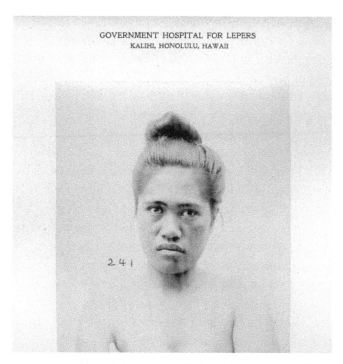

GOVERNMENT HOSPITAL FOR LEPERS
KALIHI, HONOLULU, HAWAII

FIGURE 26. Clinical photograph of Makanui Kanehe, cropped from original. Kalihi Hospital case 241, February 5, 1903, twenty-one years. Hawai'i State Archives.

The mise-en-scène of the leprosy photograph hewed to a particular choreography of poses and exposures, such as arms crossed, fingers spread, or feet flexed to best allow the physician to correlate earlier findings. Depending on the affected areas of the body, these poses could be accomplished via full-length, medium, or close-up shots of buttocks, thighs, or ulcerated feet. Capturing skin through photography did not necessarily require removal of clothing, but it subjected patients to vulnerable positions before the camera nonetheless. The suspects were posed to reveal skin on their cheeks, backs, chins, hands, or feet, even if their bodies were fully or partially "dressed" with clothing. Hands and feet transformed by nerve damage and lesions became favored subjects of the medical camera in Hawai'i.

Hawaiians assumed greatest visibility in this archive of skin, followed by Chinese and Japanese. The clinical exam and visual files became opportunities for physicians to inspect and probe raced-sexed bodies in the guise of dispassionate clinical observation. With labels indicating gender and national background, doctors learned to map race, sex, and gender onto the bodies of

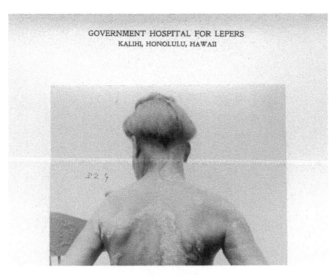

GOVERNMENT HOSPITAL FOR LEPERS
KALIHI, HONOLULU, HAWAII

FIGURE 27. Clinical photograph of Oliwaliilii, cropped from original. Kalihi Hospital case 329, September 11, 1903, eighteen years. Hawai'i State Archives.

those patients variously described as "half-Hawaiian" boy, a "Chinese" girl, or a "½ Hawaiian, ½ Japanese" woman.

Hundreds of images of Hawaiian, Chinese, Filipino, Japanese, and Portuguese suspects at their most exposed, including those identified as racially mixed, were placed in BOH files. In this archive of skin, the leprous body and racially Othered bodies became indistinguishable. Just as the female hysteric was invented via photographic tableaux of "spectacular evidence" in the Salpêtrière Hospital, convincingly theorized by Georges Didi-Huberman, so were the figures of leprous Hawaiian and Asian suspects invented in this visual archive of skin.[57]

In contrast, the bodies of white settlers, who were a statistical minority of patients overall, were not the principal objects of eroticized medical stares in the archive. In keeping with the de facto exemption of whites from incarceration at Molokai, the board visualized white suspects as innocent victims of leprosy, rather than its agents. When photographed, white European and American suspects often were imaged according to representational codes that accorded anonymity, privacy, and gendered discretion.

In 1903, the same year that the Hawaiian women Makanui Kanehe and Oliwaliilii (figures 26 and 27) were seized as suspects, another American woman was photographed using a different set of visual conventions.

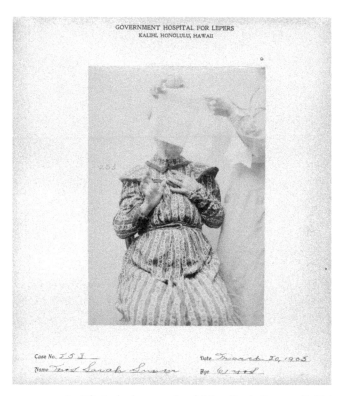

FIGURE 28. Clinical photograph of Mrs. Sarah Sunter. Kalihi Hospital case 253, March 20, 1903, sixty-one years. Hawai'i State Archives.

Sixty-one-year-old Sarah Sunter was suspected of leprosy because of shrunken digits on her hand and extensive anesthetic patches (areas without feeling and pain) on both feet and legs. These symptoms were duly noted in her 1903 clinical record. Sunter was addressed with the honorific "Mrs. Sarah Sunter" in her clinical file, although she was divorced.[58] Her hands, with their shrunken and amputated digits, are posed on her chest, similar to the clinical choreography of contemporaneous Hawaiian and Asian patients (figure 28).

However, another white woman, possibly a nurse, friend, or relation, stepped into the frame to hide Sunter's face with a cloth. With the covering of her face, Sunter's personhood was uncoupled from her diseased body. Nor did the board photograph Sunter's feet, as they did scores of other patients. Thus white womanhood was represented through the gendered visual codes of victim; Sunter was figured as the unwitting recipient of disease, rather than a culpable source of leprosy.

Sunter's photograph is the only one I have seen of a white American woman taken during a fifteen-year period in Kalihi detention. In the early 1900s, white Americans and Europeans, and American women in particular, constituted a virtual minority, if not an outright anomaly, in the settlement. When Sunter was exiled to Molokai on March 24, 1903, she entered as the sole American woman in the settlement; there is no record of any other American women living there at least two years prior to her arrival. Only four American men were incarcerated, compared to 794 Hawaiian men and women.[59]

Sunter's gendered-raced access to privacy in this photographic setting remains significant, as it represents broader legal and social protections accorded to white-identified people in territorial health policies and practices, regardless of their small numbers. Racial segregation along the axis of white/non-white was enacted and reinforced among leprosy patients in the very built environment and forms of material access.

The American-born superintendent of the settlement, Jack D. McVeigh, with the support of prominent missionary-son patrons, initiated a private charitable fund to build a separate and better-appointed home for "white foreigners" in 1908. Approved by the BOH and opened in 1910, the home created a privileged space for white inmates, so they would not have to live, sleep, and eat under the same roof as non-whites. McVeigh Home, which opened in 1910, was run by the territorial BOH and offered superior services compared to the charity-based dormitories supervised by Catholic orders.[60] Even within the sanitary arrangement that separated diseased people from the uninfected, racial-class hierarchies were fortified between disabled whites and non-whites.

In this settler-colonial context, privacy was a deeply racialized privilege accessed by white women and men of multiple classes and ranks. Sarah Sunter (née Rogers), the aforementioned woman, was the daughter of American Congregationalist missionaries. Educated at the missionary-founded Punahou School in Honolulu, Sunter had worked as a schoolteacher in Hawai'i. While Sunter's economic status may have been more precarious than the circle of haole settler missionaries from which she hailed, her relations were able to obscure her illness from greater public view. When Sunter died in Kalaupapa settlement in January 1904, her obituary in the *Friends* missionary journal omitted mention of her exile, alluding only to final years "clouded by illness."[61] Indeed, as another lasting mark of her racialized access to privacy and privilege, Sunter was not buried in Kalaupapa. Her grave is recorded at the cemetery at Kawaiahaʻo Church, the prominent Congregationalist church in Honolulu attended by Hawaiian aliʻi and foreign missionaries.

Hawaiians of chiefly and non-chiefly status could not secure this privacy, nor could Asian immigrants.[62] One leprosy suspect was the daughter of two highly regarded Hawaiian leaders. In September 1905, Moses and Emma Nakuina wrote to the BOH president surrendering their sixteen-year-old daughter Emma Kalanikupaulakea Nakuina. Moses and Emma Nakuina were widely respected kaukau aliʻi (lower-ranking chiefly status) with bicultural fluency. They held prominent positions in the Hawaiian community: Moses as a minister and member of the Hawaiian Evangelical Association, and Emma Kaʻilikapuolono Metcalf as a multilingual ethnographer, writer, and museum curator. Their daughter, Emma Kalanikupaulakea Nakuina, had developed symptoms of leprosy. Moses and Emma Nakuina implored the president, "We would take it as a favor if she is allowed to waive all the usual examinations in consideration of her perfect willingness to go. Such examinations cannot fail of being very painful to the feelings and repugnant to any young girl or modest woman."[63] Yet this courtesy was not extended to the genteel daughter and her family. Emma Kalanikupaulakea Nakuina was photographed as a suspect at Kalihi Hospital on October 2, 1905, her arms crossed over her chest and her face exposed.[64]

PAROLE AND PEDAGOGY: BEFORE AND AFTER

Archiving leprosy patients was a powerful practice of colonial governance and carceral medicine. Colonial archives were "intricate technologies of rule in themselves," as Ann Stoler has argued.[65] I consider here how the photographic archive of skin underwrote one such technology of rule: the "parole," or selective release of patients. This represented a key shift in the biopolitical management of leprosy in the early 1900s when Hawaiʻi was an incorporated territory under U.S. federal control. Territorial status brought federal resources and the arrival of U.S. public health surgeons who contributed technical expertise to the Board of Health, a former kingdom institution led by white settler physicians and businessmen.

A sense of optimism about a cure for leprosy emerged in the early 1900s. With the introduction of therapeutics like the Southeast Asian chaulmoogra oil in the early twentieth century, some patients began to show improvement and possible arrest of the disease.[66] The board adopted the language of parole to describe provisional release of such patients from Kalihi Hospital and Molokai settlement in 1911, although patient agitation had been successful in securing medical re-examination and release as early as 1908.[67] Hawai'i physician and bacteriologist J. T. McDonald went so far to announce "Leprosy Not an Incurable Disease" in a 1920 U.S. public report.[68]

Between 1912 and 1921, 242 leprosy patients, or approximately 30 percent of segregated cases, were paroled.[69] The board claimed parole was an "almost revolutionary departure from the old method of segregation for the remainder of the victim's life."[70] However, parole was not simply motivated by benevolence and effective curative treatments. Rather, it was a strategic carceral-medical shift from incarceration to self-regulation. While the board did not pinpoint its reasons for leprosy parole, increasing legal challenges to its authority may have hastened this turn toward conditional release.[71]

The arrival of American medical personnel in the territory as staff for the federal leprosy investigation laboratories in Molokai and Kalihi also may have brought attention to reform and parole. Prison reform experiments in continental United States penal institutions had begun in Michigan and New York in the 1850s–1870s. Reform was taken up by other states by the early 1900s.[72] Strikingly, conditional parole for leprosy prisoners preceded parole for prisoners convicted of felonies in the territory of Hawai'i. Leprosy parole was adopted at least six years earlier than that of prisoner parole in the islands: leprosy in 1911 and felony parole in 1917.[73]

Why this shift to conditional release? Incarceration alone had proven ineffective for the control of leprosy. Hawaiians in particular had frustrated the board since the beginning of the segregation and exile policy. They hid until their condition became severe or they were caught, possibly causing further spread of the disease. The introduction of parole was a pedagogical and visual strategy to encourage recalcitrant people to surrender voluntarily to medical detention. As with contemporaneous parole experiments in United States penal institutions, leprosy parole emphasized compassionate compliance and dangled shorter sentences as rewards for good behavior and submission to the law. Wrote the head of the U.S. Leprosy Investigation Station at Kalihi Hospital, "[Parole] has caused a considerable number of lepers to surrender themselves and receive treatment, thereby removing dangerous cases from the community."[74] Paroled cases were living illustrations aimed to shift opinion in favor of self-segregation: select improved examples were released to their communities to more effectively manage putatively "dangerous" people.[75]

Patients were photographed in different stages while being treated with experimental therapeutics during their incarceration.[76] In one such experiment in 1921–1922 with oral and injected therapies at Kalihi Hospital, photographs constituted proof of medical efficacy. The director of the hospital wrote optimistically, "The photographs show the progress of the cases better than any description that can be written."[77] Fourteen such photographs of five cases were published in a 1924 U.S. public health report outlining the effectiveness of chaulmoogra oil for leprosy. Here again, these photographs merged racial alterity with leprosy by imaging patients identified as "Japanese," "Hawaiian," and "part Hawaiian."[78]

One published photograph of case 2140 shows an unnamed Japanese woman at her intake in 1922, sitting in a chair with her legs and arms exposed for the camera. Over a year later, she was photographed in a similar position with her hands on her chest, after having been treated with intramuscular injections of chaulmoogra oil (figure 29). She did not qualify for parole, but the physician noted in the report that her "condition [was] much improved."[79] Transnational medical audiences viewed the published photographs and adopted similar therapeutic regimes.[80]

Meanwhile, the photographs obtained significant administrative and juridical influence in Hawai'i, beyond the medical demonstration of a cure. At a 1923 meeting of a leprosy parole board, the board of examining physicians relied on physical examinations and bacteriological exams before discharging nineteen patients for parole. They included a complete set of "before treatment and after parole" photographs.[81] Such photographs constituted vital evidence of whether a patient was a "menace" or no longer considered a public danger. "To see is to believe," declared the superintendent of the leprosy settlement. The photographs rendered a cure self-evident "especially to any who may still contend that leprosy is incurable," reported the board.[82]

Yet a cure was less a stable medical condition than an inventive visual staging. A cure would not be discovered until the 1940s, when sulfone antibiotics were developed at the Carville, Louisiana, national leprosarium. The carceral-medical category of parole correlated far more with the superficial appearance of a reformed body than with empirical data. Parole was only loosely based on medical categories of infection and contagion. The board did not claim that paroled patients were no longer capable of spreading infection, despite sanguine proclamations of a cure. It acknowledged that relapse occurred for parolees, resulting in re-arrest.[83]

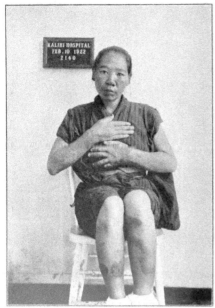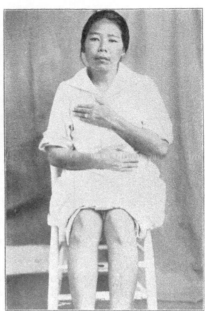

FIGURE 29.

Left: "Case 2140. Japanese. Age 32. Admitted January 21, 1922. Photograph taken February 10, 1922. Nodular type."

Right: "Case 2140. Photograph taken April 26, 1923. Treated with ethyl ester of dihydrochaulmoogric acid." Published in *Studies upon Leprosy, Public Health Bulletin* no. 141 (July 1924).

Although parolees needed to meet a baseline of bacteriological evidence—no leprosy bacilli could be present upon microscopic examination[84]—what seemed to matter more was parolees appearing clean, able-bodied, and whole. Thus, patients admitted with a milder and less visible form of leprosy were the most likely to be paroled, while cases resulting in visible disfigurement (so-called "nodular cases") were less likely.[85] Put another way, a "cure" that led to release was literally skin deep.

Placing the first clinical intake photographs in relation to ones shot during and after experimental treatments enabled the board to envision a cure. These stagings were not necessarily conscious or cynical manipulations by physicians; they believed they had effected a cure. Nonetheless, these "before" and "after" photographs encouraged favorable interpretations of somatic improvements unfolding over time. For a patient to become a parolee, his/

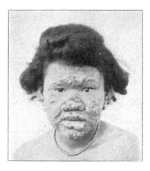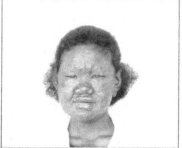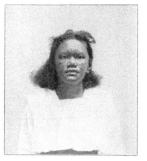

FIGURE 30.

Left: "Case 2026. Part Hawaiian. Age 13. Admitted March 18, 1921. Photograph taken March 20, 1921. Typical leprosy of nodular type."

Middle: "Case 2026. Photograph taken December 10, 1921. Treated with ethyl hydnocarpate until January 1, 1923."

Right: "Case 2026. Photograph taken May 1, 1923, after two years and two months treatment with chaulmoogra derivatives. Ethyl hydnocarpate first nine months; mixed ethyl esters remainder of period." Published in *Studies upon Leprosy, Public Health Bulletin* no. 141 (July 1924).

her photographs had to reveal a transformation from a visibly leprous body to a less marked body.

Take, for example, three published shots of case 2026, a patient identified as "Part Hawaiian," age thirteen. The visual and textual convention of before, during, and after treatment already imposes a progressive framework (figure 30). Although something may have shifted between the photographs, it is unclear what these changes are. Any differences among the shots—the subject's dress, the removal of the necklace, or her relative positioning within the frame—encourage the viewer to register them as rehabilitation.

Yet one might argue that the transformation occurring is not the shrinking of her nodules, but the girl's transformation into a normatively gendered woman who is "civilized" from the perspective of a Euro-American physician. This transformation is signified by her donning of modern clothing, as the camera shifts from a facial close-up, to a medium shot revealing a swatch of cloth, to a final shot of her fully clothed in a crisp white blouse. The captions indicating specific treatments and duration (in this case, ethyl hydnocarpate and chaulmoogra derivatives) further guide the viewer to scan for alterations in skin. However, if the third photograph were viewed singly, out of temporal sequence, the subject might easily be interpreted as a "suspect" in the leprosy archive: a Hawaiian woman with leprous nodules.

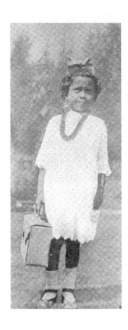

FIGURE 31. "Not Going to Molokai." Published in *Paradise of the Pacific,* December 1921.

With the adoption of "after treatment" shots and parolee release to their communities, the board and public health officials shifted the signification of leprosy photographs from *everyone is a suspect* to *some suspects can be rehabilitated*. By the early 1920s, the board was claiming its parole policy had been effective in convincing more people to self-report as suspects. Reported the physician who headed Kalihi Hospital, "Because of the widespread knowledge in the Territory of Hawaii that entrance to Kalihi Hospital does not necessarily mean a life of exile, there is now little tendency to conceal lepers and allow them to reach advanced stages before discovery. On the contrary, more and more of the arrivals are voluntary, and many of the patients are waiving the right to an examination by a board of three physicians, to which they are legally entitled, and enter the hospital quite willingly."[86]

The board publicized their success stories through local print media. "Six More Inmates Paroled, Took Chaulmoogra," read one article, while another article in the lushly illustrated tourist-oriented periodical *Paradise of the Pacific* heralded the chaulmoogra treatment and heroic scientists for having "cleansed and released" 142 leprosy patients from Kalihi Hospital.[87] A photograph of a young Hawaiian girl holding a suitcase was emblematic of the beneficent practice of parole (figure 31). Captioned as "not going to Molokai," the girl was heralded as one of the 142 "paroles" that would be able to step

"Out of the Darkness into the Light."[88] Her light-colored dress and white socks filling the frame emphasized the restoration of her clean body.

However, incarcerated people and their kin did not uniformly embrace the rationality of the board. They responded in far more complex and varied ways to parole, segregation, and experimental treatment, with hope, refusal, grudging capitulation, and warm gratitude. Parole presented a small window of opportunity for some Hawaiians to press for their release, as Rosalie Puea Blaisdell, a self-described "paroler," believed the new treatments had secured for her. She advocated for the Kalihi experiments at public meetings and in letters to newspapers, offering herself as living proof of the cure.[89]

Others never stopped trying to question their sentences and win release from the Board of Health. While detained at Kalihi Hospital, James Keao wrote in Hawaiian to the board in December 1912. Keao contested his diagnosis of "ma'i Pākē" (Chinese disease, one term for leprosy), believing he had been misdiagnosed because no one in his family or his wife's family had the disease. Keao detailed his previous experiences with puupuu (scabies) and painful urination that were treated by his doctor in Wailuku, Maui. He stated these symptoms could have been mistaken for leprosy. He also told the board his wife and six children were asking for his return home.[90]

Families also challenged the authority of the territorial Board of Health in court. Emma L. Kaipu, daughter of Mikala Kaipu, from Kaua'i, hired a prominent lawyer. They filed a writ of habeas corpus for Mikala Kaipu against the BOH in 1904, arguing that Mikala had demonstrated enough improvement to be released from Kalihi Hospital. The writ was denied by the U.S. District Court in Hawai'i in 1905. However, another Kalihi inmate named Anamalia Maunakea was discharged after filing a successful writ of habeas corpus with the First Circuit Court of Hawai'i. The BOH appealed the decision to the Supreme Court of Hawai'i, but the original order was affirmed in 1908. In the wake of this legal defeat, the board noted in 1909 that no active work to apprehend leprosy suspects had been pursued as it could not enforce the law. It only detained suspects who had turned themselves in voluntarily.[91]

During the two-year period of her mother's detention at Kalihi, Emma Kaipu visited Mikala frequently, applying for visitation permits, as did many others.[92] Kalihi Hospital, centrally located in the city of Honolulu, was much more accessible to visitors than the Makanalua peninsula. Family members, friends, and legal representatives made recurrent use of permits to visit those detained at Kalihi. At Kalihi, inmates were separated from callers by a fence and could not be touched, but they could see each other. Inmates may have felt compelled to accept medical treatment by threat of removal to the Molokai settlement, where they would be unable to see family and friends regularly, as in the case of the Wittrocks.

Frederick Wittrock, a Danish immigrant, and his Hawaiian wife Kukonaalaa (Susan) Kepano lived in Hāna, Maui. Wittrock wrote a pleading letter to the BOH president in 1913, asking for news of their two daughters, taken six months prior to Kalihi Hospital. He and some of the family had relocated near the Kalihi pineapple cannery, which allowed them to "go down and see the children every day from outside the fence." Wittrock expressed his grief: "I always feel so sad to think of these children, that I not can [sic] be able to do something for them." The president's reply to Wittrock implied that the girls would be kept in Kalihi if they complied with medical treatment: "As long as they show signs of improvement and there is hopes [sic] of doing something for them I do not think that the Board would be likely to send them to the Settlement."[93] Two months after composing his letter, Frederick Wittrock died suddenly of a stroke in Honolulu. Daughters Ella and Augusta Wittrock, jailed at Kalihi Hospital, would not have been able to attend the large funeral and burial held in Hāna.[94]

Despite the rhetoric of volunteerism, the criminalizing language of "parole" and its visual framing reveal the deeply carceral nature of leprosy management. Parole did not mean medical acquittal or declaration of innocence for suspects, but heralded a more diffuse and pervasive version of surveillance in the guise of compassionate and temporary reprieve. This period of optimism was short-lived, as many of these "parolers" relapsed. Chaulmoogra oil and radium were not cures, but palliative treatments; sulfone antibiotics would not cure leprosy until the 1940s. In June 1923, the board resumed exiling patients who had shown little improvement to Molokai.[95]

CLINICAL EROTICA AND POLITICAL CAPITAL

The Board of Health's confidence in photography as a useful scientific and juridical tool was periodically tempered by anxiety over the promiscuous circulation of leprosy images. It issued occasional missives to ban photography and rebuked physicians and visitors who took photographs without its permission.[96] When the board learned that "hideous photographs" of patients were being sold to the general public in 1893, it resolved to prohibit "photographs of lepers" at its institutions, except by express permission of the

BOH president. It even considered confiscating photographic equipment in the settlement, including that of resident patients and physicians.[97]

Why this concern over photographs? Why would board officials object to images of leprous bodies dispersed outside of the articulated confines of medical venues? If physicians relied on photography for leprosy diagnosis and empirical documentation, BOH members had different priorities. Board members had vested interests in protecting the plantation and tourist economy of Hawai'i. Physicians and bacteriologists were usually investigating leprosy as a disease and trying to prevent its spread, while BOH members prioritized the preservation of law and order and the economic investments of the white settler oligarchy. By the 1893 overthrow of the Hawaiian Kingdom, board membership was constituted of equal numbers of physicians and lay members. It was also increasingly dominated by wealthy white settlers like the attorney general, plantation owners, mercantilists, businessmen, and lawyers.[98]

Leprosy photographs, like the bodies they indexed, associated the danger of leprous infection and disability with the Hawaiian Islands, threatening the territory's economic development, white settlement, and its image culture. Significantly, Hawai'i's developing tourist economy was attached to the visual economy of an "imagined intimacy" between alluring Hawaiian women hosts and white guests.[99] In 1902, the new territorial government created the Hawaii Promotion Committee to promote tourism; its brochures relied on scenic photographs of white guests enjoying lū'au (Hawaiian feasts) and panoramic vistas.[100]

Absent from this promotional media, however, was leprosy, a disease constructed through law and medical policy as a collective disability. A strong association with raced and disabled bodies would have darkened Hawai'i's reputation as a paradise of the Pacific. Physicians and white settlers considered leprous people vectors of disease and dangerous liabilities, threatening development in multiple ways. In this view, leprous people put able-bodiedness at risk, imperiling capitalist productivity and growth. If leprosy spread, who would work on plantations? And who would invest in these ventures? Further, ideologically, leprous bodies signified immorality and erotic excess. As Indigenous people, immigrants, and white settlers mingled, was the dramatic transformation of some bodies linked to sexual and interracial transgressions? BOH physician George L. Fitch called leprous people "rotting festering loathsome persons" unfit to be seen.[101] Their uncontrollable appearance suggested something was not right in civil society, perhaps tied to aberrant desires and behavior.

Visiting writers and physicians also publicly worried about leprosy spreading from the potential Pacific territory to the United States. American physician and syphilis expert Prince A. Morrow visited the Molokai settlement in 1889 and cautioned strenuously against Hawai'i's annexation by the United States because of leprosy in the islands. Morrow wrote in 1897, "When it is considered that more than ten per cent of the Hawaiian race are affected with leprosy it becomes a serious question as to what will be the effect of the absorption of this tainted population upon the health interests of this country."[102]

The Board of Health continued to photograph all leprosy suspects at Kalihi Hospital, amassing thousands of individual patient images. Yet it maintained tight control over these clinical photographs in order to keep the disabled bodies of leprosy patients sequestered from the paradisiacal image culture of Hawai'i. Board restrictions of patient photographs were most vigorous between the 1893 overthrow and 1898 annexation by the United States, when Hawai'i's territorial status was liminal and actively debated.[103] Yet after Hawai'i was formally incorporated as a territory in 1900, the board relaxed some of its interdictions, and the archive of skin became a valuable and convenient asset for physicians and politicians in the territory and the U.S. continent. Circulated as clinical erotica to select audiences, this archive whet the appetite of policy makers and experts, and served as a vital political resource. Spectacular images dispersed from the archive mobilized arguments for territorial funding and the extension of mandatory leprosy segregation on the U.S. continent.

Photographs of leprous people elicited fear, shock, and voyeuristic pleasure. They were made to perform long after they were shot, despite official concerns over their illicit circulation and sale. Following U.S. annexation, the board sought federal funds for the management of its nearly nine hundred leprosy patients kept quarantined in the territory. The territory's best strategy to wring resources and money from the federal government was leprosy. As medical historian O. A. Bushnell put it, "[W]hat more fearsome thing could they show [Uncle Sam] than a leper?"[104]

In 1904, the president of the Hawai'i BOH, Dr. Charles B. Cooper, made such a direct appeal in Washington, DC, bringing a large collection of clinical photographs with him. These photographs of Hawai'i leprosy patients showed "disease in various forms and in its different stages." As Cooper made his rounds in Washington lobbying for leprosy funding, he displayed his photographs in large albums and as single shots.[105] He took them to a conference of health officers from the U.S. Public Health and Marine Hospital Service, the federal agency responsible for instituting quarantine.

The territory's solicitations for leprosy research and carceral-medical management resonated forcefully with U.S. public health services physicians and U.S. congressmen. In the early twentieth century, territorial officials like Dr. Cooper shrewdly capitalized on broader xenophobia in the United States to direct more funding to territorial coffers.

Cooper exhibited his photographs during a presentation on the isolation of patients on Molokai.[106] He also met with Surgeon General Wyman, the highest-ranking medical officer in the United States, to discuss a research experiment station on Molokai that would investigate a cure. The attendees' responses were revealing: "[T]he entire collection aroused a very lively interest among the physicians present . . . The physicians and health officers made many demands upon Dr. Cooper for copies of certain of those photographs." The men's erotic appetite is suggested by this scene of arousal. The images were not readily available outside of Hawai'i at the time.[107] Distributed to a select number of viewers, the photographs were an erotic resource purveyed for political consideration.

In all likelihood, Cooper curated his photographic exhibit from the Board of Health archive, a stable and convenient source of images to which he would have had immediate access. While we do not have a record of the exact photographs he exhibited, the photographs were likely similar to, if not the same as, those of four Hawai'i patients published within a 1902 U.S. Senate report about the prevention of leprosy in the United States.[108] Nearly hidden within dry administrative prose about medical quarantine, photographs of Hawai'i leprosy patients offered an intimate, voyeuristic peek at leprosy in racialized-sexualized bodies: clawed hands, missing toes and fingers, facial lesions, and large breasts with mottled skin. Four photographs of people published in the 1902 Senate report were taken originally during their 1898 detention at Kalihi Hospital. They are unidentified in the report, but I have traced them back to their original Hawai'i clinical records. They are of an eighteen-year-old Hawaiian woman, Halauwai (figure 32); Kaupe, a fifty-year-old Hawaiian woman whose breasts are exposed; a fifty-three-year-old Portuguese man, Juan de Freitas; and a seventeen-year-old Hawaiian man, Henry K. Apolo.[109] Each photograph was printed on a full page at the back of the report, with only clinical symptoms as captions.

Health agents and politicians relied on photographs as a cornerstone of alarmist, commonsense arguments about the protection of U.S. citizens from leprous bodies in Hawai'i. The 1902 report documented only 278 confirmed cases of leprosy in the United States proper, while tuberculosis killed nearly two hundred thousand. Despite these modest mortality figures, the U.S.

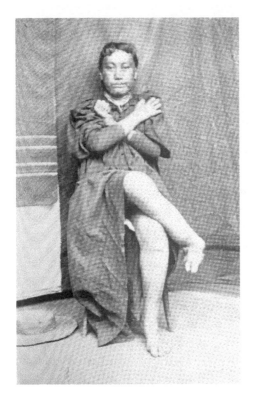

FIGURE 32. "No. 2. Anaesthetic Leprosy—Loss of Fingers and Toes." Published in U.S. Senate report on the origin and prevalence of leprosy in the United States. S. Doc. No. 57-269 (1902). Unidentified in the report, the photograph's subject was Halauwai; the photograph was taken on May 11, 1898, when she was about twenty years old. Kalihi Hospital case 05172, Hawai'i State Archives.

Committee on Public Health and National Quarantine recommended that the federal government establish at least one, preferably two, federally funded leprosaria to isolate patients within the continental U.S.

Three years after this report's recommendations, leprosy appropriations were still under discussion by Congress. Cooper left an album of similar leprosy photographs as a personal gift for Surgeon General Wyman, the official he needed most in his corner for territorial funding. Letters exchanged between the two men suggest that Wyman appreciated the photographs.[110] While we can only speculate about the concrete effects of the album, the following year Surgeon Wyman supported the Hawai'i territorial request for leprosy research funds, and Congress approved the bill in 1905.[111] This U.S. congressional appropriation had material effects: it funded a federal leprosy investigation station at Kalawao, Molokai, that operated between 1909 and 1913. Federal monies also brought government scientists to Hawai'i who proceeded to conduct biomedical experiments and the imaging of patients at the Molokai leprosy investigation station and Kalihi Hospital.[112]

ETHNOGRAPHIC MEDICINE AND
RACIAL-SEXUAL TYPES

Just as the photographic archive provided rich material for health authorities to draw upon, so too did medical writers dip in regularly to highlight clinical cases and the practice of leprosy segregation. When the colonial medical file traveled to transnational medical contexts, the publications stripped the patient's specific medical history and resignified the clinical image as a racial-sexual pathological type. The original clinical file embedded the patient in a particular location and time, notating names, dates, family histories, and symptoms. However, articles represented the clinical image as an ethnographic icon of tropical leprosy and Native and Asian disability. I offer here two examples of medical print culture that merged ethnography with medical illustration.

An occasional American tourist and physician, J. Chris O'Day had difficulty gaining access to the Molokai settlement because the board wished to strictly limit publicity of leprosy. After several years of entreaties to the board, O'Day was only allowed to visit Molokai after operating successfully on the son of a prominent Hawaiian politician. O'Day proceeded to publish accounts of his tour to the Molokai settlement in U.S. medical journals between 1911 and 1919. In these articles and other illustrated lectures delivered to American audiences, O'Day offered narrative and visual portraits of incarcerated patients, bridging the ethnographic and medical.[113]

He argued that leprosy was "not a contagious nor an infectious disease," sympathizing with the pathetic experience of these "poor outcasts" whose children were taken from them.[114] Nevertheless, his articles sensationalized the disease using copious images of leprous bodies. Equipped with clinical images from the archive of skin, O'Day chose two people with dramatically transformed bodies to represent "typical" leprosy inmates (figure 33). Nodules on these subjects' cheeks, brows, and foreheads were highly visible.

Not only was each person's photograph captioned with the type of leprous infection, but each was identified by race and gender. The first image was captioned "Hawaiian boy, age 17. Typical tubercular leprosy," and the second photograph was captioned "Half Chinese and Hawaiian woman. Tubercular leprosy." Untethered from the archive, medical photographs like these were implicitly ethnographic and instructional. They staged racial-sexual pathology in the guise of medical illustration. The photographs encouraged viewers to peer at bodies as spectacular pathogens.

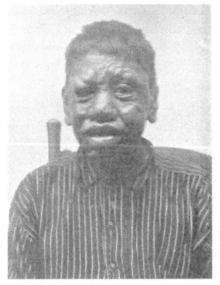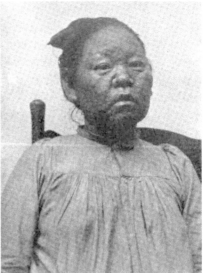

FIGURE 33.

Left: Clinical photograph of Puaiku Iokepa. Kalihi Hospital case 760, April 16, 1908, fifteen years.

Right: Clinical photograph of Wari Goto. Kalihi Hospital case 755, April 16, 1908, thirty years. Hawai'i State Archives.

These photographs were published in O'Day, "A Visit to the Leper Colony of Molokai, Hawaii" (May 1915).

Ironically, despite the author's attempt to assert ethnographic authority, the woman patient identified as "half Chinese and Hawaiian," was in fact, neither Chinese nor Hawaiian. Her name was Wari Goto, a Japanese immigrant living in Wahiawa, Kaua'i. When she was seized in April 1908, she was thirty years old, married, and pregnant. The "Hawaiian boy" who stood as the visual example of tubercular leprosy was not seventeen years old, as described, but a fifteen-year-old boy named Puaiku Iokepa. He had been apprehended with his father and older brother in Kawaihae, Hawai'i in 1908, and one of his sisters had already been exiled to the Molokai settlement.[115] Yet these discrepancies mattered little—Goto and Iokepa's mediated images were still associated with the infectious peril of leprosy emanating from Hawai'i.

Euro-American doctors working in Hawai'i offered even more elaborate cultural ethnographies to explain the physical and moral demise of their patients. Writing as a BOH physician posted on Maui island, the American physician Edward S. Goodhue offered an insider's view of those indigent natives, Chinese, negroes, and "stray individuals from all countries" affected by social and sexual chaos and terrible diseases in Hawai'i. In a lushly illustrated 1900 *Journal of the American Medical Association* piece called "The Physician in Hawaii," Goodhue positioned the white physician as an underpaid savior encountering the immoral choices and unclean habits of his Hawai'i patients. He provided brief ethnographic sketches of the strange and smelly Japanese and Chinese laborers who lived surrounded by refuse and pickled vegetables in sugar plantation tenements.

One of Edward Goodhue's most confounding patients was a young and immodest Native girl who became pregnant after a sexual liaison with the scion of a good white family. Goodhue describes attending the birth of the illegitimate child and providing counsel to the mother, ultimately concluding his "effort at reforming native girls was rather a failure."[116] The unruly crossing of racial, sex, and class boundaries in the islands, as suggested by the baby's birth, could produce bodily decay in the form of contagious disease, it was thought.

When the article appeared in this leading medical journal in 1900, Hawai'i was already globally famous for harboring leprosy. Though Goodhue made but a passing reference to leprosy, the unnerving images embedded in his piece are those of two Hawaiian leprosy patients (figure 34). These photographs are the only clinical portraits in the article, appearing among ethnographic scenes of Hawaiians preparing cooked taro root and sitting by grass houses.

Goodhue relied on two of the earliest images from the Hawai'i archive of skin to link race, gender, infection, and deformity. The production of these particular photographs was well documented when the Board of Health commissioned them in June 1878. A Honolulu-based photographer, Henry L. Chase, had been hired by the board to photograph twelve patients during its inspection visit of the Kalawao, Molokai, settlement. Chase produced twelve wet plate negatives of advanced leprosy cases during this trip. Per his contract, Chase was not allowed to make additional prints of the negatives without the explicit permission of the BOH president, and this restrictive agreement was published in a daily Honolulu newspaper.[117]

Yet twenty-two years after the portraits were first taken, they reappeared side by side in a major medical journal to bolster Goodhue's study of Hawai'i as a site of disability. The woman is blind and her hands are missing fingers; the second person, a man, holds swollen hands to his chest, and nodules are apparent across his face.[118] No further textual explanation was necessary, for these leprosy images attached disability and difference to Goodhue's narra-

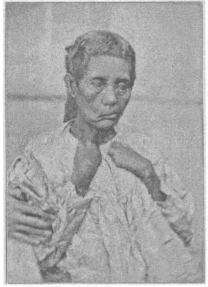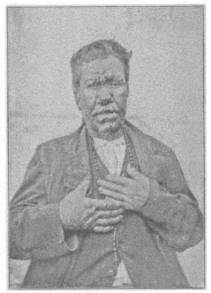

NERVE LEPROSY.   TUBERCULAR LEPROSY.

FIGURE 34. Clinical photographs of two Hawaiian patients published in Goodhue, "The Physician in Hawaii," *Journal of the American Medical Association,* January 20, 1900. They were taken by Henry L. Chase at Kalawao, Molokai, in June 1878. Although unidentified when published, they were of Kalamau from Honolulu, age fifty, and Naluaai, age fifty-six, from Kalihi. Both had been exiled in Kalawao for five years.

tive depictions of improvident and morally suspect behavior. The racial-sexual pathology of Hawai'i's people thus manifested on the surface of the epidermis and the photographic grain.

After territorial incorporation in 1900, photographs from the archive of skin surfaced with greater frequency in prominent medical journals and public health reports. Photographs in journals also appeared more regularly by 1900 because technological developments made them far less costly to print.[119] BOH officials permitted the publication of some clinical photographs, granting access to physicians, scientists, and health officials in the continental United States. Years after the original clinical photographs were shot at Kalihi Hospital, they were reissued in publications like the *United States Naval Medical Bulletin* (1902), the *Journal of the American Medical Association* (1903), *American Medicine* (1913), the *New York Medical Journal* (1913), and *U.S. Public Health Bulletin* (1924).[120] Their audiences were not confined to the United States; these articles were read and discussed by scientists in Europe, Japan, and the Philippines.

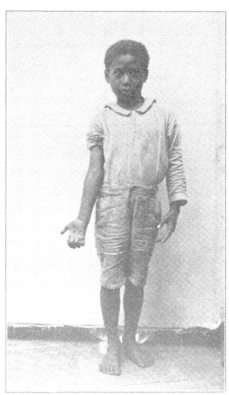

Fig. 1. Anesthetic Leprosy.

FIGURE 35. Clinical photograph of "Anesthetic Leprosy" published in Goodhue, "The Cure of Leprosy an Established Fact" (March 1913). Its subject is William Eli Hodge, age eight, who was photographed on September 29, 1902. Kalihi Hospital case 211, Hawai'i State Archives.

Doctors also created slide presentations on leprosy and public health using clinical images from the Hawai'i archive. The voyeuristic image of the young Hawaiian woman Oliwaliilii (figure 27), along with several other clinical patient photographs from Hawai'i, was featured in the lantern slide collection of Dr. George McCoy. McCoy was a director of the U.S. Leprosy Investigation Station in Hawai'i and later became head of the Hygienic Laboratory of the U.S. Public Health Service, now the National Institutes of Health.[121] These images usually lacked attribution to their origin in the Hawai'i government hospital, but still identified patients by their race and/ or gender (e.g., "Part Hawaiian, age 13"; "girl aged 8 years"). Some, like William Eli Hodge, an eight-year-old Hawaiian boy originally captured in 1902, made multiple appearances in print in 1912 and 1913 (figure 35).[122]

What was the net effect of detaching photographs from the archive of skin and displaying them in American medical print culture? Whereas individuals in Hawai'i had been inspected, photographed, and catalogued for potential incarceration and tracking of suspects, the appearance of clinical cases in national and transnational media resignified individual leprosy cases as a broader racial-sexual contagion emerging from the Hawaiian Islands. Individual patients were made highly visible, yet evaporated into racial-gendered types from Hawai'i who were darker skinned and often deformed and disabled. In the guise of a clinically neutral gaze, photographs instructed clinicians to "see" race and sexual difference as attached to disease and bodily decay. Thus, the leprous body and the racialized body melted into one.

IMAGING COMPASSIONATE REHABILITATION

Were there other contemporaneous modes of representing leprosy? Were all bodies with leprosy subject to these prevailing primitivist and Orientalist associations? At the same time clinical photographs from Hawai'i attached leprosy to Indigenous and Asian bodies and behavior, debates about a potential federal leprosarium and their wards took a distinct turn away from carceral medicine. These discussions relied on a different set of visual and discursive representations to decriminalize leprosy for U.S. citizen-subjects.

John Early, a white American veteran who had served in the Philippine-American War, had been diagnosed with leprosy in 1908 and quarantined off and on for five years. Early traveled to Washington, DC, in 1914 and was isolated and confined again in a house in the capital, as there was no central facility on the continent where he could receive treatment in isolation. Photographs of Early published in the popular illustrated *Munsey's Magazine* were non-clinical, representing him as an ordinary person in everyday settings. Dressed neatly, Early was shown playing music and dining in a tent, separated from his wife and young children.[123]

Early became a touchstone during congressional debates about the need for a leprosarium on the U.S. continent. Senators cited Early's case as an example of the "sad" and inhumane treatment of Americans afflicted with leprosy.[124] Early himself wrote a letter to Congress, stirring support for care of deserving U.S. citizens and leprosy patients like himself. As historian Michelle Moran has argued, "[T]he face of the leprosy patient became 'American'" within these political discussions.[125] The person in need of compassionate isolation and treatment was imagined as a white American beneficiary. For such citizen-subjects, the carceral-medical model of Molokai, and its successor in the Philippines, the Culion leprosy colony, would have been inappropriate and cruel.

Like John Early, who had served overseas in the U.S. Army, soldiers, missionaries, and commercial workers who had traversed into tropical areas and contracted leprosy became viewed as unwitting victims. A U.S. Senate bill passed in 1917 established both segregation and permanent care for people with leprosy in the United States at federal expense. It funded the National Leprosarium, which opened in 1921 on the site of the Louisiana Leper Home in Carville, Louisiana.

Indeed, when Carville opened as a modern care facility for the care and treatment of leprous people on the U.S. continent, it did not image its charges as criminal suspects or inmates, as the Hawai'i Board of Health did at least until the 1950s. In contrast to the colonial model of carceral medicine and exile exemplified by Molokai, the Carville leprosarium championed a humane rehabilitative model of quarantine. Therefore the U.S. Public Health Service generally eschewed clinical mug shots in its publicity material, borrowing instead from patient-produced images of leisure activities in the Carville residential compound.[126]

The shift to the decriminalization of leprosy at Carville for American patients, however, did not mean leprosy became detached from indigeneity and racial and sexual difference. In the 1940s, the sulfone drug Promin, developed at Carville, was confirmed as a cure for leprosy and became known as the "miracle at Carville."[127] Yet at least until the 1970s, medical atlases and textbooks continued to utilize leprosy photographs taken at Hawai'i institutions to illustrate the "presulfone era." A canonical tropical disease atlas published in 1976, for example, relied on clinical photographs originally taken in 1931 of a "13 year old Hawaiian" boy with advanced lepromatous leprosy and deformities.[128] For nearly a century, photographs sealed leprosy to Hawaiian corporeality.

CONCLUSION: AFFECTIVE EXCESS

On February 28, 1907, a Hawaiian girl named Nailima Lishman was admitted to Kalihi Hospital at the age of nine (figure 36). She was photographed sometime after her medical examination in June. She sits solo in a chair, her arms crossed over her chest in the convention of the leprosy portrait—to best reveal her "slightly enlarged" hands and fingers. Imaged alone, Nailima was

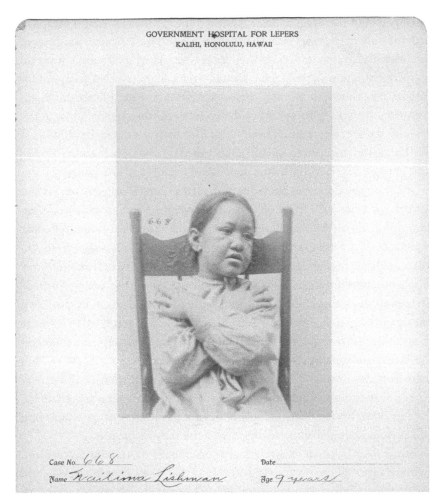

GOVERNMENT HOSPITAL FOR LEPERS
KALIHI, HONOLULU, HAWAII

Case No. 668
Name Nailima Lishman
Date
Age 9 years

FIGURE 36. Clinical photograph of Nailima Lishman. Kalihi Hospital case 668, 1907, nine years. Hawai'i State Archives.

the only one of her immediate family, including seven siblings, to be medically incarcerated, and she declared no other leprous relative during the exam.

Yet the visitors' permission log from Kalihi Hospital tells a far more intimate experience of collectivity after she was incarcerated—her family refused to abandon her. The very next day after Nailima was admitted—on March 1, 1907—"Mr. and Mrs. Lishman," as her parents' names were recorded, went to see her at the receiving station. Thereafter, from March 1907 through August 15, 1908, they applied repeatedly for thirty visitation permits that covered themselves and their relations to see Nailima during two-week allotments.[129]

Only one of these logs appears to have been retained by Kalihi Hospital, with the bulk of the visits in the years from 1904 to 1908, but it is a register of persistent aloha: women visiting their lovers, daughters their mothers, brothers their siblings, neighbors their friends, and a score of other relationships that are not known to us today. Before fourteen-year old Elizabeth Francis Napoleon was sent to Molokai in July 1906, her mother applied for a permit to see her daughter "twice each week" until Elizabeth was moved to Molokai.[130] The Kalihi inmates, young and old alike, were far from unbefriended, as they continued to be comforted by the presence of friends and loved ones.[131]

The experience of being photographed at this hospital suggests similar caregiving that exceeds the frame of medical incarceration and surveillance. What was it like to sit on the other side of the medical lens and be captured? Patient performances in front of the medical camera disrupted the exposure of surveillance. Medical photographs, despite their archival authority, did not uniformly support the interpretation of its subjects as loathsome, threatening suspects. Patients appropriated clinical photographic settings and poses for their own discrepant authorizing systems. As the Board of Health attempted to organize its archive of Native and immigrant populations into knowable and manageable collectives and dispersed them to new audiences, the photographs within these files also unwittingly unsettled this process with what I call *affective excess*. The process of visual identification and prediction was more aspirational than actualized by the Board of Health, and not just because of epistemological and methodological weaknesses internal to the archival process.

British and German anthropologists attempted to visually capture and measure races of men beginning in the 1870s. They recommended rigid anthropometric systems for photographing Native subjects in the nineteenth century, including photographing them nude against a measuring grid in full-length frontal and side views.[132] In his criminological practice of imaging somatic difference, Alphonse Bertillon recommended consistent camera focal length, even lighting, and a fixed distance for criminal identification portraits in Paris.[133]

However, photographers at the leprosy receiving station were not trained in physical anthropology, criminology, or medical photography; they did not consistently conform to uniform settings. In fact, the photographer was a local studio photographer hired by the Board of Health; he could have been any one of about sixty photographers working in Hawai'i at the turn of the century.[134] This photographer incorporated some visual anthropological conventions like positioning the body for maximum exposure.

Yet other clinical images resemble commercial studio portraits available to working-class and more affluent people in Hawai'i. Subjects without obvious markings were allowed to keep their clothes on and pose with a range of significant adornments. For many Hawaiians and immigrant workers, this would be their first experience being photographed. The sitting was not always approached as an abject experience. Some patients offer oblique looks. Others look straight at the camera; others off to the side. Some smile, while others seem to flirt with the camera.[135] Though expected to reveal their bodies and diseased parts for the camera, suspects also insisted on adorning themselves in discrepant ways. Men and women of all classes and birthrights often dressed their finest for the camera; some men wear suits, and women their best dresses and jewelry, even if they were required to remove some clothing for the photograph.

A Hawaiian patient exiled to Molokai around 1920 elaborated on the relationship between being photographed and being declared a "leper": "Even though we were poor, my father said he wanted me to be dressed nicely when I was taken to Kalihi to be declared a leper. They took my picture for the official record of the Board of Health wearing that new suit of clothes. When the picture was taken, my father broke down again and cried. So, I became a leper."[136] From the perspective of this patient, the memory of this photographic moment merged both the pain of being rendered socially dead *and* the loving care of his father to have him look his best in the photograph.

Photographs in the leprosy archive reveal the emergence of such affective care within visual economies of abjection and objectification. More than a repressive site of knowledge production or thanatopolitics, they also perform as "affective archives," or archives animated by desires, attachments, and feelings that may be ephemeral and prone to forgetting.[137] Not simply a piece of scientific evidence, these photographs represented a chance for patients to maintain their personhood apart from the signification of bodily distress.[138]

Embedded within the archive of skin are scenes of people socializing in the clinic. The six images of leprosy suspects shown in figures 37–42 were taken on the same intake day, September 11, 1903. Herman Kuhilani, Kauluhinano, Hattie Kekai, Kealaaea, Cecelia Kalili Naea, and Kalema Kaaukai had arrived from varied island districts and were admitted to the receiving station on different days. People who completed their medical examinations were usually photographed in succession on a single day. Within a week of being photographed, at least three were sent to Molokai on the same boat.[139] They were neither related to each other nor appear to have known each other prior to their detention. However, on this day, they dressed

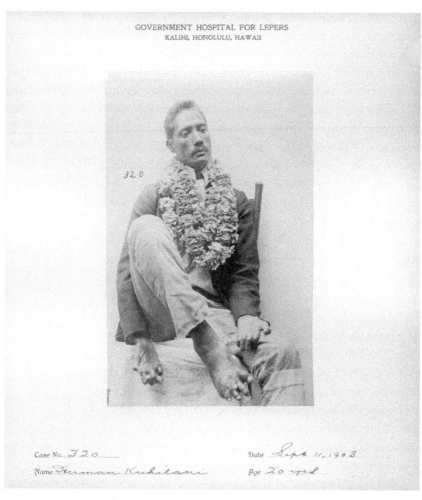

GOVERNMENT HOSPITAL FOR LEPERS
KALIHI, HONOLULU, HAWAII

320

Case No. *320*   Date *Sept 11, 1903*

Name *Herman Kuhilani*   Age *20 yrs*

FIGURE 37. Clinical photograph of Herman Kuhilani. Kalihi Hospital case 320, September 11, 1903, twenty years. Hawai'i State Archives.

themselves for the camera and perhaps even helped each other prepare for their medical portraits.

In these portraits, the patients wear lei po'o (lei worn on the head) or lei 'awapuhi, strands of fresh ginger blossoms (*Hedychium Coronarium*) around their necks. Although they were made to reveal afflicted parts for the camera, such as Herman Kuhilani with ulcerated hands and feet (figure 37), the flowers radiate within the frame. The lei disrupts the encounter between patient and omniscient physician by inserting other affective relationships. Though suspects were not allowed to touch their family members while under medi-

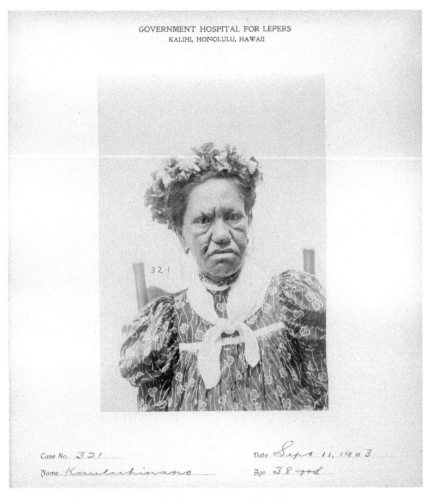

FIGURE 38. Clinical photograph of Kauluhinano. Kalihi Hospital case 321, September 11, 1903, thirty-eight years. Hawai'i State Archives.

cal arrest, family or friends may have brought the lei to the station, or they may have woven lei from flowers cultivated on the hospital grounds.[140]

Lei are a Hawaiian adornment for the head and the body, but they are not simply ornamental. They are placed on heads and over the shoulders, parts of the body that contain mana, or sacred power. Giving lei, then, bestows respect and honor upon the adorned body. Acts of giving and wearing lei are further suggestive of affective labor, care, and touch. The lei 'awapuhi (figures 37, 39, 40, 41) were strung together by hand from fresh blossoms that have to be handpicked, usually in the evening hours when the buds are just

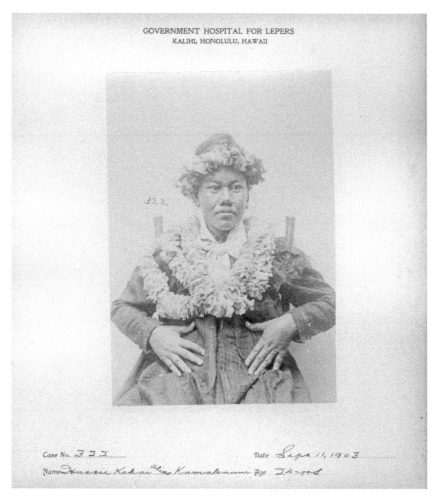

GOVERNMENT HOSPITAL FOR LEPERS
KALIHI, HONOLULU, HAWAII

Case No. 322   Date Sept 11, 1903
Name Hattie Kekai alias Kamakanui Age 24 yrs

FIGURE 39. Clinical photograph of Hattie Kekai, alias Kamakanui. Kalihi Hospital case 322, September 11, 1903, twenty-four years. Hawai'i State Archives.

beginning to open. Crafting these heavy garlands would have taken hundreds of blossoms and many hours of careful work.

Furthermore, lei must be given and received through close contact, often with an embrace or honi (nose to nose contact)—acts verboten between "clean" and "leprous" bodies because of potential contagion and social prohibitions. The Hawaiian saying, "E lei no au i ko aloha" (I will wear your love as a wreath), communicates the aloha, or love, associated with giving and receiving lei. Variations of this refrain are woven through numerous mele (songs) and hula repertoire in the twentieth century.[141] Family and friends

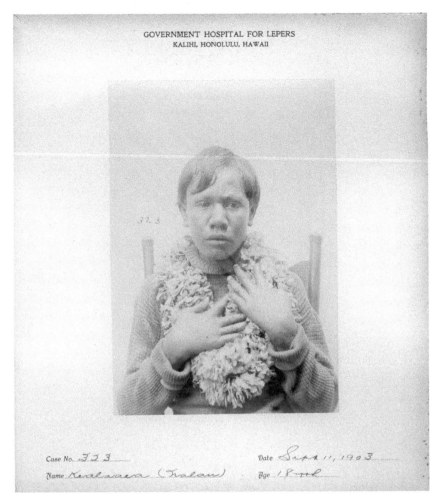

GOVERNMENT HOSPITAL FOR LEPERS
KALIHI, HONOLULU, HAWAII

Case No. _323_   Date _Sept 11, 1903_
Name _Kealaaea (Nalau)_   Age _18 yrs_

FIGURE 40. Clinical photograph of Kealaaea (Nalau). Kalihi Hospital case 323, September 11, 1903, eighteen years. Hawai'i State Archives.

of inmates gave lei to loved ones departing for Molokai at Honolulu Harbor, knowing they were unlikely to see each other again.

Once learning of the death of a beloved person at the leprosy settlement, people grieved by composing kanikau (poetic dirges) and sending them to newspapers to be published.[142] These kanikau were poetic lei that strung together loving remembrances of the person; in many, the deceased person often was likened to favorite lei. One kanikau lamented a precious daughter exiled to Kalaupapa, "He hiwahiwa oe na ka makua, he lei mamo laha ole" (You are an adornment for the parent, a rare lei of mamo feathers). Mrs.

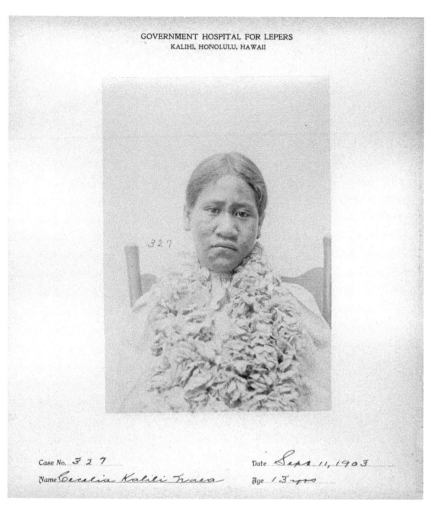

GOVERNMENT HOSPITAL FOR LEPERS
KALIHI, HONOLULU, HAWAII

Case No. 3 2 7   Date Sept. 11, 1903
Name Cecelia Kalili Naea   Age 13 yrs

FIGURE 41. Clinical photograph of Cecelia Kalili Naea. Kalihi Hospital case 327, September 11, 1903, thirteen years. Hawai'i State Archives.

Kealualu and Mrs. Mary Keaka composed this for Mary Nohinohiana, who had entered the settlement on May 9, 1899. She died in July 1899, and their kanikau was published less than a month later.[143] This abundant draping of literal and figurative lei on leprous bodies suggests Hawaiians were more than willing to touch and claim afflicted bodies, and in contradistinction to Western medicine and law, to view them as worthy of care.

Hawaiians relied on numerous names for leprosy that ranged from more dispassionate, neutral descriptions like "ka pilikia" (the trouble), to emotionally charged expressions of terror, agony, despair, and sadness. Among its

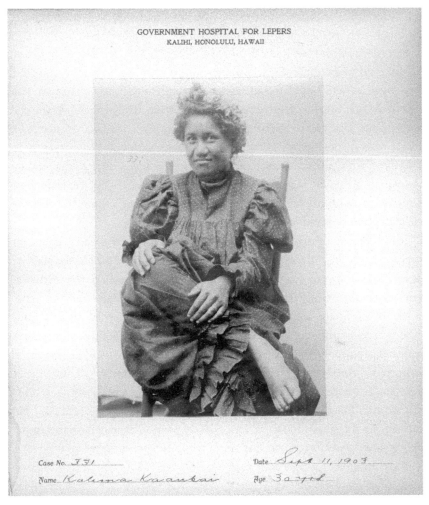

GOVERNMENT HOSPITAL FOR LEPERS
KALIHI, HONOLULU, HAWAII

Case No. 331   Date Sept. 11, 1903
Name Kalema Kaaukai   Age 30 yrs

FIGURE 42. Clinical photograph of Kalema Kaaukai. Kalihi Hospital case 331, September 11, 1903, thirty years. Hawai'i State Archives.

evocative and poetic names were "mai makamaka ole" (disease that leaves one friendless), mai hoehaeha kino (disease that agonizes the body), mai hookae a ka lehelehu (disease despised by the public), and mai aloha ole (disease without mercy). While these names acknowledge the powerful and painful effects of the illness upon the physical body and social relationships, these appellations tend not to disparage the person with leprosy. In Euro-American contexts, leprous bodies provoked fear and were often pronounced as "loathsome," a term that places emphasis on the disgusted reaction of an external viewer.[144] Photographs in the archive of skin usually exposed the most dramatically altered features of bodies and amplified such fearful responses.

This is not to say Hawaiians uniformly embraced leprous people, but they did not tend to attribute somatic changes as repulsive or disgusting, nor did they linger on revulsion. After a diagnosis of leprosy, they demonstrated that their loved ones were worthy of touch and affection. They continued to provide intimate care and to live with each other against the admonishments of government agents. Some hid their kin from authorities or refused to report symptoms, while others chose to accompany their loved ones to the leprosy settlement as unpaid mea kōkua (caregivers), as I discuss in the following chapter.[145] And, like Nailima Lishman's parents, many visited imprisoned friends, neighbors, and lovers at Kalihi Hospital.

Just as these quotidian acts disrupted the presumed criminality of leprosy suspects, so the lei in the photographs also convey love and care in the alienating criminal archive of skin. The lei within are not Barthesian punctum; while they may mobilize and arouse the viewer, they do not offer a masculinist "prick" of the image, nor do they wound.[146] Rather, they offer affective and sensory excess, suffusing the image with ephemeral scents. The photograph could not capture the fragrance of these flowers and bountiful affection shared between the inmates that day. Anyone who has ever worn such lei knows that lei 'awapuhi are fragile and ephemeral, lasting at most a day before their blossoms wither. But to those who gifted them and those who wore them, this transient nature likely mattered little; the lei would have been treasured for their onaona (sweet fragrance) and the enduring love they signified.[147]

These strands of ginger blossoms would have filled the clinic with perfume, offering a sensory experience of the wet valleys that produce these flowers. For thirteen-year old Cecelia Kalili Naea (figure 41), who hailed from such a lush locale, Kapena in Nu'uanu Valley, the scent would have recalled her own home and her kin, but a few miles away from the clinic.[148] Because of the apparent similarity of the lei in this series of photographs, these six people may have shared the garlands, perhaps passing them on to one another before each was photographed separately. Their portraits, then, documented each individual's imminent emergence as a criminal suspect, as well as growing bonds with one another—a new collectivity born out of violent dislocation. These gestures within and just outside the frame were acts of love, connection, and farewell prior to exile. The photographs anticipate the affective possibilities of touch and physical proximity that patients would experience and re-create at the leprosy settlement.

THREE

Dressing the Body

LAUNDRY AND THE INTIMACY OF CARE

ALICE KAELEMAKULE AND HATTIE PIIPIILANI KALUA likely did not know each other prior to their first meeting at Kalihi Hospital in Honolulu. Hailing from different ahupua'a (districts) on the island of O'ahu, they were captured and detained by medical authorities around the same time in 1905. Alice was twenty, while Hattie was thirty years old. On January 20, 1905, the women sat separately for clinical photographs that highlighted the state of suspicious hands that might have been symptoms of leprosy (figures 43 and 44). Determined to be leprous by the examination board, they were sent on the same ship to the Molokai leprosy settlement later that month.[1] The older woman, Hattie Kalua, was married at the time. It appears Hattie's husband was not under medical investigation, meaning she would have been separated from her non-leprous husband. Hattie's clinical record does not note whether she had any children, but if she did, she would have had to leave them behind as well.

A year or two after their exile to Molokai, Alice and Hattie staged themselves for a photographic portrait strikingly different from their clinical photographs (figure 45). They chose to be photographed together instead of individually. On this day, Alice and Hattie dressed and styled their hair nearly identically for this joint portrait. In numerous portraits taken by Catholic medical missionaries in the leprosy settlement, patients and caregivers sat for photographs like this one between ca. 1901 and 1925.[2]

The women nestle close to one other. Hattie sits confidently, squarely facing the camera. Alice stands next to her, half-smiling. Instead of her hands crossed across her chest to reveal enlarged fingers, Alice places her hand against Hattie's sleeve. Their choice of clothing—mu'umu'u (long gowns) cut from the same patterned cloth—was no accident.[3] The patterned material

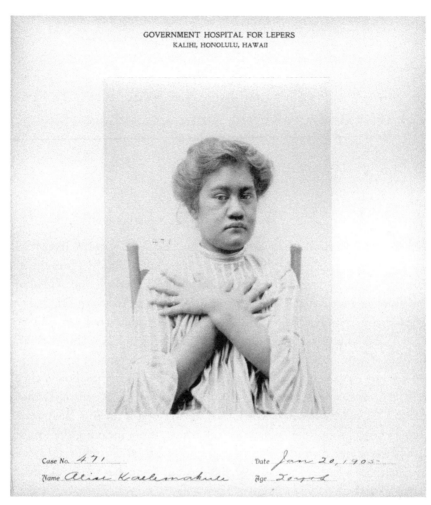

GOVERNMENT HOSPITAL FOR LEPERS
KALIHI, HONOLULU, HAWAII

Case No. *4 7 1*

Date *Jan 20, 1905*

Name *Alice Kaelemakule*

Age *20 yrs*

FIGURE 43. Clinical photograph of Alice Kaelemakule. Kalihi Hospital case 471, January 20, 1905, twenty years. Hawai'i State Archives.

enveloped both of their bodies and brought the women into a cohesive unit. Their experiences in the settlement are not known fully, as with many thousands of people exiled in this period, but Alice's and Hattie's clothing reveal their deliberate choice to be seen and understood relationally. With their sartorial choice and proximate choreography, two women wove themselves into a single composition: an interdependent pair.

Without clinical records identifying Hattie and Alice as exiled people with leprosy, it is not obvious these two women were patients. Any telltale stigmata of leprosy that might have been present on their skin—lesions,

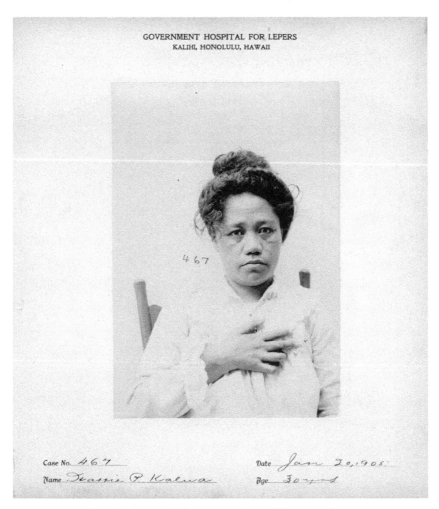

467

Case No. *467*

Date *Jan 20, 1905*

Name *Hattie P. Kalua*

Age *30 yrs*

FIGURE 44. Clinical photograph of Hattie P. Kalua. Kalihi Hospital case 467, January 20, 1905, thirty years. Hawai'i State Archives.

sores, or spots—are not visible under voluminous folds of cotton. Groomed and dressed carefully, they are not immediately apprehended as incarcerated people. The photograph makes visible their interdependence, but the tidy dresses also gesture toward much more outside of the photograph frame— the care, comfort, and sustenance of clothing beyond the momentary temporality of the photograph.

This chapter turns to a critical, yet frequently overlooked, aspect of caregiving for sick and disabled patients: the material, affective, and often gendered labor of laundry and dressing. Who washed these dresses and how?

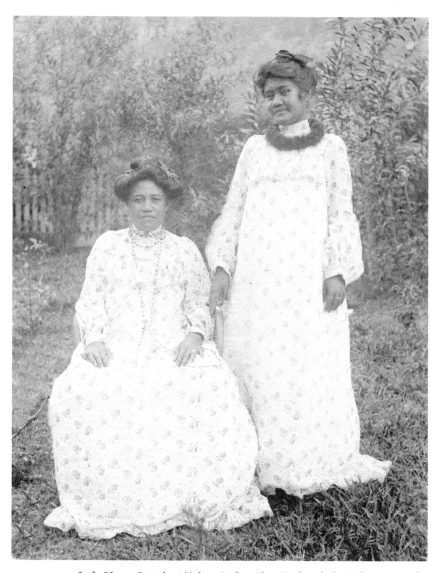

FIGURE 45. Left: Hattie Piipiilani Kalua. Right: Alice Kaelemakule. Kalaupapa settlement, ca. 1906. Photograph may have been taken by Father Joseph Julliotte of Congregation of the Sacred Hearts. SG 283, Congregation of the Sacred Hearts of Jesus and Mary U.S.A Province.

Who scrubbed out stains, the material traces of bodily distress? Who laundered and wrapped the bandages that covered bleeding sores and pustules? Who touched the bodies and skin underneath the cloth? Who provided care as patients experienced disability, pain, and distress? Who sought intimacy with patients at the risk of becoming ill and morally contaminated? In order to apprehend the persistent material and affective registers of life-making and kinship, I turn to a counter-archive of kinship emerging from the materiality of illness and caregiving. These often unheralded and denigrated practices of care sustained the carceral-medical institution, as well as intimate ties between biological and non-biological kin. This chapter begins and ends with photographic portraits, but the archive of kin exceeds visual epistemes and may not readily noticed.

The people who provided the bulk of this labor were unpaid caregivers, often kin of exiled patients. As we have seen in previous chapters, Kānaka ʻŌiwi were vulnerable yet visible medical and political subjects, as Western physicians and health agents backed by influential and wealthy settlers executed the medical incarceration of people with leprosy. Kānaka ʻŌiwi composed the majority of incarcerated patients in the nineteenth and early twentieth centuries. Once exiled to the settlement, patients experiencing increased disability and pain received care from relations that became known as "mea kōkua" or "kōkua." Kōkua were non-leprous family members and friends who chose to accompany their loved ones in exile.[4] In Hawaiian, kōkua is a verb, literally meaning "to help" and suggesting reciprocal practices of care. However, by Board of Health definitions, "kōkua" were treated as an administrative category of labor and personhood—those willing to live with diseased outcasts and provide necessary, but reviled, care. These kōkua became quasi-incarcerated in order to care for relatives and friends at Molokai.

At the same time kōkua provided vital, unpaid care under carceral conditions, Catholic missionaries in the settlement nursed, sheltered, and ministered to patients. However, the interpretation of the care provided by kōkua contrasted sharply with that furnished by medical missionaries: kōkua were undermined as debauched malingers by colonial health authorities, while Catholic caregivers were valorized as saintly and selfless.[5] These categories of caregivers coexisted, but diverged, as I reveal.

If we consider "dressing the body" as deliberate acts of self-presentation and attiring by patients like Hattie and Alice, "dressing" in an expansive sense also references quotidian, yet essential, caregiving bestowed upon the distressed and disabled body: the laundering of soiled clothing and the frequent changing of dressings and bandages that kept skin and sores comfortable. Laundry is far from straightforward, however; it is, literally and metaphorically, a mess. For laundry involved not only the changing and cleaning of clothes in the colonial leprosy settlement. As we shall see, laundry mingled the materiality of water, soap, stains, and skin with colonial anxieties about boundaries between hygiene and contagion, the able-bodied and the disabled, the morally pure and the illicit, Hawaiian and non-Hawaiian, patient and caregiver.

The colonial commodity of soap, as Anne McClintock has argued, offered a Victorian domestic ritual that policed and restored racial-sexual imperial order, while the dirty laundry of leprous people in the colonial Pacific represents perhaps the epitome of the *abject,* an impure element expelled from society.[6] Yet the abject can never really be eradicated; it returns to haunt modernity and threaten the dissolution of Western civilization. Hawaiian laundresses who washed soiled linens and provided intimate care for the sick perform as abject figures—consigned to the margins of colonial life, while unable to be fully discarded.

By touching soiled laundry and bodies, these women trespassed social-medical categories of cleanliness and defilement and exposed themselves to moral disapprobation and social pollution. They haunt and pervade Western medical discourse as alluring, yet dangerous, figures that were founts of moral and bacteriological contagion. Western physicians' lingering fascination with these women would further open their bodies to biomedical experimentation in the age of bacteriology. After taking these messy turns through laundering, we will reconsider Hattie and Alice's photograph and their clean dresses at the end of the chapter.

THE MATERIALITY OF LAUNDRY

How and why did laundry constitute an essential part of care for leprosy patients? Leprosy affects the peripheral nervous system and skin. Prior to the discovery of an effective antibiotic cure in the mid-twentieth century, leprosy produced dramatic and painful changes in skin, including open sores and ulcers. With neither cure nor effective treatments available to him, Ambrose Kanoealii Hutchison, a Kanaka ʻŌiwi man exiled to Kalaupapa settlement in 1879, described the painful transformation of his body as "the wasting of the ball of my right thumb . . . sores and deep ulcers down to the bone, which healed with difficulty."[7] When the Belgian priest Damien de Veuster arrived to establish a Catholic mission at Molokai in 1873, he found patients covered with scabs, "ugly sores" and "fearful ulcers."[8] These open sores festered and smelled, attracting flies and rodents, and required careful dressing. A resident doctor was not installed until 1878, so for the first twelve years of the settlement, patients largely were dependent on one other and unpaid kin for their daily dressings. This community numbered around seven hundred people.

In the first decades of the settlement, patients tended to be in advanced stages of the disease, but received the barest of food rations and clothing allowances from the Board of Health. Men received a pair of blankets, a hat, and a pair of pants, while women got a blanket, a cotton shirt, and one calico dress for the entire year.[9] Most patients were so sick they could not farm, feed themselves, or launder their clothes. In advanced cases of leprosy, fingers and toes shorten as a result of nerve damage, infection, tissue loss, and cartilage absorption. Damaged feet and hands made daily tasks almost impossible.

Laundry, in its most basic sense, requires water, labor, and able bodies. None of these were consistently accessible or available in the first few decades of the settlement. Clean water was scarce and difficult to procure on both sides of the peninsula where patients resided. In the earliest days of the eastern Kalawao settlement, residents had to gather water in large cans from a valley stream and carry them on their shoulders or on horses. Although the Board of Health eventually built a reservoir and water pipes around 1882, these narrow pipes could become clogged by sand and mud, forcing patients to walk a long distance to obtain water.[10]

Soap was also a scarce resource. In 1878, Hawaiian patients provided forceful testimony about terrible settlement conditions directly to a visiting sanitary committee; this committee of prominent Hawaiian and white men were conducting a board inspection. Three male patients wrote a detailed petition in Hawaiian about insufficient food, clothing, and water buckets. They further specified, "During several months past, we have been entirely deprived of soap with which to wash our clothes."[11]

Even if patients had access to soap, those who had hands with shortened or missing fingers could not wash their meager wardrobes in streams, where laundering was usually done.[12] An exiled Hawaiian man named John W. Nakuino lamented in a letter to an English-language newspaper in 1878 that sickly patients experienced particular hardship with their washing: "Some are very painfully affected by the water. I have tried several times to wash my own clothes, but I cannot do it, for as soon as I put my hands in the water it chilled me dreadfully, and I had to go and wrap myself up in blankets to get warm . . . the destitute ones with no fingers—it is pitiful to see them trying to wash their own clothes. All they can do is let them soak over night and in the morning let them dry, without any scrubbing."[13]

Nakuino's letter, however, also expresses great appreciation for the kōkua who provided essential tasks in the community for disabled people unable to walk or work. While kōkua means "to help or assist" in Hawaiian, the labor kōkua provided was vast and included all manner of medical, non-medical, affective, and material caregiving for patients. While their precise number is unknown, many hundreds of these helpers, usually kin or friends of patients, volunteered to go into exile at the settlement with loved ones.[14] These kōkua lent their hands to wash clothes when patients could not. They provided indispensable forms of labor like domestic and manual tasks necessary for the basic functioning of the settlement: nursing and feeding patients, burying of bodies, and the growing and preparation of food. Without kōkua, the board would not have been able to run the settlement at all.

A man named Hao testifying before the Sanitary Committee in 1878 credited kōkua for bolstering the survival of patients: ". . . were it not for the faithful help between parent and child, husband and wife, brother and sister, and between friend and friend," many would have perished. Hao praised his own wife, Luka Kaakau, for dedicating herself to his care for four years of exile. As reported by the committee, Hao said that "he had wanted his wife to abandon his wretched carcass long ago, as she was sound and well . . . but Luka said she was content and happy to wait on the man she loved until his last moments, rather than go back to her friends."[15]

Some members of the board grudgingly recognized how important kōkua were. Board physician, American missionary son, and future BOH president Nathaniel B. Emerson acknowledged kōkua for making the settlement functional. He wrote in 1882: "The kokuas are an indispensable arm of service at the settlement. Without them it would be a very difficult task to carry on the establishment. They climb the pali [cliffs] and drive down the cattle, they fetch the wood from the mountains and carry water from the valleys, they go into the water and cultivate and pull the kalo [taro] . . . They do the work which only sound hands and fingers can do. In fact this important and necessary class of people supply hands and feet for the leper when his own give out."[16]

Congregate institutions in the nineteenth and twentieth centuries in North America, Asia, and other locales greatly depended on labor and materials contributed by residents or their kin. Adequate food and clothing were not provided in many prisons, off-reservation boarding schools, custodial institutions, asylums, and hospitals. Instead, family members often furnished meals, clothing, produce, and daily necessities for loved ones, as was the case in precolonial Vietnam.[17] The Molokai settlement's boundaries proved far less porous, however, as family and friends seeking to provide comforts to patient-prisoners had little choice but to submit to exile and social exclusion as quasi-prisoners.

KŌKUA AND INTIMATE CAREGIVING

Who were the kōkua in the Molokai settlement? The people who provided this uncompensated labor of care were men, women, and even children of diverse ages. The earliest shipments of patients were permitted to bring male and female spouses and grown sons or daughters with them as caregivers.[18] Dr. Emerson estimated that there were ninety-four kōkua and about eight hundred patients on the peninsula in 1879, making the ratio of kōkua to patients about 1 to 8.[19] His contemporary, Dr. Arthur Mouritz, counted a larger number of kōkua men and women residing at the settlement in the early 1880s, at 225 kōkua.[20] In the twentieth century, patients continued to submit petitions to the Board of Health for family members to enter as their kōkua.[21]

The vast majority of these kōkua were Kānaka 'Ōiwi, as were exiled patients, but a smaller number of Asian immigrant descendants became kōkua in the twentieth century. Kōkua were a regulated class of "clean" (that is, non-leprous) residents who were granted permits by the Board of Health to live in the settlement.[22] They were expected to work by caring for the leprous patient, live in an orderly manner, and depart the settlement upon the patient's death if they did not contract leprosy themselves.[23] By becoming kōkua, they became quasi-prisoners who had to submit to printed and unofficial regulations. Agreeing to relinquish their claims in civil society, many adult kōkua sold their property and expected to die in the settlement. In a juridical sense, this class of caregivers was non-leprous, but subject to periodic medical inspection and clearance by the settlement physician.

Eligibility to become kōkua was narrow by the board's criteria; it recognized heterosexual marriage and lineal forms of kinship, such as children and male and female spouses of patients.[24] This was the case although Hawaiian social relations were built on much more expansive practices of kinship, including lineal and collateral descent, as well as non-heterosexual, polyandrous, and polygamous unions, and other forms of non-biological kinship and informal adoption.

These kōkua willingly served as able-bodied proxies for friends, lovers, and family members. However, kōkua were far more than prosthetics lending their "sound hands and fingers," as Emerson described them, because kōkua lived, loved, and labored in the same households as leprous patients. These helpers were deeply disturbing to many settler physicians and other observers. As much as they were necessary, kōkua constituted a problematic social and administrative category. Indigenous caregivers occupying marginal spaces between the healthy and diseased presented an epistemological conundrum for settler-colonial health agents. Emerson characterized the potential medical danger posed by kōkua: living "on terms of unrestricted and fearless intimacy" in the settlement, these caregivers could carry "away with them the germs of leprosy" and distribute them to other islands.[25] Yet in a far more troubling sense beyond trafficking in bacteria, intimate bonds between caregivers and patients trespassed the very boundaries between sick/diseased, leprous/non-leprous, clean/foul bodies that medical incarceration sought to establish.

Wrote Dr. Emerson: "The kokuas ... live on terms of the most perfect and unguarded intimacy with their leper friends, among whom they find their wives, husbands, and lovers. They wash and dress, feed and nourish their leper friends and relatives, when necessary, and come daily in contact with their loathsome ulcers and their garments soiled with the foul exhalations and secretions of their diseased bodies ..."[26] His pejorative language aside, Emerson was not wrong to assess sex and washing as key components of Hawaiian caregiving.

Having sex with a person with leprosy was an important form of providing care—it was an intimate act to breathe with someone and share a bed, especially as Western biomedicine mandated strict separation. Close contact of any kind between "clean" and "leprous" bodies was verboten due to the risk of social and medical contagion. Sex and laundry were practices symbolically and materially linked through the intimate mingling of fluids, skin, and cloth in domestic spaces. Emerson did not gender kōkua in this baroque passage; he found male and female kōkua equally culpable for intimate contact with diseased people. Men and women alike had sex with loved ones and washed their soiled garments.

However, in broader medical scrutiny and lay representations of Hawaiian leprosy, this suspicion narrowed and was specifically cast onto female figures.

Among kōkua, Hawaiian female laundresses became perhaps the most troubling and alarming group of caregivers for medical agents. Dirty laundry and those who handled it became spectacular, suspicious sites of leprosy transmission, though this would be shown to be scientifically unfounded. Leprosy bacilli are not transmitted through soiled cloth, blood, sexual intercourse, or intravenous injection, but through respiratory droplets over long periods of time, as was discovered in the twentieth century.

The laundresses' willingness to engage in intimate forms of labor and living arrangements—valued in a Hawaiian context, but considered indecent to most Euro-Americans[27]—made them highly visible to medical authorities. Touching fluids, tissue, effluvia, bloody cloth, and the bodies of leprous patients, Native women caregivers were imagined as receptacles of bacteria and immorality. Unmarked, beautiful, and seemingly impervious to normative Western standards of propriety, they both fascinated and repelled observers and became culpable for acts of caregiving.

THE LICENTIOUS LAUNDRESS

Who were these infamous laundresses? Why and how did Hawaiian women symbolically and materially mark the boundaries between clean and filth, moral and illicit behavior? Within Western medical literature and Hawai'i Board of Health reports published from the 1880s to 1905, a figure I call the licentious laundress appeared with increasing regularity.[28] As cast by medical observers, the licentious laundress was an attractive Hawaiian woman who washed the filthiest linens of leprosy patients and had sex with leprous partners, yet did not become infected with the disease herself. The laundress became an unacknowledged obsession for non-Hawaiian physicians and health agents, whether they were residing in the islands or observing leprosy from afar.

The licentious laundress first made her appearance in 1885 in reports written by resident physicians at the settlement, all foreigners. The washerwoman at the Kalawao settlement hospital took on grotesque contours in these accounts. Medical superintendent George Fitch identified her as a Hawaiian kōkua named Kalehua who did the "washing of the blood and pus saturated garments of the inmates."[29] Kalehua had accompanied her leprous husband to Kalawao in 1868 and had multiple liaisons after her husband died. Fitch described Kalehua as a "common strumpet" who lived "a most licentious life with the inmates of the hospital, lepers in the last stages of the disease."[30]

Despite this extensive contact with fluids and flesh, Kalehua remained "a remarkably fine looking healthy woman, showing no trace of the disease."[31] Kalehua performed valuable domestic labor, but disturbed Fitch by engaging in promiscuous sexual behavior with leprous bodies.

British physician Arthur Mouritz, who subsequently served as setttlement resident physician, also reported on the curious case of the Kalawao washer-woman. "Any one who has seen advanced cases of tubercular leprosy knows the condition this soiled linen will present; nor is this her only contact with the disease, she has lepers living in her house, and to crown all, her husbands, two in number, were lepers for years before they died; and yet, in spite of all this contact, this said woman to-day is hale, hearty and plump, and as fine as specimen of womanhood as any in the islands . . ."[32] Mouritz's laundress was in all likelihood the woman Kalehua discussed by his colleague Fitch.

The laundress traveled far beyond Hawai'i public health reports to numerous transnational medical reports and journals. She took on spectacular contours in the 1888 *American Lancet;* 1889 *Medical Record;* 1889 *New York Medical Journal;* a 1894 textbook on syphilis and dermatology; a 1902 U.S. congressional report on leprosy, and the 1903 Proceedings of the Connecticut Medical Society.[33]

By 1904, a laundress named Hoolemakani appeared in a U.S. Public Health and Marine-Hospital report. Similar to Kalehua, Hoolemakani was a kōkua who had chosen to accompany her husband to the settlement in 1868. After this husband died, she had married a kōkua. Widowed a second time, she then married another leprous man. Hoolemakani had been doing the washing for some of the "worst cases" in the settlement for twenty years, but was "still in a healthy condition."[34]

The laundress was likely an amalgam of several different women like Hoolemakani and Kalehua who represented a broader cohort of Hawaiian female caregivers. While male kōkua with multiple spouses were mentioned in medical and public health literature, the laundress appeared more frequently and with far more dramatic and salacious details. In these reports, the laundress willingly touched all kinds of filth, cared for, and had sex and lived with leprous people, yet remained unmarked. Her unblemished skin opened her up to more scrutiny and wonder—how could someone touch sick people and their stained clothes, but still appear "clean"? Was the laundress indeed clean beneath her skin? Was she actually immune to leprosy?

On the one hand, doctors marveled at her robustness and beauty and wanted to understand it. Yet flaunting the boundaries between purity and impurity made the laundress liable as licentious and morally dissolute. Physicians' disgust with and suspicion of laundresses cathect around two central anxieties. First, as perceived by medical authorities, the laundress was essential for sanitary regimes, but did not practice hygiene herself. She seemed to have no regard for the danger of infection. Laundresses welcomed, even desired, intimacy with leprous bodies. Unlike Westerners, many of whom pushed for strict segregation, kōkua were neither disgusted nor fearful of leprous bodies, fearing separation from loved ones far more. They were socially troubling for not shunning diseased and disfigured kin. More than lending their limbs, they willingly joined leprous communities, affectively co-mingling, living together, loving, and washing the clothes of people Western observers eschewed as loathsome.

Further, laundresses remained unmarked, healthy, and clean despite extensive contact with soiled linens and bodies. Though the laundress willfully traversed boundaries between the pristine and filthy, she did not become sick herself. If the laundress was immune and there were no somatic consequences for intimate co-mingling, then perhaps segregation itself made no sense. Why would anyone need to abide by strict and punishing laws of medical segregation? The entire system which demanded the removal of the diseased could be exposed as unstable.

Laundry in key ways serves as a proxy for skin. Laundry is a layer that touches the skin. It is a membrane that protects, but it is also porous and leaky. Like skin, laundry is perceived as a boundary between cleanliness and disease. Laundry holds and retains stains excreted from and by distressed bodies, and those who touch these stains may become contaminated, whether socially or bacteriologically. Mary Douglas notes how "excretory functions of the body" can become particularly fraught and associated with the bodies that labor to clean, groom, mop, or manage these excretions.[35] Having intimate contact with abject people consigned to the furthest margins of society, the laundress absorbed stigma through the laundry she touched.

Laundry has been a highly racialized and gendered site of regulation in domestic and urban zones of contact. In San Francisco's Chinatown, laundries operated by Chinese immigrants were monitored as a public health menace, as the filth of Chinese—moral and bacteriological—was believed to seep through the clothes they laundered.[36] Ethnic white immigrant and working-class women who had access to households as cooks, cleaners, and domestic help in the continental United States would similarly come under suspicion for spreading contagious diseases. In the early twentieth century, the Irish cook Mary Mallon became infamous as "Typhoid Mary," an asymptomatic carrier of typhoid bacteria. Mallon infected people while cooking food in the kitchens of her wealthy employers.

Women in particular mark boundaries between purity and danger due to their privileged relationship to social and biological reproduction. Douglas writes of the Hindu caste in India, "Females are correctly seen as, literally, the entry by which the pure content may be adulterated. Males are treated as pores through which the precious stuff may ooze out and be lost ..."[37] Anne McClintock extends this argument to theorize the Victorian obsession with "boundary sanitation" during imperial expansion. Women's bodies and sexuality were permeable "body boundaries" that required purification to control racial and cultural contagion. Women "ambiguously placed on the imperial divide" such as prostitutes, nurses, and servants were "especially fetishized as dangerously ambiguous and contaminating," McClintock argues.[38] In late-nineteenth century Hawai'i, Hawaiian women denoted the raced-sexed boundaries between the clean and defiled, settler and Native, and were monitored and indicted for labor and sexual practices that physicians believed led to disease.

Taking on successive leprous partners and loads of unsanitary linen, the laundress troubled categories of purity: her behavior did not result in disease or signs of leprosy. Could something be hidden underneath her veneer of beauty? There were two possibilities: she could harbor and spread bacteria as a so-called immune carrier, or she could spread immorality through illicit sexual intercourse. Therefore, doctors would spend a considerable amount of effort puzzling over these confounding questions. Her promiscuity and sexual habits were probed discursively, while her body was poked with needles.

THE LAUNDRESS AS EXPERIMENTAL MATERIAL

How leprosy bacilli was transmitted from person to person was unknown and debated. As government physicians observed cases of leprosy in Hawai'i, they debated overlapping theories of transmission, such as a hereditary disease or a racial susceptibility among Hawaiians and Asian immigrants.[39] The most common thread, however, was excessive sexual contact and behavior among Hawaiians: leprosy as a disease transmitted via sexual intercourse, an advanced stage of the venereal disease syphilis, or, more generally, an infection spread by sexual promiscuity. Thus, in these assessments, despite leprosy being bacteriological in nature, Hawaiians were culpable for spreading contagion through what Westerners perceived as promiscuous behavior. European premodern medicine and religion also saw leprosy as a result of sinful behavior that included illicit sex, but these ideas were re-animated in a late nineteenth-century colonial context, melding gender and racialized sexuality in a nexus of sin and bacteriological infection.

Historian Regina Kunzel has described the American prison as a "laboratory of sexual deviance" upon which researchers relied for its "literally captive subject pool" in the twentieth century. She observes how the sexual life of prisoners became "the subject of intense anxiety, fascination, and scrutiny even as it was treated as a closely guarded secret of carceral life."[40] In the U.S. imperial archipelago, leprosy institutions also gave researchers wide access to thousands of colonized and incarcerated people for the imaging of and experimentation on racialized sexuality. In the guise of mapping a contagious disease, leprosy provided an alibi and unique opportunity for a series of physicians to probe race and sex.

The American doctor and syphilis researcher Prince A. Morrow offered these conclusions after visiting the Molokai settlement as a medical tourist in 1889: "[T]he disease is propagated through sexual intercourse."[41] Morrow linked leprosy contagion with promiscuity, writing: "It is this total absence of fear, this ignorant contempt of its contagiousness combined with the promiscuous and intimate intercourse between the healthy and the diseased which accounts for the rapid and unexampled spread of the disease in these islands."[42] Physicians attributed leprosy's spread to the sexual excess of Hawaiians.

Dr. George Fitch, resident physician at Kalawao, wrote that the "disorder has been allowed to run on unchecked and uncontrolled ... undoubtedly [because of] their uncontrolled licentiousness."[43] Fitch became obsessed with the conjugal lives, sexuality, and kinship of patients. In his clinical data collection on leprosy, Fitch obsessively catalogued patients, their sexual partners, non-monogamous children, and affinal kin. His reports are a veritable gossip column, rife with wondrous amazement at polyamorous Hawaiians, and to a lesser degree, the white men who chose to go native and take up with Hawaiian women.[44]

Physicians like Fitch blamed Hawaiian people and pathologized their behavior as excessively sexual. How could leprosy be controlled among such unruly, polyamorous people? By these assessments, they were disgusting, led dissolute lives, and could not abide monogamous relationships. American settler physician Nathaniel B. Emerson summarized the culpable behavior of Hawaiians: they were infected with leprosy at a much higher rate than whites "because white people are much more careful than Hawaiians in their choice of companions."[45]

Connecting Hawaiian promiscuity to leprosy did not end with rhetorical assertions, however. Most infamously, the hypothesized relationship between sex and leprosy culminated in a series of biomedical experiments on kōkua by British physician and leprologist Arthur Mouritz, who worked as a resident physician at the Molokai settlement. Mouritz was not testing the sexual transmission of leprosy, but he wished to understand why some people who engaged in intimate activities with patients did not get infected. The sexual practices and permeability of female kōkua made them suitable as Mouritz's human subjects. Mouritz selected a total of fifteen uninfected kōkua, men and women, for "experimental inoculation" between 1884 and 1887. Wanting to determine if leprosy bacilli could be grown in their uninfected tissue, he inoculated them with a solution of "leprous serum" taken from the blisters of patients.[46] In these fifteen experiments, none contracted leprosy. Of these cases, Mouritz's most elaborated subject was a Hawaiian laundress he called patient "Q."

Mouritz had originally become familiar with Q when he engaged her to wash his clothing at Kalawao. Q worked as a laundress and performed other domestic labor in the settlement, including hat making, sewing, and mat weaving. According to Mouritz, the thirty-five-year-old Q was "petite, and very comely and graceful" and had attracted one husband after another.[47] Q, like Kalehua and other scandalous laundresses that became medical curiosities, did not get sick.[48] Each of Q's husbands contracted leprosy and died, as did her three children, but she herself remained beautiful and "free from blemish."

Mouritz described Q as a willing participant in his inoculation experiments. Contradicting his observation of Q's assiduous labor, Mouritz characterized kōkua as malingers "perfectly willing to acquire leprosy if that could be brought about," because they desperately wanted to secure free government rations as patients. Q suffered a terrible reaction to his injections— headache, chills, fever, nausea, sweating, and bodily pains over four days—so she refused further injections. Q did not contract leprosy and Mouritz ruled her to be immune despite twenty-nine years of exposure. Although Mouritz conducted contemporaneous experiments on ten male kōkua, he honed his experimental and clinical gaze much more on women kōkua, their supposed immoral character, and sexual practices. Furthermore, though he tallied Europeans and Americans engaging in non-monogamous sexual contact with Hawaiian women and becoming sick, his experiments were chiefly focused on Hawaiian women.

Mouritz inoculated four other female kōkua in addition to Q: all supposedly engaged in suspect sexual habits, whether evidenced in actual practices or symptoms of venereal disease. He published florid details of these kōkua cases in a 1916 quasi-medical memoir and treatise on leprosy thirty years after he had left Molokai. Patient "O" was married to a male patient, but led "a very dissolute life" as a prostitute who had sex with leprous patients for pocket money. She had gonorrhea that had erupted in venereal warts. Patient "P" was married; she was not a prostitute, but had cervical ulcers. Patient "R" had multiple leprous husbands; she had ulcers on her anus and labia resembling syphilis. Patient "S" was married to a kōkua and had gonorrhea.[49] Mouritz's case notes betray an obsession with the conjugal lives and sexual practices of Hawaiian women.

What made these kōkua so "suitable in every respect as subjects," as he suggested, was not only their uninfected tissue and availability as human subjects, but also the imagined permeability and vigor of the Hawaiian female body.[50] They were a receptacle of bacteria, but could not become infected. They were hardy stock, ideal as clinical material. In these experiments, two seemingly contradictory imaginaries were brought together: 1) Hawaiians were dirty/infected/diseased and conduits of disease, and 2) Hawaiians were so resilient, they could not become sick. Patient Q cleaned clothes and looked clean, but under her "clean" skin, perhaps she was just as filthy. Beauty and horror were married in a single duplicitous female body.

This intense preoccupation with female sexual pathology in Hawai'i leprosy institutions overlapped with scientific investigations into the biological roots of female delinquency at the turn of the century. The Italian proto-criminologist and physician Cesare Lombroso attempted to uncover the biological basis of prostitution, female criminality, and female degeneracy by probing the bodies and sexual behavior of imprisoned Italian women in the 1880s. His theories of female criminality became immensely influential in Europe and English-speaking countries throughout much of the twentieth century.[51]

Experiments on colonized and incarcerated kōkua—little remarked upon in bioethics or the field formations of microbiology, venereal diseases, or infectious diseases—place Hawaiian women in a long line of non-white, colonized, and enslaved women readily utilized as clinical material in Western biomedicine.[52] Laura Briggs has discussed how non-white women, particularly enslaved African American women, were ideologically constructed in Western biomedicine as fertile and strong. This made them handy, disposable subjects for dangerous and unethical gynecological experiments like cesarean sections and fistula repairs in the nineteenth century.[53] The laundress and female kōkua were similarly useful biocommodities— marvelously impervious to leprosy and Western social conventions. While their laundering practices were devalued and discredited, doctors relied on their bodies to test hypotheses about Native female sexuality and contagion.

These figurations of Native women as immune conduits of contagion spread outside of Hawai'i. By 1895, a story on Hawai'i leprosy was printed in a San Francisco newspaper. The article associated female sexual promiscuity with immunity: "While leprosy is held to be contagious, and even infectious in some cases, there are women in the leper settlement who have had one, two, and in one case even three leper husbands who have died of their affliction, and yet these women are unaffected."[54]

The narrative of patient Q and other Hawaiian women as unmarked carriers and potentially unknown vectors of infection amplified medical and popular anxieties over the unstable bodies of domestic caregivers. Although the non-leprous laundress has nearly disappeared from medical and popular literature today, she pre-dates the early twentieth-century medical cause célèbre of "Typhoid Mary" by at least twenty years. The 1907 case of Mary Mallon, the immigrant Irish cook who purportedly spread deadly typhoid germs through the food she handled in New York households, is much better known and claimed to be the first United States case of an asymptomatic carrier.[55] However, on the borders of the U.S. empire, debates over gender and healthy carriers of disease were already well under way due to Hawaiian laundresses and kōkua.

What did the laundress look like? The laundress was described narratively with adjectives like "fine looking," "comely," "clean and neat," but was she ever photographed? There was no photograph of patient Q in Mouritz's reports or of a laundress in other medical literature describing her. Yet Mouritz did offer a significant visual proxy that amply associated Native female sexuality with disease. He inserted a seemingly incongruous, nonclinical photograph of a young Hawaiian woman in his 1916 treatise on leprosy, *The Path of the Destroyer*.[56] Captioned "Hawaiian Type. Pure Hawaiian

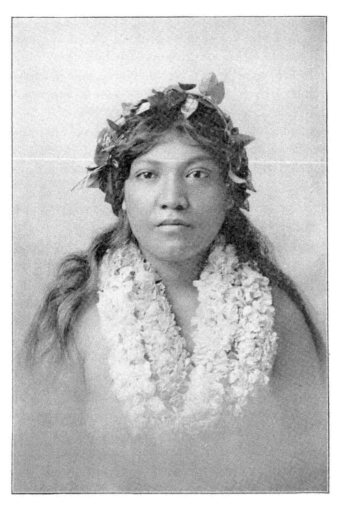

HAWAIIAN TYPE.
Pure Hawaiian Girl.

FIGURE 46. "Hawaiian Type. Pure Hawaiian Girl." Published in Mouritz, *Path of the Destroyer* (1916).

Girl," the photograph is of a woman in a three-quarter length portrait (figure 46). She wears no clothing; instead, double strands of lei ʻawapuhi (ginger lei) strategically cover her breasts and hint at her sexual difference and availability. Mouritz's voluble description of the "comely and graceful" patient Q became linked to this image of a young, healthful-looking woman.

This iconography of bare-breasted Hawaiian women had already been in circulation in American print media, fascinating Euro-American viewers since the late nineteenth century, as I have analyzed elsewhere.[57] The visual staging and coding of this woman is similar to that of contemporaneous female hula dancers, and indeed there is little to tie her to leprosy. Yet Mouritz seems to have purposely placed this photograph in relation to leprosy, and possibly even the laundress patient Q. While associated with the hidden and invisible danger of leprosy bacilli, the photograph of this beauteous woman stood in direct contrast to the lush, colored clinical images of Hawaiian people with leprosy that Mouritz also published in his book. These included pathological slides and photographs of Hawaiian patients in mild to advanced stages of leprosy.

The photograph of the "pure Hawaiian girl" thus suggested connections between Mouritz's narrative of patient Q, a sexually available, non-leprous Native woman, and people ravaged by leprosy. The image of the girl served as a proxy for kōkua like patient Q, who appeared clean and neat, but remained a suspicious vector of leprosy. "Pure Hawaiian" ostensibly signified racial purity or a non-mixed-race person, but because the term was placed in a medical volume, it also signified cleanliness of the body—a state of non-infection. As suggested by the caption "Hawaiian type," the non-leprous carrier was a "type" of a Hawaiian woman who, though of pure Hawaiian blood, could harbor germs in this blood.

The phrase "Hawaiian type" thus remained ambiguous. It ostensibly referred to a racial type, but it also marked alluring Hawaiian women as a type of unmarked carrier whose "purity" could not be trusted despite an outwardly attractive appearance. In a different ideological regime perhaps, observations and related data about kōkua who did not get sick might have led scientists to conclude that leprosy is difficult to contract. However, in this anxious colonial setting, doctors like Mouritz instead interpreted the non-infection of Hawaiian women as evidence of their fearful duplicity and sexual pathology.

MORAL HYGIENE

As the bodies of Hawaiian women were probed and experimented on by Euro-American physicians searching for infection, they were being scrutinized in other arenas of the leprosy settlement: the intimate spaces of Catholic dormitories. In this photograph taken some time after 1905, three sisters from the Catholic order of Saint Francis stand in the center of the

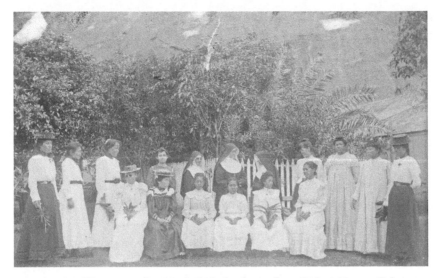

FIGURE 47. Women residents and Catholic sisters from Bishop Home, Kalaupapa, Molokai settlement, ca. 1906. Sisters from the Saint Francis order stand in the second row, left to right: Sister Elizabeth Gomes, Sister Leopoldina Burns, and Mother Marianne Cope. Seated third from left: Julia Kuokala, from Laupāhoehoe, Hawai'i, who was exiled to Molokai in November 1905 at age eighteen with other family members. She died in 1908. Kalihi Hospital case 342, Hawai'i State Archives. SG 351, Congregation of the Sacred Hearts of Jesus and Mary U.S.A Province.

photograph (figure 47). The sisters managed the Charles R. Bishop Home for Unprotected Leper Girls and Women, known as Bishop Home, which opened in Kalaupapa settlement in 1888. The Franciscan sisters belonged to an order based in Syracuse, New York; they first arrived in Hawai'i in 1883 to care for leprous patients in Honolulu.

The sisters' location in the exact center of the portrait, flanked by four Hawaiian women on both sides, marks them as authorities over their Hawaiian female wards. Although their bodies are turned at an angle and their faces not fully visible, the three Euro-American women dressed in black habits and white veils exude authority. Their habits and veils are immediately recognizable as symbols signifying the women's chastity, discipline, and dedication to God.

In contrast, the young female residents are arranged formally in orderly rows around the sisters. They wear full-length dresses or skirts, but they are subordinate and worldly in relation to the sisters. Some of the patient-residents clasp flowers, branches, or foliage in their hands and laps, further associating the Hawaiian women with the mountains and lush foliage that form the photograph's natural backdrop. The Hawaiian women are terrestrial and earth-bound, while the sisters are sacred. The residents do not make eye contact with one another or with the Catholic sisters, nor do they touch each other. They are staged as a group, but their exact relationships with one another are not signaled by the portrait's composition.

Catholic sisters and priests served in the settlement as increasingly important adjuncts to BOH agents and physicians in the 1880s, providing medical and social welfare for patients. Catholic missionaries from Western Europe and North America who ministered to leprous people in the Hawaiian Islands and other colonies acquired spiritual prestige. They had been inspired by the martyrdom of Father Damien de Veuster, a Belgian medical missionary, who arrived in Molokai in 1873 and died of leprosy in 1889.

Catholic priests residing in the settlement took photographs of patients and missionaries there, perhaps as early as the turn of the nineteenth century. One photographer-priest whose photographic work can be confirmed was Father Paul-Marie (Joseph) Julliotte. Julliotte, who hailed from France, was stationed in Kalaupapa between 1901 and 1907 as a medical missionary. He had an interest in photography and science; he took several hundred wet glass plate photographs of patients and their chosen kin in makeshift studio settings at the Kalaupapa and Kalawao settlements. He also made wax molds of the limbs of Molokai patients.[58] Other priests who followed Julliotte in the twentieth century also appear to have taken photographs.[59]

While doctors were trading images and information on a medical circuit, resident Catholic missionaries took photographs of incarcerated people at Molokai, which were then reproduced and disseminated through transnational Catholic circuits over the next several decades. The technological shift of photography to mechanical reproduction, as theorized by Walter Benjamin, thus enabled a diverse afterlife of patient images among religious audiences.[60] Catholic fathers and brothers serving in the settlement pasted photographs into elaborate personal albums, perhaps as souvenirs of their time in the settlement. These albums contain portraits of people the men may not have known or cared for personally. The portrait of Alice and Hattie (figure 45), for instance, was one of many images enclosed in a Catholic album.[61]

Yet beyond personal keepsakes, patient photographs were distributed through Catholic institutions and seen far beyond the settlement. The European centers of the Congregation of the Sacred Hearts of Jesus and Mary (the Catholic congregation that dispatched generations of missionaries to Molokai), located then in Aachen, Germany, and Brussels, Belgium, printed postcards and lantern slides with photographs of Molokai patients. Related Catholic missionary publishers in Paris and the United States also produced ethnographic lantern slide sets of Molokai and its patients, which likely were projected as illustrated lectures for Catholic audiences.[62]

Images of Molokai leprosy inmates perhaps received the widest distribution through Catholic missionary journals before World War I, however. These influential mass-market publications were mouthpieces of the French missionary organization Oeuvre de la Propagation de la Foi, based in Lyon, France. Oeuvre's bimonthly and weekly publications were some of the most widely read in the French-speaking world, exceeding the readership of the era's most popular daily.[63] Printed in a large tabloid format with photographs, etchings, and narrative reports, these missionary journals dramatized front-line Catholic evangelizing from nearly every corner of the globe. They supported fund-raising and inspired recruitment and evangelization.[64]

A photograph of young women residents at Bishop Home was published with four other photographs in the Oeuvre's weekly French-language journal, *Les Missions Catholiques,* in 1907 (figure 48).[65] The photographs accompanied a letter written by Ildephonse Alazard, a Catholic father. Alazard described a fire that had destroyed St. Francis Catholic Church at Kalaupapa settlement the year before. Captioned as "Un Groupe de Premières Communiantes au Bishop Home de Kalaupapa" (A group of first communicants at Kalaupapa's Bishop home), the photograph shows women dressed in white dresses, presumably on the occasion of their first communion. The photograph reveals leprous nodules on their faces. However, the women's white clothing signified chastity, purity, and commitment to God, as well as the moral discipline and religious conversion of the Native "filles lépreuses" that had been made possible by the charitable works of the Catholic Church.

The letter writer issued "appeals to charity" for a new church. This fund-raising proved extremely successful. In the months that followed, monetary contributions for a new church came from far and wide, from Pope St. Pius X, King Edward VII of England, and ordinary Catholic adherents.[66] Donors from England, Poland, Germany, and France earmarked funds specifically for the reconstruction of "l'église" at Molokai that had burned down, suggesting that photographs of leprous Catholic converts from Hawai'i were effective instruments for financial solicitations. The new St. Francis Church was rebuilt with stone in 1908, equipped with a bell tower, Gothic arches, and stained-glass windows.

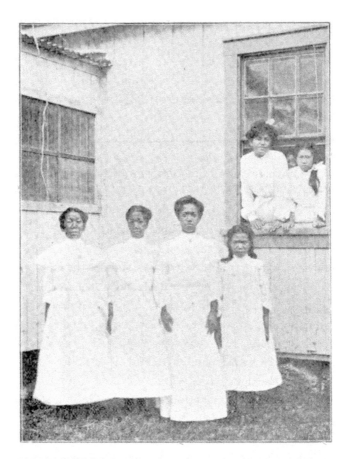

ILE MOLOKAI (Sandwich). — UN GROUPE DE PREMIÈRES
COMMUNIANTES AU BISHOP HOME DE KALAUPAPA

FIGURE 48. "Un Groupe de Premières Communiantes au Bishop
Home de Kalaupapa" (A group of first communicants at Kalaupapa's
Bishop Home). Published in Alazard, *Les Missions Catholiques,*
January 4, 1907.

These photographic subjects and their broad distribution and reception
through Catholic media suggest how the intimate spaces of settlement
dormitories were opened and placed on display for Western audiences.
The domestic space of the dormitory and its charges became privy to
inspection and visual scrutiny by curious Western audiences. The surface
tidiness of the women's clothing and hair signified what could not be
seen: the moral and sexual hygiene being inculcated in "jeunes filles
lépreuses."[67]

Far more than their male counterparts, these young unmarried Hawaiian girls and women with leprosy were believed to be particularly vulnerable to moral and sexual corruption in the settlement. As its full name suggests, Bishop Home for Unprotected Leper Girls and Women was intended to shelter unmarried girls from sexual predation. Under the direction of virginal sisters, the home was to inculcate moral and sexual hygiene in girls who did not come from male-headed, nuclear families. In keeping with the rigorous gender segregation instituted in the settlement, a separate home for boys was opened six years later on the opposite side of the peninsula. The Baldwin Home for Boys was run by brothers from a different Catholic order.[68]

In the religious home, the body was a register of virtue, and patient-inmates were expected to wear their virtue and sexual purity on their bodies.[69] As medical historian Alison Bashford has discussed, hygienic practices were more than a set of medical or governmental mandates; Victorian civility demanded the incorporation of hygienic practices into one's entire subjectivity and soul.[70] Bishop Home, a cordon sanitaire that overlapped with medicalized leprosy segregation, implemented regimes of sexual and moral hygiene in its Hawaiian female subjects. Whereas doctors and health agents segregated "clean" bodies from "unclean" bodies through clinical records, published edicts, and physical gates and fences, religious caregivers undertook benevolent forms of sanitary discipline through moral education and domestic arts in the group home. Cleanliness of the body and soul was a colonial modality to which the women were expected to conform, going beyond medical protection from infection and disease to discipline within the intimate corridors and bedrooms of the dormitory. For "clean" denoted not just a non-infectious state of the body, but a range of subjective judgments about a person's conformity to Euro-American standards of ability, appearance, beauty, morality, comportment, and disposition.

Acting in loco parentis for girls and unmarried women in the home were the mother superior, assistant superior, and sisters. About eighty-six young girls and women lived together during this period, closely watched over by their new surrogate kin.[71] The titles of "Mother Superior" and "Sisters" are suggestive of the hierarchical authority that was to substitute for the collective kin relations many girls left behind. They were expected to conform to the sisters' standards of cleanliness, chastity, and morality through dress and behavior.

As represented in a photograph staged in the interior of the Bishop Home around 1910 (figure 49), domestic arts are vital parts of gendered domestic

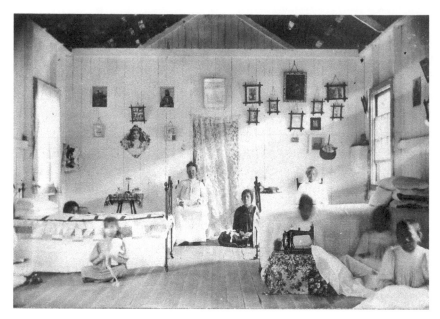

FIGURE 49. Interior of Bishop Home, Kalaupapa settlement, ca. 1910. Box 1012, p. 2, Congregation of the Sacred Hearts of Jesus and Mary U.S.A Province.

order and colonial sanitary discipline for Hawaiian girls. In this spotless dormitory occupied by girls and women, the beds are made and line up evenly with their occupants next to them. The carefully dressed girls and women sit up straight, looking toward the camera.

The domestic chores required of the girls and women, such as sewing, cleaning, and housekeeping, fill the entire frame. The quilts atop the beds are smooth, the pillows stacked tidily, and the floors scrubbed. Framed images of saints and Jesus Christ are arranged prominently on the walls, as if watching over their wards. Feminine crafts are suggested by the arrangement of baskets and a lace curtain. Within the photograph, the women and girls appear occupied with their labor. At least four of the occupants appear to be sewing—the girl seated to the left holds a doll, while the sewing machine was likely in motion, as the countenance of the machine's operator is blurred. As in federally run Indian boarding schools, which trained American Indian children to behave like industrious civilized workers, the girls' dormitory inculcated domesticity in female bodies.[72]

Some girls sentenced without family members appreciated the shelter and security the sisters provided in the settlement. Yet an unspoken and central part of moral cleanliness was the maintenance of sexual purity—the expectation to refrain from sexual contact and preserve chastity. One Bishop Home resident, Mary Kaehukulani (later known as Mary Sing), who had arrived in 1917 at age seventeen, described how their freedom was curtailed: "It was very strict. You cannot come out and talk to anybody; you have to have permission to talk to anybody."[73] Mingling with boys and men was verboten, and the girls were chaperoned and monitored. Some young women bucked this regime. Mary Kaehukulani left the home two years after her arrival to marry her first husband. Immorality and promiscuous behavior could be punished by expulsion from the home by the Mother Superior, though this did not occur very often.[74]

It would have been very difficult for Hawaiian girls and women to uphold mission standards of moral and somatic cleanliness. Hawaiians were already believed generally to be ontologically different from whites, more susceptible to disease (or not susceptible enough, in the perplexing case of the laundress); to belong to a lower evolutionary order; to be uncivilized; and to have unhealthy eating, sleeping, and birthing practices outside of heteronuclear households. Native people had to meet higher standards in order to be considered "clean," healthy, without disease, or morally righteous. Even if they performed the same actions as their white counterparts, Native women were criticized or discredited, and this was acutely the case for caregiving performed by kōkua as compared to the caregiving furnished by the Catholic sisters.

Both groups provided important unpaid care and most seemed undaunted by close contact with disabled patients. Sister Leopoldina Burns, for instance, became known as an expert "soredresser," or bandage wrapper, for women patients.[75] However, the sisters' labor was valorized while the equivalent labor of kōkua was denigrated. Dr. Fitch, medical superintendent, extolled the Franciscan Sisters' exemplary nursing of sick leprosy inmates at Kakaʻako Branch Hospital in 1884. Some of these women would later bring their mission to the Molokai settlement. Fitch wrote of the sisters, "Only those who have seen the devotion of these noble women to their work, and the blessed results of their labor, can form any conception of the worth of their efforts to the poor suffering creatures in their charge."

Female kōkua were held up to the standard of the sisters—virginal, charitable white women—and failed by this inequitable measure. Rather than being viewed as generous or self-sacrificing, kōkua were characterized as selfish, promiscuous, greedy, able-bodied parasites. Only a few paragraphs later in the same report in which Dr. Fitch praised the "noble" sisters, he described kōkua in the settlement as debauched people who "live off the rations provided by Government for the sick, and, as a rule, only add to the unparalleled licentiousness of that hideous brothel."[76]

Doing laundry and wearing clean clothes would have been quotidian requirements for residents and the supervising sisters in Bishop Home. White Catholic sisters touching and washing abject bodies and stained laundry endowed saintliness and spiritual rewards, but their wards did not gain praise for undertaking these duties. The most abject material and practices— diseased Native bodies and the care of their soiled clothes—indeed could be safely transformed into hygienic domesticity and religious piety when brought into the sanitized confines of the Christian care home. The abject and unclean were redeemed and restored through the saintly alchemy of the sisters and Mother Superior, while outside the dormitory, Native kōkua gained sexual notoriety for sustained contact with leprous bodies.

EUGENICS AND SEXUAL REGULATION

Aside from Catholic-run homes, gendered segregation and moral hygiene were also surveilled at the detention compound in Kalihi, Honolulu. Kalihi Hospital (also known as the Detention Station and Receiving Station) processed, detained, and housed people of all ages suspected of leprosy in the twentieth century. People ruled leprous by the board were kept at Kalihi until they could be sent to Molokai, while some with less severe cases received medical treatment until doctors determined they could not improve.

In the Progressive era, eugenics ideas judged normative bodies and conduct and encouraged the breeding of better humans. These concerns ramped up in Hawai'i among elite haole citizens, and to some degree, high-ranking Hawaiians. Married women reformers in elite society became so alarmed that they petitioned the BOH to investigate and correct conditions at Kalihi Hospital in 1918. One of these leaders was Alice Kamokilaikawai Campbell, also known as Kamokila or Mrs. F. Walter MacFarlane. Kamokila had ali'i (chiefly) lineage and was an heir to the Campbell Estate; her father was haole sugar industrialist James Campbell.[77] Kamokila hosted the concerned women's petition meeting and then joined the special investigative committee, composed of BOH and Chamber of Commerce members.

Many of the committee's concerns focused on better fences and physical barriers to protect the public from patient-inmates, preventing escapes into town, and instilling stricter moral codes. Kalihi Hospital separated patients into different living quarters by gender, but supervision was not constant, and there were allegations that male patients had managed to have overnight visits with female patients in their rooms. In October 1917, several male patients appeared to have spent an evening with female patients, with "immoral relations . . .between those patients."[78]

Relying on the contemporary language of eugenics, race improvement, and the elimination of disability, the committee also went a step beyond sex segregation to advocate for the sterilization of patients: "In permitting the physically diseased to breed and propagate their kind, we are vitiating and blocking the likeliest of all paths of human progress, and if individuals that are diseased could be made to remain childless, nothing would be irretrievably lost to the race."[79] It is not clear whether sterilization was formally adopted by the BOH in the 1920s, but some exiled patients in the mid-twentieth century disclosed they and others had been encouraged to submit to sterilization.[80]

How did people respond to these eugenicist sexual regulations? Women patients and caregivers in carceral institutions, especially those without kin relations, were faced with impossible mandates and expectations to participate in a virtuous bodily economy. Yet Indigenous people also consumed commodities like soap and clothing in unexpected and discrepant ways, as scholars have discussed in studies of colonial hygiene.[81] Despite the strict forms of hygienic and domestic order suggested in the photographs of Bishop Home, life and discipline were far more unruly and inexact. Women and girls managed to slip out of their chaste clothing and run away from the Bishop Home to meet boys. During what became known as fits of "The Spring Fever," girls snuck out for evening assignations, sometimes not to return.[82]

At Kalihi Hospital in Honolulu in the early 1900s, women also arranged for friends and lovers to slip into the five-acre hospital grounds, perhaps even with the night watchman's tacit permission.[83] A fourteen-year-old girl named Kahawaii from Makiki, Oʻahu, was incarcerated at Kalihi Hospital as a suspect in January 1905. Three months later she was caught with her lover Edward Alapai inside the grounds, along with fellow inmate Mary Akakao and Mary's lover, a man named Keahi. Alapai and Keahi, who were non-patients, were arrested. Kahawaii gave testimony in Hawaiian which the First Circuit Court of Hawaiʻi translated into English. The Hawaiian-language document was not retained, but she notarized the following statement: "He [Eddie] has been inside four times counting last night. We arrange to meet inside at a certain time and this arrangement is made early in the evening. We

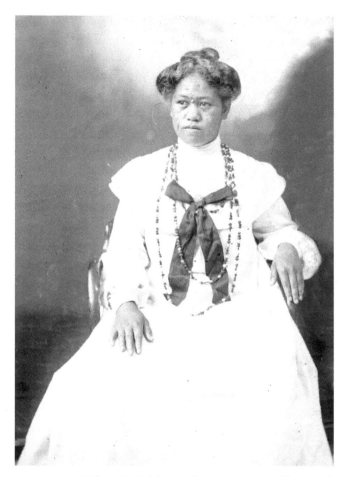

FIGURE 50. Kahawaii, Molokai settlement, ca. 1906. Photograph may have been taken by Father Joseph Julliotte of Congregation of the Sacred Hearts. SG 229, Congregation of the Sacred Hearts of Jesus and Mary U.S.A Province.

slept together sometimes in the house and sometimes out in the yard and each time he was inside we had connection."[84]

Although all four parties were subject to punitive measures for their transgressive sexuality and violating the boundaries between infected and clean people, their smuggling evokes the determined coordination to evade medical and prison authorities and act on their desires. Kahawaii was exiled to Molokai not long after this incident, while it is unclear what happened to her lover and her friends. In the settlement she posed for a photographic portrait in a handsome white dress and long shell lei (garlands) (figure 50).[85] Kahawaii's white gown signifies a deft way to present herself publicly according to gendered norms of respectability, though she may have continued to reject them through her own private conduct beyond the eyes of her peers and authorities.

Women who lived in group dormitories in the settlement found their own ways to develop and stage their own interpretations of kinship and collectivity. They smuggled in their own caregiving practices into gendered group homes and outside of them. As we will see, they also dressed and adorned their bodies for their own discrepant purposes. Women and men kōkua would assert their own domestic arrangements, kinship, and affinities within and outside of institutional spaces.

SEEKING INTIMATE CARE

As practitioners of allopathic medicine, Western doctors in Hawai'i focused on leprosy cures, disease containment, and the proliferation of scientific knowledge, while patients and their kōkua focused on treatment, comfort, and care. These divergent aims came into conflict in the settlement, and kōkua found comfort hard fought.

Wanting to live in the settlement made kōkua contemptible. BOH agents believed kōkua were lazy people who instrumentalized caregiving for their own selfish purposes: to go on patient rolls and collect rations. Dr. Arthur Mouritz, for instance, called them "artificially made" patients—malingers, rather than workers or noble martyrs. Mouritz described kōkua so "ready and willing to be experimented on by inoculation, serums, or any other means likely to develop leprosy" because they wanted to "obtain board and lodging, for the remainder of their lives."[86]

The actual rules issued by the BOH suggest, however, that unpaid kōkua sustained the operations of the carceral-medical institution. Labor was extracted regularly from kōkua with little compensation. The board had tightened rules regulating caregivers' labor, travel, and entry/exit permits by the early 1890s.[87] One such rule was that every "able-bodied male kokua" was to contribute one day's labor to the board per week in exchange for "privileges and benefits of the place."[88] Seven sections of twenty-two newly published settlement rules in 1893 pertained to kōkua, including "21) Kokuas shall not be entitled to rations of any kind. . . . Food rations, however, may be issued to them in lieu of services rendered to the board . . .; and, 22) Kokuas shall not leave the settlement without the written consent of the superintendent."

After these rules were published in 1893, kōkua were also periodically expelled from the settlement; one set of arbitrary expulsions was published in a Hawaiian newspaper in 1894 and later in 1909.[89]

The board's rules for kōkua permits were inconsistent. At the turn of the century, decisions to allow a family member to stay or enter as kōkua appeared to depend on whether a person seemed industrious, productive, lazy, morally upright, or residing in a legibly heteronormative relationship. In one 1893 consideration of permits for spouses, one permit was granted to a woman to accompany her husband, while a similar petition by a married woman was not.[90] These inhumane and arbitrary decisions led one newspaper editor to call for the "strongest censure" of the BOH president.

After resident superintendent John "Jack" D. McVeigh arrived at the settlement in 1902, his verdicts reigned supreme.[91] One kōkua, a man named Kopena, was ordered to leave the settlement in 1903, perhaps after the death of his family member. Kopena responded by telling the board, "Ko ka hele" (Go to hell). Superintendent McVeigh claimed Kopena refused to work. Kopena had sold all his possessions before entering Kalaupapa and said he had nothing left to which to return.[92] This was at least the second time Kopena had been expelled from the settlement back to his hometown of Honolulu; the previous occasion was in 1894. Kopena's indignant rebuke makes visible the vulnerable economic and social status, as well as quasi-incarceration, kōkua endured in exchange for proximity to their kin.

What were Hawaiians' responses to the stringent regulations that governed their intimate lives? In one of the most documented and public accounts of resistance, a Hawaiian family on Kaua'i took up arms against authorities that tried to separate them in 1893.[93] The dramatic episode of Kaluaiko'olau and Pi'ilani's opposition to the colonial state captured the imagination, yet everyday acts of care and comfort sustained the lives of imprisoned people in less visible, but significant, ways.

Lahela Kanewa and her family took deliberate actions to remain in close contact. Lahela Kanewa entered Kalihi Hospital on November 10, 1907. She was forty years old. Lahela, her husband Joseph Kanewa, and seven of their children resided in La'aloa in Kona, Hawai'i, over 150 miles of ocean south of O'ahu. Despite this distance, her family followed Lahela's movements through the detention system. The day after she was incarcerated at the clinic, Lahela's husband and seven children applied for and received a permit to visit her at Kalihi Hospital. At least two of her daughters remained in Honolulu that month, and they applied for three more visitation permits that November.

The board removed Lahela Kanewa to Molokai on April 17, 1908. A week later, Lahela sent a request for her husband to be allowed in as her kōkua. This petition was approved and a permit issued for Joseph. He joined her at the settlement on May 21, 1908.[94] The Kanewa family was but one of many who made similar choices to remain together. During this period, from 1908 through 1910, a substantial portion of the BOH's meetings was spent deliberating kōkua petitions.[95] Whether as patients or family members, Hawaiians kept pressing the board to allow loved ones to enter or remain in the settlement as caregivers.

In June 1909, after petitioning territorial legislators for clinical re-examinations, a group of eleven people were determined to be non-leprous and released from the settlement. However, within two weeks of their medical and legal clearance, six men from this cohort petitioned the board to be allowed to return to the settlement as kōkua to their wives. Only one of them, a twenty-seven-year-old Hawaiian man named John Kaapuni who received a favorable character endorsement from Superintendent McVeigh, was permitted to return.[96]

Outside of their direct entreaties to the board, patients, kōkua, and would-be kōkua amplified their sorrow in print media. They shared their abiding love, grief, and mourning in writing, poetry, and published remembrances. When a W. M. Riner was told by the board he could not become a kōkua for his wife and accompany her to Kalaupapa in 1896, he published a mournful lament in a Hawaiian-language newspaper. Calling his wife Sela "kuu lei aloha" (my dear beloved lei), Riner wrote that he was not able to choke the love he had for his dear companion.[97] Sela had not died, so Riner's public lament was not formally a kanikau (mourning chant), but an expression of grief and love.

Patients who willingly provided care for other patients, even if they were not acknowledged formally as kōkua or kin, also recorded their aloha (love) and sorrow. In 1912, a woman named Mrs. H. P. Paniani wrote to a newspaper in Hawaiian about the death of her loved one, a Mrs. Kalamau she had cared for in Bishop Home, where both resided in Kalaupapa. They had lived in the same dormitory for about six months, and Mrs. Paniani wished to announce her fond remembrance (hoomanao) publicly for her companion. Similar inscriptions of remembrances were carved on stone grave markers upon the death of patients, and these can still be found in the settlement cemeteries.[98] The important lateral relationship between patients engaged in mutual care and comfort is also suggested in the photograph of Alice Kaelemakule and Hattie Piipiilani Kalua (figure 45).

CONCLUSION: FASHIONING AN EXTENDED
SOCIAL BODY

On the same occasion in 1903 when the kōkua Kopena was expelled, two women patients successfully petitioned to have their husbands join them in the settlement as kōkua. Contrary to the predominant Euro-American notion that kōkua were a class of freeloading women with loose morals moving from lover to lover, these men served as kōkua for their female spouses. Jessie Kaena's husband Kalani Joseph Kaena was one able-bodied man who served as a kōkua.

After Jessie Kaena was apprehended by health agents, she was photographed in 1903 at Kalihi Hospital with her foot exposed as a fetish for the medical camera. Her foot ulcers indicated nerve damage from leprosy (figure 51).[99] However, in contradistinction to her individual clinical image, Jessie posed with her husband and kōkua Kalani Joseph Kaena at the Molokai settlement around 1905, sometime after he was allowed to join her as a kōkua (figure 52). In this portrait, Jessie's status as a patient is suggested by her seated position in a chair. Wearing a long gown, Jessie assumes a seated position of honor and Kalani that of an attendant, similar to how Hawaiian attendants were imaged in photographs watching over and protecting their ali'i (chief).[100]

Another portrait taken around the same time in the settlement complicates the normative hierarchal relationship of patient and caregiver/attendant. In this portrait, two women flank a seated Kalani Joseph Kaena and place their hands on his body (figure 53) The two women, Jessie Kaena and Malaea Hakalau, were unrelated patients who did not know each other prior to exile. Kaena and Hakalau hailed from different islands and were exiled in different years. Kaena was sent from Hanamaulu, Kaua'i, in 1903, and Hakalau from Pu'uhale, O'ahu, in 1904.[101] Standing above Kalani, the women position themselves as more than patients, but as agents of care for Kalani. Physicians had excoriated kōkua for their willingness to touch and be touched by loathsome patients, but Jessie's hand on her husband's shoulder reveals how kōkua welcomed the touch of patients. In contrast, the girls and women staged in the photographs of Bishop Home do not touch each other, nor do the Sisters touch the girls (figures 47–49). We do not and cannot know the domestic triangulation of Kalani, Jessie, and Malaea, but in this photographic setting patients and kōkua performed relationships of mutual care and interdependence.

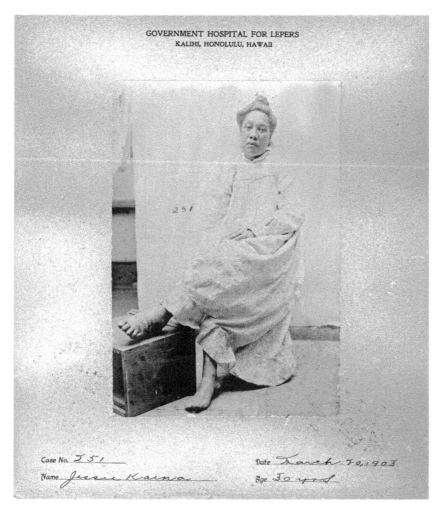

GOVERNMENT HOSPITAL FOR LEPERS
KALIHI, HONOLULU, HAWAII

251

Case No. 251

Date March 70, 1903

Name Jessie Kaina

Age 30 yrd

FIGURE 51. Clinical photograph of Jessie Kaena. Kalihi Hospital case 251, March 20, 1903, thirty years. Hawai'i State Archives.

Why and how did settlement patients and kōkua dress their bodies elaborately and present themselves in such portraits? Answering this question brings us back to the deep materiality of laundry in these photographs. The best current evidence about these portraits' provenance is that they may have been shot by Father Joseph Julliotte between 1901 and 1907. Julliotte did not leave manuscript records, so we know little today about the conditions under which these photographs were shot and developed; he did not leave specific dates for these portrait of Kaena, or for that matter, the portrait he may have taken of Alice and Hattie (figure 45).

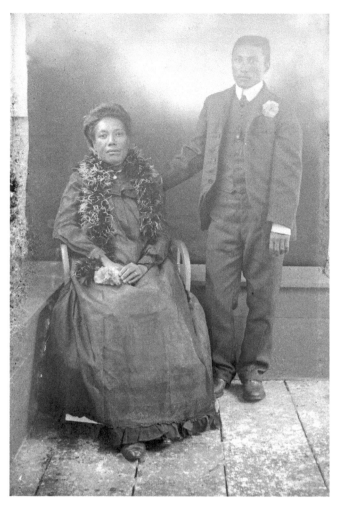

FIGURE 52. Jessie Kaena and her husband Kalani Joseph Kaena. Kalaupapa, Molokai settlement, ca. 1905. Photograph may have been taken by Father Joseph Julliotte of Congregation of the Sacred Hearts. SG 358, Congregation of the Sacred Hearts of Jesus and Mary U.S.A Province.

Although taken by a priest, the photographs appear to have been co-produced with active participation from the subjects within. For across the majority of these approximately eight hundred images, patients and kōkua dressed themselves in their very finest—hats, gloves, lei (garlands made of feathers, flowers, or foliage), three-piece suits, pocket watches, and cummerbunds. How and why did they do so?

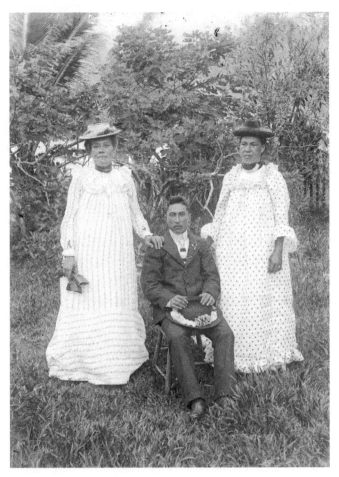

FIGURE 53. Left to right: Jessie Kaena, Kalani Joseph Kaena, Malaea Hakalau. Kalaupapa, Molokai settlement, ca. 1905. Photograph may have been taken by Father Joseph Julliotte of Congregation of the Sacred Hearts. SG 154, Congregation of the Sacred Hearts of Jesus and Mary U.S.A Province.

While discrepant and discredited relationships of care were often invisible in or achieved outside of official state documents like marriage certificates, clinical records, or kōkua permits, Jessie and Malaea chose to be imaged as chosen kin flanking Kalani. Wearing hats encircled with lei hulu (feather garlands) and high-collared, voluminous gowns cut from similar patterned cloth, the two women assert their relatedness and affinity through this photographic medium. Jessie, Kalani, and Malaea importantly project non-heterosexual (and possibly non-monogamous) domesticity apart from an authoritative religious-sanitary order. Their arrangement, while captured with the technological expertise of a French Catholic father, is neither situated in a group home nor anchored in the care of missionaries.

Exiled patients and their non-leprous kin were wards and prisoners of the Board of Health, as we have seen. How much they could eat and drink, how often their houses were to be whitewashed, how loud they could be at night, where they could plant crops, the partners with whom they lived, had sex, or raised children—these and many other aspects of their social and material existence were regulated and monitored by medical and religious authorities. However, clothing was one arena, albeit a circumscribed one, in which patient-inmates could exercise some measure of choice, autonomy, and self-expression within a colonial sanitizing regime. Many adopted hybrid idioms of indigenized Victorian fashion—the missionary-inspired calico gowns paired with feather lei, for instance, as their limited circumstances would permit.

Even when the face became disorganized and unrecognizable because of the progress of the illness, one's clothing could be neatly pressed, conveying that one was surviving and receiving care. Contemporaneous Hawaiian women, some who almost certainly had kin imprisoned at the leprosy settlement, exercised political prerogatives and autonomy over their bodies in the form of fashionable gowns, hats, and jewelry. As they toured Europe and North America, women hula performers laboring on performance circuits outside of the Hawaiian colony adopted modern fashion in ways that worked counter to U.S. empire-building.[102]

The prospect of social engagement with kin also may have prompted people to participate in portraiture. Beyond the dictates of Western religious and medical hygiene, patients invested in immaculate modes of self-presentation that communicated their survival, wellness, and continued sociality to loved ones outside of the medical settlement. There are strong clues suggesting patients intended to send these portraits to their relations. In a modality that might be called *refracted portraiture,* people pose with photographs of loved ones in order to refract the first set of images back to intended viewers. These refracted portraits display images back to anticipated viewers within a new frame.

In one such refracted portrait, a man poses with two cabinet cards attached to his clothing—one card pinned to his chest, and another tucked in his belt (figure 54). Although it is not possible to identify the subjects of the two cabinet cards, they appear to be of five or six young children taken in a studio setting. They may have been the man's own children. If so, the man's

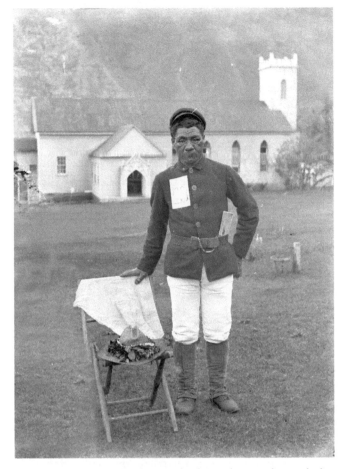

FIGURE 54. Unknown subject with cabinet photographs attached to his chest and belt. Kalawao, Molokai, ca. 1905. Photograph may have been taken by Father Joseph Julliotte of Congregation of the Sacred Hearts. SG 050, Congregation of the Sacred Hearts of Jesus and Mary U.S.A Province.

current state and his relationship with the children are represented simultaneously within the new photographic frame. These refracted portraits attempt to achieve reunification across temporal and geographic divides.[103]

Knowing it was unlikely they would get to see their loved ones face to face, patients show themselves wearing and looking their best. Jessie and Malaea both died within a decade of their photograph—Jessie in 1913 and Malaea in 1915—a reminder of how many incarcerated subjects enjoyed only a brief window in which to display themselves dressed for the camera. After separation, family members expressed concern about whether their exiled kin were receiving adequate clothing and sent money for clothing to the settlement. While there are few extant records of these exchanges, a Hawaiian man named John wrote to a Catholic interlocutor in 1889 to ask whether his grandson Kapeliela had clothes; in the same letter, John also passed along his aloha (love) to the child.[104]

Sitting for these social portraits required clean and pristine clothing for patients like Hattie, Alice, Jessie, and Malaea (figures 45 and 53). Returning to this chapter's opening photograph of Hattie and Alice, I underscore that portraits like these were made possible through laundry and affective caregiving by kōkua. The clothing worn in hundreds of these portraits is remarkably impeccable, spotless, and unsoiled. Prior to the installation of steam laundry facilities in July 1907, clothing had to have been washed and hung by hand by able-bodied kōkua.[105] Jessie had a disabled foot and Malaea disabled hands and feet, for example, and Hattie and Alice's hands were also likely in pain, preventing them from washing their own clothes.

You may also notice that Hattie, Alice, Kahawaii, Jessie, and Malaea (figures 45, 50, 53) wear light-colored or white dresses. Exiled leprosy patients adopted white clothing in subversive ways that flouted anxious Victorian hygienic rituals imposed by medico-religious authorities. On the one hand, white clothing donned for communion rituals symbolized virginal purity and godly dedication (figure 48). Yet white clothes also assert relationships beyond those forged through the church and clinic: they were people connected through touch and skin.

White gowns would have been a particularly challenging and intrepid sartorial selection for these women. Molokai is known as an island that radiates heat; tight collars and long sleeves are impractical choices, for most people cannot help but sweat in the hot weather. The settlements had unpaved dirt roads, and long dresses risked getting tamped and stained with dirt and mud. Beyond perspiration and dirt, there were other dire pragmatic considerations. In untreated cases of leprosy, ulcerated skin could bleed profusely and seep through clothes, making light-colored clothing unfeasible. Henry Nalaielua, a Kanaka ʻŌiwi patient incarcerated a few decades later, remarked that only with the late-1940s introduction of sulfone antibiotics, which healed open sores and ulcers, were patients able to wear white clothes.[106]

Yet these portraits were taken forty years prior to effective antibiotic treatments. Poised before the camera, women whose skin might have swelled in unpredictable sores dare to don light clothing, cleaned and prepared by kōkua and chosen kin. Even if their skin might bleed under or through the cloth, they stand confidently, assured they will have aloha and affective care bestowed upon them. They wear this care on their skin in the form of laundered cloth.

Perhaps these portraits present a version of the "fearless intimacy" between kōkua and patients decried by the settler physician Nathaniel Emerson, though not the troubling spoilage of "clean" bodies by disabled leprous bodies he so dreaded. It was fearless intimacy that emboldened these subjects—patients and kōkua alike—to stage themselves as connected bodies worthy of giving and receiving care.

FOUR

————

Dreaming in Pictures

QUEER KINSHIP AND SUBALTERN FAMILY ALBUMS

IN A PHOTOGRAPH NESTLED WITHIN an album of similar images, a group of young men fish and cook on an island coast. It is a familiar scene of youthful frivolity, a casual snapshot perhaps taken during a camping expedition (figure 55). Despite the ordinariness of this scene, the teenage boys and men were inmates at the Molokai leprosy settlement in the 1930s. The cliffs visible in the background of the photograph provide a clue to their location. These mountainous walls were part of the settlement's purposeful design, creating a natural prison.

The compiler of this album, a Chinese immigrant descendant from Oʻahu named Franklin Mark, was one of an estimated eight thousand people exiled to Molokai settlement between 1866 and 1969. In this chapter, I consider snapshots taken and collected by patients incarcerated at Hawaiʻi leprosy institutions. In vernacular photography albums, what I call life-making albums, exiled patients forged visions of uncertain futures in the face of death, removal, and instability.

While leprosy colonies have been analyzed as necropolitical institutions that established quarantine regimes and social death in the age of empire, the Hawaiʻi leprosy system did more than consign death—it produced and rearranged life.[1] Far more than a graveyard, the settlement was a life-making institution where babies were born, children resettled, and kinship reconstructed, albeit in ways that did not align with heteronormative, able-bodied expectations of biological time and kinship.

Thousands of babies may have been born to patients in the Molokai settlement during its hundred-year history, with the majority of "non-leprous children" removed and placed in institutional homes or foster households.[2] At the same time, leprous children and young people also were detained and incarcer-

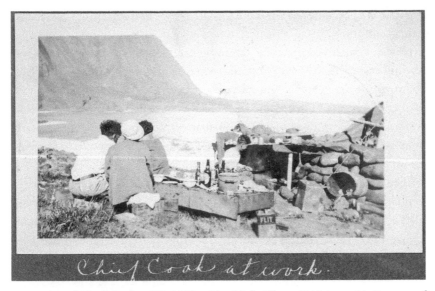

Chief Cook at work.

FIGURE 55. "Chief Cook at Work." Franklin Mark Album, KALA-00366. Courtesy of Kalaupapa National Historical Park.

ated at Kalihi Hospital and Molokai settlement, often unaccompanied by caregivers or family members. In the absence of a cure, many of these young people believed they could die within a few years of arriving. However, some lived long lives with chronic illness and disabilities, especially after the introduction of effective antibiotics in the 1940s. To their own surprise, some lived long enough to be granted temporary medical release beginning in the 1950s.

The Molokai settlement might be called a "queer time and place," to borrow from Jack Halberstam. Queerness here does not refer to homosexual practices or identities, but a differential temporality.[3] Exiled people did not and could not expect normative linear experiences paced by childhood, adulthood, marriage, reproduction, and death. Their lives were marked by the "strange temporalities" of queer and "crip time": the unpredictable possibilities of lives unfolding with senescence and disablement.[4] Medical exile produced a peculiar temporality outside of curative time. The state required a person to live out a death sentence with other incarcerated people, but the executioner would be the patient's own unpredictable body. There were no effective treatments or cures, nor anticipation of release. People lived with various degrees of disability. Rather than biological children, the relief of a cure, or reunification with loved ones, they focused on companionship in the present moment with delight and despair. One patient recalled passing the time drinking because she felt there was little hope and few things to occupy their attention.[5]

How did patients' vernacular albums visualize intimate forms of recognition and companionship as queer and crip time unfolded? I approach these albums as subaltern archives of queer kinship. I propose looking at them as subaltern archives of kin because their creators were pressing, however tentatively, against dominant views of normative biological kinship, somatic progress, and longevity. They and their subjects were not expected to survive, nor were these private albums intended to enter public view.

Their albums are unremarkable and hardly stand out, saturated with familiar and ordinary scenes of friendship, pleasure, and leisure perhaps typical of other twentieth-century albums. Yet their *anti-spectacular* ordinariness is what makes these albums extraordinary—they presented quiet intimacies between people who were usually spectacularized as abominations, pitiful wards, and curiosities in medical and religious media. As a subaltern "archive of feelings" or "affective archive," the albums stirred subjugated knowledges, subjectivities, and feelings as their creators were being observed, treated, and managed within leprosy institutions.[6] While gesturing toward normative forms of claiming and connection, the photographs expressed ambiguous and negative affects of loss and loneliness that were left unresolved.

What contradictory dreams, desires, and affective relations did these albums bring to life? How did albums and scrapbooks reimagine a-filial caregiving and queer kinship outside of normative biological or curative time? How did patient-photographers represent extraordinary bodies and disabilities as ordinary sights in public and private spaces? Why and how men readily took up the "kin work" of domestic photography—aesthetic, affective, and archival practices associated with women's labor and which strengthen kinship ties—are questions I also pursue.[7]

INTRODUCING THE FAMILY ALBUMS

While medical photographs spectacularized disabled leprosy patients in what I have termed an archive of skin, some men incarcerated in carceral-medical institutions eagerly adopted photography and created vernacular albums. These men had access to cameras and the time to pursue photography as a leisure activity during decades-long detention and exile from the 1930s to the 1990s, unlike most institutionalized and incarcerated people in the twentieth century.[8]

The photograph collections of three men reveal visual kinship practices undertaken at Kalihi Hospital and the Kalaupapa, Molokai, settlement. These vernacular albums were created by Franklin Mark, a second-generation Chinese descendant detained at Kalihi in 1927 and exiled to Kalaupapa in 1929, and Edward Kato, a second-generation Japanese man detained at Kalihi in 1936 and exiled to Kalaupapa in 1938. The third was a second-generation Portuguese man who entered Kalihi Hospital in 1920 and was exiled in 1924. I refer to this man by the pseudonym Alfred Costa. All three were born in Hawai'i as children of immigrant settlers. Their incarceration at the settlement overlapped, but I have no evidence they collaborated on their photographic work. I have chosen them because of their collections' depth and aesthetic practices, as well as biographical information that can be corroborated via textual records. However, there are at least five other patient collections that display similar impulses from the 1920s to 1990s.

Although women patients assembled albums, photographic collections by men appear to have been more extensive in the mid-twentieth century, with images numbering in the thousands. This may be because women patients chose other aesthetic avenues like painting, sewing, or crocheting during exile, but it also because fewer women than men were exiled overall. More men contracted leprosy than women, and the ratio of leprosy cases was as high as two men to one woman in Hawai'i.[9]

In the 1920s and 1930s, when these young men entered the settlement, there were approximately four to five hundred patient-inmates living at Kalaupapa, a small village carved out and governed by the Hawai'i territorial Board of Health. With the U.S. incorporation of Hawai'i as a territory in 1900, immigration from East Asia, the Philippines, Portugal, and Puerto Rico supplied the territory's agricultural plantation labor force. Kalaupapa's exiled patients, in turn, became a more heterogeneous mix of Indigenous and non-Indigenous peoples. During this period, Kānaka 'Ōiwi (Native Hawaiians) remained the largest group of patients, while Filipino, Japanese, Portuguese, Chinese, and Korean settlers and their descendants, as well as many who were of mixed racial backgrounds, also were exiled to Kalaupapa.[10]

Leprosy patients were subject to numerous laws, rules, and restrictions. For example, they could marry another patient, vote, and receive visitors, but they could not leave the settlement without permission, touch visitors, or raise their own children. A diagnosis of leprosy also gave a non-leprous spouse legal grounds to seek uncontested divorce.[11] Men and women did marry and sometimes more than once during medical incarceration, but it was not unusual for some men to remain longtime bachelors or to live much of their adulthood as divorced men or unpartnered widowers. Prior to the introduction of sulfone antibiotics here in 1946, people died abruptly, leaving lovers and partners abandoned. Social life at the Kalaupapa settlement was not organized around the conventional rhythms of normative reproduction; reproduction was socially risky and exposed people to further loss. Some men and women were sterilized, chose not to reproduce, or were forced to surrender their children to the Board of Health.[12]

In a patient community where bachelors and non-reproductivity were commonplace, photographic albums enabled bachelors to pursue aspirational and affective kinship through homosocial or non-normative relationships that did not conform to cycles of heteroreproduction. I do not use "bachelor" in the strict sense of men who never married, nor do I rely on this term as a euphemism for closeted queer men. Bachelorhood instead references unpartnered men without children who had strong social attachments with other men in the public and private spaces of the settlement and beyond. Bachelorhood thus encompassed unmarried men, widowers, and those temporarily or permanently unpartnered. It is inclusive of men who were unpartnered for a range of reasons often tied to leprosy diagnoses: they chose not to marry, were denied opportunities to live with those they loved, lost partners to the illness, or were separated from non-leprous partners. Marriages and relationships dissolved for many reasons, but exile and death hastened the dissolution of relationships.

PHOTOGRAPHY AND LEPROSY INCARCERATION

How widespread was the practice of photography at leprosy detention facilities? Leprosy suspects were photographed after medical examinations. As elaborated in chapter 2, thousands of clinical photographs were shot at Kalihi Hospital, the islands' central medical detention facility, beginning at least as early as 1895. These were filed in an archive of leprosy patients and suspects. Concurrently, the Board of Health regulated the use of cameras in its leprosy facilities. Beginning in 1893, the Hawai'i BOH required special permission for camera use in leprosy institutions, because they did not want unauthorized images of disfigured patients circulating to the general public. The board even considered confiscating the photographic equipment of patient-residents and physicians in the settlement.

Scientific purposes constituted the sole justification for cameras. Resident physicians and medical missionaries have been able to take photographs in the settlement since the early 1900s, even creating darkrooms on-site. While occasionally relying on patient privacy as justification for its restrictions, BOH officials at the turn of the century were primarily motivated by the need to protect Hawai'i's plantation and tourist economy from associations with uncontrollable racialized disease and disability.

Today photography remains restricted in Kalaupapa settlement by the Hawai'i State Department of Health.[13] Tourists, workers, and visitors may not take photographs of patients or their private residences. This curtailed access to photographic technology evokes the board's historic oscillation between optimism about photography as a diagnostic tool and ambivalence toward the circulation of patient images.

More importantly, patients taking up photography were well aware of how they were being captured by the medical camera, for each had been photographed upon entry to Kalihi Hospital. At least one patient, a Chinese immigrant named Jack Sing Kong, who was sent to Kalaupapa in 1919, was hired and paid to take clinical photographs of patients, euphemistically referred to as "progress photos." Sing Kong worked for resident medical superintendent William J. Goodhue.[14] Some patients thus may have had access to the clinic's darkroom or learned photography while working for physicians; others may have learned photography prior to exile. Although medical photographs often marked a violent break in the lives of incarcerated patients, some adopted photography enthusiastically.

Disparities in racialized class status, political authority, and education between Asian and Portuguese settlers and Native Hawaiian patients may have influenced access to and interest in photographic technology and equipment during medical exile. Of the twentieth-century photographs currently known from Kalaupapa settlement, more appear to have been produced by non-Native Hawaiians who were Portuguese, Chinese, Japanese, and Filipino. However, it would be premature to conclude that Native Hawaiian and Native Pacific Islander patients did not pursue photography or that their collections were less extensive. Kanaka 'Ōiwi patients and those with multiracial genealogies did take and collect photographs during their institutionalization, and I speculate that more of these will be found and enter public view in the future.[15]

By the 1930s, when Franklin Mark, Alfred Costa, and Edward Kato were crafting their albums, the board appears to have allowed patients increased access to their own camera equipment. Kato's friend and contemporary Kenso

Seki owned a portable consumer camera in the 1950s and sent his film to drugstore photo labs in Honolulu to be developed into prints.[16] Photographer-patients at Kalaupapa did not leave robust written records or manuscript collections that could tell us more firsthand about their photography.[17] What were their aesthetic pursuits, social lives, and affective relations during exile?

"SAINT MARK" AND HIS PICNIC GANG

Franklin Mark, who was also known as Frank Mark, was Chinese and a resident of Kalihi, Honolulu, on the island of Oʻahu. While little is known about his life and biography, Mark was born in Honolulu in 1905 and baptized En Fan Mark at St. Andrew's Cathedral, an Episcopal church. His parents were immigrants from China. He was sent to Kalihi Hospital in January 1927 as a leprosy suspect and spent two and a half years there in medical detention. He was twenty-three years old when he was sent to Kalaupapa in August 1929.[18] Mark died in 1977 and is buried in the settlement's Protestant cemetery. He took photographs of friends, visitors, and staff, compiling them in an album spanning about a decade from the early 1930s to ca. 1940. To my knowledge, his album is one of the two earliest extant albums created by incarcerated patients there.

It is clear from this album that Mark had an exuberant sense of humor. He exercised a ready command of colloquial English and laced his album with playful handwritten commentary. In contrast to medical images taken of leprosy patients in public health and government reports, Mark's informal photographs of friends and loved ones were of a profoundly different, private register of production and circulation. Mark produced them for himself and perhaps his closest group of friends, who were also exiled youth. Mark's photographs do not offer the dignity or repose of a classically composed family portrait, nor was he interested in producing an edifying "wholesome" normative body as an antidote to the individual surveillance shot. In a self-portrait, one of several in which he grinned for the camera, Mark adopts the irreverent ascription of "Saint Mark" who was "Busting the Lense [sic]" (figure 56).

Calling himself "Saint Mark" was a boldly impudent posture to adopt in a community where medical philanthropy performed by Catholic priests and sisters had been bedrock since the late 1800s. Contemporaneous with Mark's album was the 1936 exhumation of the body of Damien de Veuster, from his crypt in Kalawao, Molokai. Father Damien had contracted leprosy and died

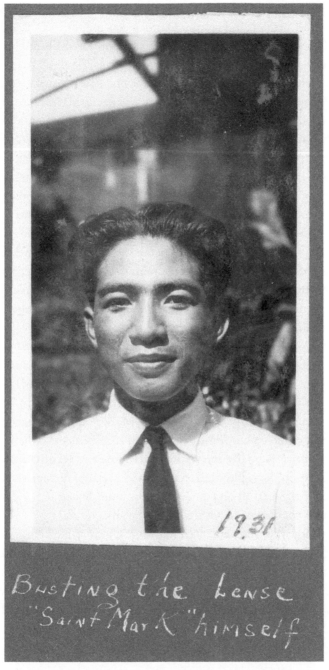

FIGURE 56. "Busting the Lense, 'Saint Mark' himself." Franklin
Mark, ca. 1931. Franklin Mark Album, KALA-00366. Courtesy of
Kalaupapa National Historical Park.

while caring for patients at Kalawao in 1889. Famed worldwide for his devotion to outcast patients in Hawai'i, Damien was reinterred in Belgium as a martyr of the Catholic Church, but Mark's inscription deliberately inverted the hierarchy of priest and ward by naming himself a "Saint."

Formed during their shared incarceration, Mark's social circle also eschewed hierarchies and leaders. He called this group his "picnic gang." This loosely a-filial, mixed-gender gang of friends, potential romantic partners, and peers did not have parents, grandparents, matrons, social workers, or doctors regularly monitoring them. Nor did they have children. While a youth gang can refer to a group that commits violent or delinquent acts, Mark's "gang" was hardly menacing. His friends shared common interests and circumstances, as in the American saying, "The gang's all here."

Mark's vision of exile features his gang of young men and women enjoying relative freedom outside institutional spaces and surveillance. Kalaupapa settlement is a village with about a dozen small roads, but the rugged undeveloped lands, coasts, and ocean of the wider peninsula offered ample opportunities for Mark and his gang to roam and explore. The settlement that first meant exile and separation afforded some freedom and mobility. In Mark's album, we see young men camping, fishing, and cooking on the peninsular coasts, as in figure 55. They cavort, drink beer, and enjoy picnics away from the constraints of the hospital or church, institutions that exerted much control over patients and demanded compliance from individual bodies and souls. For example, on page 38 of the album, Mark's caption noted the hospital dispensary unit—a key feature of medical confinement—where patients received treatments and had sores bandaged (figure 57). Yet on the same page, in two images to the right, Mark represented sociality outside the hospital with men sitting around and enjoying a cookout. Social life and affective kinship were not contained within hospital walls.

Some youth who were sentenced felt more comfortable being with their peers in the settlement than with family members outside. Edwin Lelepali was not part of Frank Mark's picnic gang, but a later group that was moved to the settlement in 1942 after the bombing of Pearl Harbor. Fourteen-year-old Lelepali was one of about fifteen other juveniles sent in a group of thirty-eight patients, and he spent the rest of his life in Kalaupapa. Lelepali described in Pidgin (Hawai'i Creole) how he came to prefer living with his new friends:

> At first I had [grudges]. I was a little kid. Who would like live away from your family? No way you like leave your family. Who would like come this kine

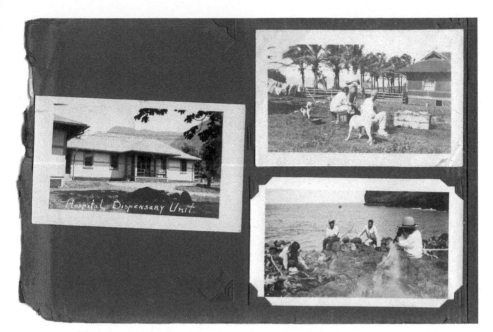

FIGURE 57. "Hospital Dispensary Unit." Franklin Mark Album, KALA-00366. Courtesy of Kalaupapa National Historical Park.

place where they tell you this the last place you going come, you going die? Make you scared. I never like come this place for nothing. I tell you, I hate this place. Take me away from my family. But when I came over here and stayed over here only two months, now, not even my father can pull me away from here. Honest! Never! He said, "You know, time for you come home." I said, "Papa, if you no mind, I like stay Kalaupapa." He said, "Why you like stay the kine place, Ed?" I said, "I can go fishing, I can go hunting, I get car for go ride, I get horse for go ride. The things that us kids like enjoy, that's what we have over here today. Honolulu, I no more that, Papa." [19]

Lelepali relished the festive socializing of his adolescence: "The joy that we had. Oh, I tell you. We just know when to get together to enjoy each other's company. That's the main thing, we enjoy everybody's company." [20]

LONELY TOGETHER

At first view, Mark's album seems almost incidentally situated in a leprosy institution, displaying the generic desires and pursuits of similarly energetic

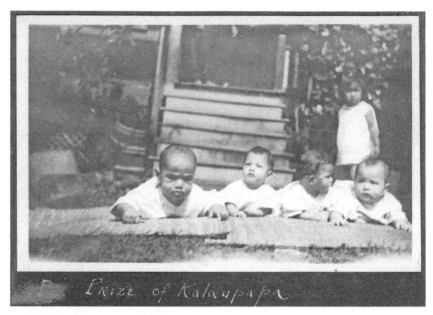

Prize of Kalaupapa

FIGURE 58. "Prize of Kalaupapa." Franklin Mark Album, KALA-00366. Courtesy of Kalaupapa National Historical Park.

heterosexual men. Mark positioned himself as a potential suitor, expressing oblique romantic longings for a young woman who appears throughout the album as Mark's muse. At times it is easy to forget that Mark likely did not expect to live longer than a few years, while he carefully pasted his photographs into albums and captioned them.

Yet the carceral conditions and unpredictable mortality that constrained Mark and his peers are never far away in the album. In his photograph of babies from the Kalaupapa nursery, Mark signaled social disruption, longing, and ambivalent desires for filial kinship. Captioned "Prize of Kalaupapa," the photo shows four infants on their stomachs and a toddler standing in the background (figure 58). These children born to patients were indeed the prize and pride of the settlement, though they were not permitted to grow up there.

Mark shot this photograph in the early 1930s, a period of child removal and increased placement into foster care. After birth in the maternity hospital, these "clean" babies would have been removed from their parents and placed behind glass as part of a sanitary regime. The babies would be cared for by nurses and never handled by patients. At around age one, the babies would be removed from the settlement. They were sent to relatives, institutional homes for children, or foster care outside of Molokai.[21] Naming the babies as a "prize" designated their preciousness and hope for the future of the Kalaupapa community. The snapshot expresses an aspirational, though temporary, filial connection with these infants. Mark knew they would be sent away not long after, and indeed the babies do not reappear in his album.

Mark married a woman named Clara Kelehiwa in 1933, and perhaps they contemplated having children.[22] Others in Mark's "picnic gang" endured separations from their partners and children. A friend of Mark's, who appears as one of the vibrant bachelors in the album, had been separated from his wife when he was removed to Kalaupapa.[23] Other friends may have had their own children, only to have them taken from their care.

This "prize" photograph anticipates the interruption and loss of filial connection.[24] Mark, like these infants' parents, would not have been able to touch the babies when he knelt on the grass to shoot this photograph at close range. The infants are near, but still untouchable, in this photograph's proximate staging. One of the few occasions a parent could be reunited with a non-leprous child was upon burial together in a settlement gravesite. This may have been the near future of one infant in this photograph, as their surname matches one on a 1932 gravesite next to their father.[25]

Mark's album may be interpreted as queer in terms of its production of non-normative affect, communicating non-normative feelings "in relationship to normative family formations."[26] Being lonely is one of these queer feelings that suffuse the album as Mark envisions an uncertain present and future. The intertextual assembly of inscriptions and photographs guide the interpretation of being lonely while together. The captions call attention to isolation and separation, even as snapshots of groups represent sociality. A shot of two small islands—the rock islets of Mōkapu and ʻŌkala—photographed from shore, for example, is inscribed, "Two Lonely Islands."[27] Next to it, on the same page, a photograph of smiling figures atop horses reads, "Mother & Dad gone to Heaven."

Death and loss are interspersed in the album's lively scenes. Mark self-consciously indicated friends who had died and "gone to Heaven."[28] Mark also relayed the presence of death via a snapshot of a marble and granite works store that displayed a neat row of headstone samples in a verisimilitudinous cemetery. At least two of the Mark's intimates in the album—a man named "Lookie" and a young woman named Mary Ann Apana—died not long after Mark had photographed them or while Mark was compiling the album.[29] Mark would outlive many friends during his five decades of medical incarceration.

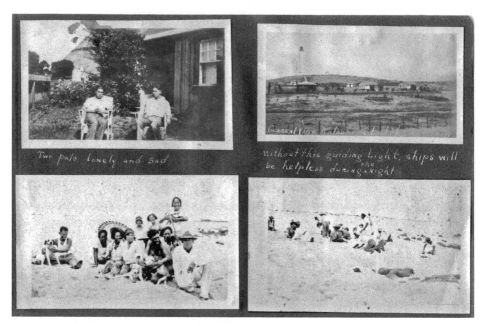

FIGURE 59. Top left: "Two pals, lonely and sad." Top right: Kalaupapa lighthouse. Franklin Mark Album, KALA-00366. Courtesy of Kalaupapa National Historical Park.

Mark's visions mingled joyous occasions with mourning for relationships aborted or unfulfilled. On another album page, men and women laugh on a beach in a scene bathed in light, and the overexposure of the photo also increases this effect (figure 59). However, above on the same page, Mark sits next to another male friend in a far darker and moodier scene. The young men wear light-colored shirts, but the composition is dense with shadowy detail—a dark wood-paneled house and foliage frames them. Both wear sober expressions; Mark inscribed, "Two pals, lonely and sad." Mark further accented this theme of darkness and light, loss and joy with a photograph of the Kalaupapa lighthouse perched above the coast. As he wrote, "Without this guiding light, ships will be helpless during the night," Mark may have identified with the motif of a ship far out at sea searching for light. Sitting on their chairs "lonely and sad," Mark and his companion appear to bear their wounds side by side, taking comfort in their proximity. After Mark died in 1977, an unknown friend remembered Mark and their sustaining relationship. At the head of Mark's tombstone at Kalaupapa, a grave marker reads, "To my best friend, Franklin Mark."

A contemporary of Frank Mark crafted a different kind of photographic scrapbook. A man whom I'll call Alfred Costa was born on the island of Hawai'i in 1903. The son of Portuguese immigrants, Costa was raised in Honolulu until he was detained as a leprosy suspect at Kalihi Hospital at the age of sixteen. He spent a few years at Kalihi and was sent to Kalaupapa in 1923. He married a Hawaiian woman, another patient in the settlement, in 1925, when they were about twenty-one and twenty-two years old.[30] He appears to have been widowed within a few years of their marriage. When he died at the settlement at the age of eighty-four, Costa had lived more than sixty years at Kalaupapa.

Costa's images appear to date from the 1920s during or perhaps prior to this period of detention. I am not able to show Costa's photographs, as the executor of his estate has not allowed me or others to publish them. To my knowledge, this executor has not published the images, so they exist as a vital, but elusive, presence between the archives, the written page, and my own recollection. In lieu of reproducing his photographs, I am describing them textually, leaving a blank frame on the page to signify the images' absent presence. The empty frame also anticipates a possible future when the photographs may be seen in relationship to this discussion.

Costa's eight-page album is a photographic collage that relied on a vernacular scrapbooking aesthetic: he hand-cut snapshots into smaller geometric shapes and pasted them into uneven rows. Each shape contains an individual or groups of people—they appear to be cherished intimates from his pre- and post-exilic life. The pages are rhythmically patterned: rectangles, hearts, and rough ovals accrue into scenes generously populated with men, women, and children. On one of these pages, he constructed four rough rows with seven to nine shapes pasted next to each other.[31] The rough-cut edges and the stickiness of the glue call attention to its maker's efforts and aesthetic process.

Katrina Hof has made this observation about the meaning of scrapbooking: "On a small scale, life can be cropped, embellished and laid out according to available resources, aesthetic preferences and as contemplations on the past and dreams for the future."[32] Piecing together communities disrupted by medical segregation, Costa's scrapbook achieved such a dream-like state. It reassembled social relations that were frayed or perhaps never co-existed in the same space or time. Thus, we might approach this family album as a

Blank frame representing Alfred Costa's scrapbook, ca. 1925.

chronotope, a "fictional fusion of time and space," as photography scholar Martha Langford conceptualizes.[33]

A photographic chronotope might animate the imagined hierarchy of a family, yet Costa's album resisted the linearity and legibility of the family tree. A viewer cannot discern who's related to whom, who is a leprosy patient and who is not. Costa provided no labels, names, or captions; it is an organized presentation, but non-hierarchical and disorderly in sociological, ethnographic, clinical, and genealogical senses. The people he assembled in his collection may or may not be related at all to Costa or to one another. Some of his loved ones were patients, or perhaps not at all.

Why is it significant that Costa conjured *proximal kinship* instead of lineal kinship in his album? In order to answer this, I turn briefly to the lineal kinship conventions that mapped, visualized, and categorized leprous people. During medical intakes, family and family ties were criminalized. Those who were "clean" were separated from those who were "unclean." The logic of colonial medical segregation sought to distinguish and separate clean and "dirty," infected and salvageable. The Kalihi Hospital examiner asked: "Any relative or intimate association past or present leprous?" The preprinted clinical form included space for the examiner to notate conditions of the leprosy suspect's mother and father. Admitting to having kin at Molokai or sharing food with a relative or lover who was leprous precipitated suspicion and potential incarceration during a health inspection.

Relying on family trees and kinship diagrams, physicians scrutinized filial relations for clues to the etiology and spread of leprosy. A kinship chart of the imprisoned Hawaiian man Keanu (discussed in chapter 1), for example, was published in the 1890 *Occidental Medical Times* along with lithographs of his kin, to demonstrate the family's susceptibility to leprosy. The family tree was a useful visual system for scientists to map racialized sexuality, kinship, and disease. In clinical records, interviews, and health reports throughout the twentieth century, the intimate relationships of inmates were charted and analyzed.[34] These approaches continued apace in the 1930s, with the Board of Health championing a social scientific method of using a patient's life histories to trace the path of infection.[35]

Costa's scrapbook subverted these biological and bacteriological "family trees." His collage avoided solid trunks of descent and distinct branches of relationships. While sanitary regimes sought to establish hierarchies of clean/unclean, doctor/patient, white/non-white, and infected/uninfected, the scrapbook disregarded these, offering an unrestrained mingling of these hygienic and social categories. Snapshots of people of different ages, genders, and generations are nestled together closely on the page, and it is not possible to tell who is a patient, doctor, friend, or kin or how they might be related. His album is "messy" in a sociological sense, eluding and refusing to explain who is imaged and how they might be related. There is no "key" to unlock the mystery of the album; it is for an intimate audience, perhaps only for Costa himself.[36]

Some were people with whom Costa likely was detained at Kalihi Hospital, the Honolulu leprosy compound. Death, removal, and instability marked the social worlds of leprosy institutionalization. While family albums always require imaginative labor to craft stable visions of the past or future, Costa's exilic album required even more creative labor when he perhaps did not occupy the same space with these loved ones or had to re-imagine himself into relation with them years later. As Langford has suggested, "A photographic album formed in a crucible of instability may by intent seem more normal than any other family album, and its vision will be just as enduring."[37] Costa cut and pasted shots of people whom he was no longer allowed to touch or accompany, constructing a chronotope from paper.

This fictional chronotope of Costa's is intertwined with queer and crip temporality. Queer studies scholars Jack Halberstam, Kathryn Bond Stockton, and others have analyzed how queer subjects grow sideways, not up.[38] They resist ascending heterosexual modes of development. Amplifying the interrelated status of queerness and disability, Alison Kafer contends queer time is already imbued with disability, as people with disabilities are written out of normative, curative time and biological reproduction.[39] Moving through queer and crip time, Costa's subjects favor lateral, parallel, or a-filial relationality in the non-nuclear family album: they do not grow older, nor do they move toward maturation, able-bodied development, or heterosexual parenting.

Costa's subjects fit together imperfectly on the page and in a shared chronotope. This differential relationship to time is suggested by another anti-development practice among some of Costa's peers at the settlement. Some elderly patients, both male and female, collected stuffed animals through the late twentieth century and 2000s. They amassed large collections, decorating their homes, porches, and vehicles with assemblages of soft toys. While a practice usually associated with young children, patients well into their eighties treasured their stuffed toys, with some jealously coveting each other's special friends.[40] As evoked by Costa's scrapbook pages, the lifeworlds of exiled people cannot be measured by conventional adult milestones.

BACHELOR INTIMACIES

The images of photographer-patient Edward (Ed) Kato span the black-and-white era to color 35 mm film. Kato's first album begins the same decade as Costa's and Mark's, but his albums continue into the 1990s. The son of Japanese immigrants, Edward Yutaka Kato was born in rural Nāhiku, Hāna, on the island of Maui in 1917. He appears to have been the only one in his immediate family of two brothers and four sisters to contract leprosy. Kato entered Kalihi Hospital as a leprosy patient in 1936 at the age of nineteen. Two years later, in 1938, he was exiled to Molokai at the age of twenty-one. Kato died in Kalaupapa in 1998, after sixty years of residence.[41]

Kato represents a cohort of patients who were incarcerated when no cure was available, but whose lives changed after the introduction of sulfone antibiotics in the 1940s. Those who took these new sulfone drugs experienced the healing of ulcers, improved vision, reduction of skin nodules, and the elimination of leprosy bacilli.[42] Drugs improved patients' quality of life, but it also shifted their carceral status and their own sense of time. William Malo, a Hawaiian contemporary of Kato's at Kalaupapa settlement, explained the improved health and longer life expectancy that accompanied sulfone drug therapy: "We were able to discard crutches and did not have as many bandages. Our sores were all healed so we were able to participate in a lot of sports programs. There was volleyball, softball, hunting and fishing, all of which became possible because the drugs were introduced."[43]

After securing a series of negative bacteriological tests for the leprosy bacilli over several years, patients could obtain temporary medical release to travel or work outside of Kalaupapa. After securing temporary release in 1956, Kato embraced the pleasures of mass tourism. He maintained Kalaupapa as his home, but toured places like Hong Kong, Thailand, Japan, France, Las Vegas, Mexico, New Zealand, and New York City with other patients. Men and women patients, Native Hawaiian and non-Native islanders alike, also traveled during this period, though perhaps not as widely as Kato.

This period of temporary medical release in the late 1950s overlaps with Asian American and Japanese American political ascendancy in the territory and Hawai'i statehood in 1959. The admission of the territory of Hawai'i as the fiftieth state of the union sedimented ongoing American violations of Kanaka 'Ōiwi sovereignty and the expropriation of Native lands for military and tourist development.[44] While there is little evidence that Kato and Asian settler patients in the settlement sympathized with statehood and its promise of liberal racial inclusion, Asian Americans and Japanese Americans in Hawai'i generally supported statehood efforts, becoming "beneficiaries of U.S. settler colonialism," albeit in uneven ways.[45] Kato's keen participation in middle-class commercial tourism and photographic technologies suggests that he and some non-Hawaiian patients were better positioned to take advantage of consumer capital and opportunities in their new roles as released patients in the fiftieth state, as Native Hawaiians remained structurally subordinate in their homeland and Hawai'i's "militourist complex" expanded in the wake of U.S. statehood.[46]

Although relationships to land, capital, and opportunity structured Native, immigrant, and settler communities differently, the most palpable racial divide in the leprosy settlement was between white and non-white patients. This division was built into the carceral-medical environment and produced through preferential policies. Haole (white foreigner) patients, while the fewest in number, were accorded better accommodations and treatment by the territorial BOH and its agents. The McVeigh Home had been built and set aside exclusively for "white" patients to segregate them from Hawaiian and Asian patients in the early 1900s. This facility eventually housed so few white male patients that it began to allow Asian and Native Hawaiian men entry by the early 1920s.[47] Kato entered McVeigh Home as an

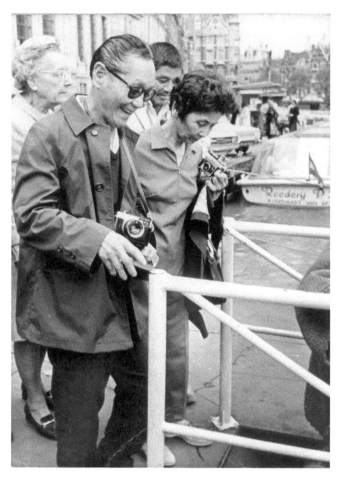

FIGURE 60. Edward Kato with his camera on European tour, ca. 1972. Page 26-1, Edward Kato Album 14. Edward Kato Papers, KALA 17804. Courtesy of Kalaupapa National Historical Park.

unmarried man in 1938, joining a multiracial male cohort of men from different hometowns.

Kato appeared in some photographs with a point-and-shoot 35 mm camera around his neck (figure 60). He took photographs after entering Kalihi Hospital and the McVeigh Home, suggesting he was already familiar with photography in his youth. Kato had received formal schooling prior to medical detention at the age of nineteen, while some of his Hawaiian peers were too young or impoverished to attend school. At least one Hawaiian boy could not read when he was sent to Kalaupapa. Kato was a more educated and older arrival relative to juvenile patients. He worked at Kalaupapa Store, which supplied groceries and staples to patient-residents, eventually becoming store manager. This employment provided Kato with a modest but steady income with which to pursue his artistic and civic interests, including painting, photography, and leadership positions in the settlement's Japanese Society and Lions Club. When he retired from the store, Kato likely had no dependents; he would have received a state pension and social security income that stretched enough to allow him to travel outside Kalaupapa.

The twenty albums in Kato's extensive collection are centered mostly on male friends and travel. Throughout the albums, Kato serves as a folksy tour guide, adopting the jocular rhetoric and presentation of a slide show narrator. Kato's earliest album begins with his segregation in Kalihi Hospital, where he was detained as a leprosy suspect in 1936. Homosocial bonding is figured in this album through an image of Kato draping his arm around a younger Hawaiian boy. Kato captioned this photograph "Pete and Me, 1936" (figure 61). As the albums continue through the 1990s, they are populated with bachelors, patients, and non-patients alike who pursue homosocial hobbies like sports and fishing.

One might miss altogether that Ed Kato had been married to another Kalaupapa patient, Roselyn Makae Wong. They married in 1943 and lived together for a period of time in the settlement, though they do not seem to have been living together for some years prior to her death. Roselyn (aka "Rose") makes but a few brief appearances in Kato's albums, most prominently in a posthumous image: a snapshot of her gravestone. Rose died at the National Leprosarium in Carville, Louisiana, in August 1973 while receiving medical treatment there. Patients from Hawaiʻi traveled to Carville to obtain more advanced surgery and therapy.

In 1977, Kato made a visit to the Carville leprosarium. Reunions at Carville presented occasions for partying, singing, and socializing for men and women patients from Hawaiʻi, as captured by Kato's camera and that of other patients. However, these scenes were interrupted by a snapshot of Rose's gravestone flanked by a contingent of Hawaiʻi friends (figure 62). The shot of Rose's grave at the Carville leprosarium cemetery appears immediately prior to tourist shots of the New Orleans Superdome and the nearby Mississippi River. There are no images of Ed Kato's domestic co-habitation with Rose in the albums that overlap with the period of their marriage; perhaps they had separated. Rose remains a mysterious and fleeting presence. While it is not possible to draw a conclusion about their marital status, images of homosocial bachelor relationships freight Kato's albums.

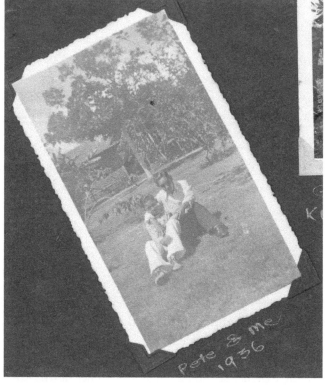

FIGURE 61. "Pete and Me, 1936." Page 32-1, Edward Kato Album 6.
Edward Kato Papers, KALA 17804. Courtesy of Kalaupapa National
Historical Park.

As Franklin Mark relied on "picnic gang" to describe his youthful social
circle in the 1930s, Kato similarly referred to his various companions as "gangs,"
and these taglines are interwoven through different albums. Kato's "Aloha
Gang," for instance, was a mixed-gender group of patients and non-patients
who took a tour to Europe in 1972. He called the younger men with whom he
fished and drank beer the "Haleiwa Gang." These men appear to have visited
occasionally from Haleʻiwa, Oʻahu, for outdoor sporting and relaxation, suggesting the primacy of Kato's friendships with male contemporaries.[48]

One fellow male patient, Kenso Seki, surfaces in the albums as a primary
member of Kato's bachelor gang. Seki was about seven years older than Kato,
and a child of Japanese immigrants to Hawaiʻi. Seki had been detained in his
early teens at Kalihi Hospital and arrived in the settlement in 1928. Kato and
Seki had been born on different islands and did not know each other before

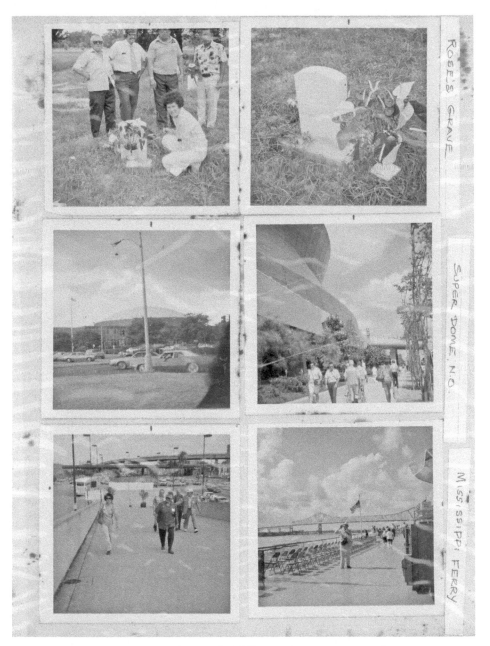

FIGURE 62. Top Row: "Rose's Grave." Middle Row: "Super Dome, N.O." Bottom Row: "Mississippi Ferry." Page 3-1, Edward Kato Album 2, 1977. Edward Kato Papers, KALA 17804. Courtesy of Kalaupapa National Historical Park.

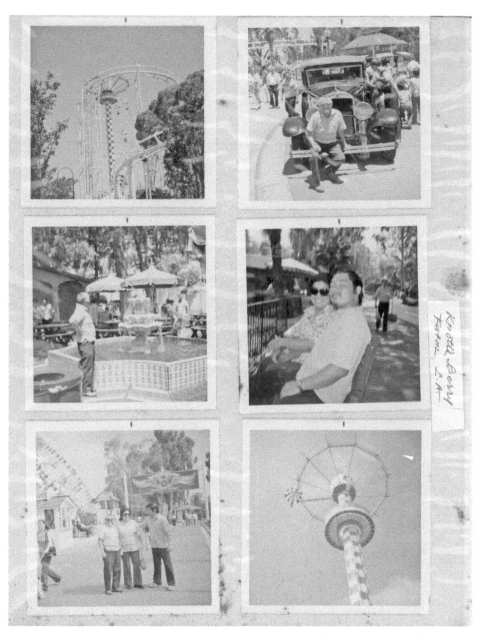

FIGURE 63. Knott's Berry Farm. Page 14-1, Edward Kato Album 2, 1977. Edward Kato Papers, KALA 17804. Courtesy of Kalaupapa National Historical Park.

Molokai, but they became good friends and regular traveling companions. Kato humorously captioned a two-shot of himself and Kenso Seki from 1987 as "The Odd Couple"; their relationship becomes ubiquitous in scenes of homosocial companionship.[49]

Seki also made the trip to Carville, Louisiana, in 1977 and appears regularly in this album. After visiting Roselyn's grave at Carville, Kato and Seki visited Southern California and Seattle, among many other stops. Their a-filial kinship emerges in a series of quotidian interior scenes and tourist shots: Seki flopped on a hotel bed, in front of Hoover Dam, and at Knott's Berry Farm (figure 63).

The homosocial relationships visible in Kato's albums did not emerge naturally; in many ways, these gendered worlds were already dictated by the settlement's infrastructure and its medical and religious practices. Like jails and prisons, Kalihi Hospital and Molokai settlement practiced gender regulation from the late nineteenth century. The BOH and medical missionaries sought to separate men and women in order to discourage reproduction, limit heterosexual contact, and instill moral standards, especially in unmarried girls and women, as explained in chapter 3.[50]

After arriving at Molokai, patients were assigned to one of four group homes organized by gender and located in different sections of the peninsula: Bishop Home for "unprotected" girls and unmarried young women, which was run by the Franciscan Sisters; Baldwin Home for younger boys, which was run by Catholic lay brothers; and the McVeigh and Bay View Homes for unmarried men. As Kato's residence, McVeigh Home, housed mostly young men, it is not surprising that his early photographs of Kalaupapa sociality feature men and boys in gender-segregated groups.

MOTHER'S DAY WITHOUT CHILDREN

The conventional family album performs a deeply conservative function by enshrining idealized domesticity and eugenical heteropatriarchal order, photography scholars have demonstrated.[51] Kato's albums, however, unfold according to different rhythms: there are almost no weddings, formal studio portraits, or babies. Ed and Roselyn Kato, like many married people in Kalaupapa, either did not have children or had been separated from biological children. Children are largely absent in the schema of his albums; when they do appear, they are in school or graduation portraits sent to Kato by relatives or friends. His albums of Kalaupapa life are instead usually paced and structured by the occasion of outside visitors arriving at and departing from the settlement's airstrip, organized by sights to be photographed and compiled by Kato.

Yet Kato also appears to aspire to the coherent organization of the hetero-patriarchal family album in a series of more formal snapshots he took on Mother's Day in 1956 (figure 64). Kato was serving as an officer of the Kalaupapa chapter of the Lions Club, an international community service organization. On Mother's Day, Lions Club members, all of whom were male patients at the time, ceremoniously hand flower bouquets to women residents to honor mothers in the settlement. The flower ritual captured by Kato is fraught with contradictory sentiments and structures. On the one hand, the photographs seem to stage normative families based on biological reproduction and patriarchal chivalry. The tug of idealized patriarchy can be felt in Kato's choreography of men temporarily playing heteronormative roles as fathers, husbands, economic providers, and heads of households.

Perhaps all family albums are unfinished and fraught fictions that require one not to peer beyond the surface of the image or outside its frame.[52] Kato's Mother's Day snapshots generate a fragile and unstable vision of family by

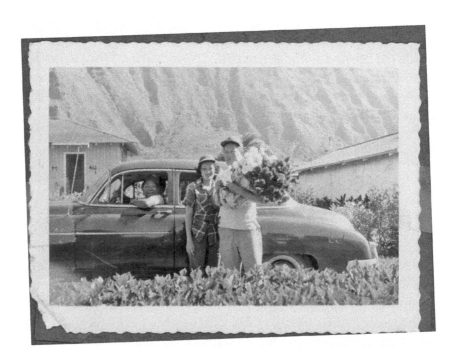

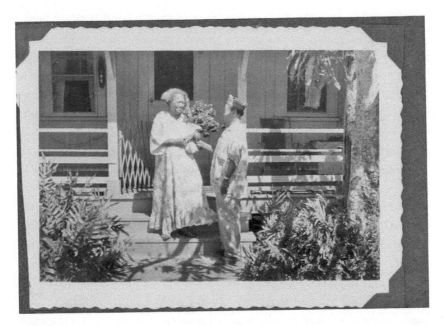

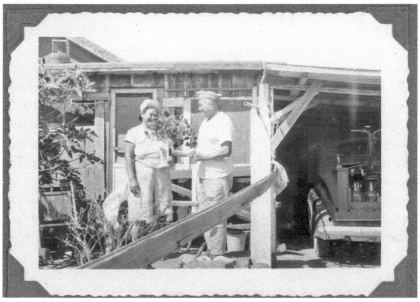

FIGURE 64. "Lions Presenting Flowers—Mother's Day '56." Page 19-1, Edward Kato Album 6. Edward Kato Papers, KALA 17804. Courtesy of Kalaupapa National Historical Park.

unwittingly invoking the absence of children. There are no children commemorating their mothers in these holiday scenarios; these women were mothers who no longer had access to their children. Thus, the snapshots project confidence in family, while straining to smooth over wrinkles in a scene that lacks constitutive elements of heteronormative families. In a community without children or ancestral forebears, Kato's task of staging biological family was far more difficult.

A more careful examination suggests how Kato's photographic practices contributed to social reproduction and unsettled a gendered division of labor. The all-male Lions Club strengthened homosocial lateral relationships between men, but also promoted a-filial kinship ties across households and heterosexual partnerships. Through the staging and production of these Mother's Day scenes, Kato initiated the maintenance and celebration of kinship ties, what Micaela di Leonardo has called "the work of kinship"[53]— affective and material labor performed by women to maintain a sense of family. Kato and fellow Lions Club officers cooked communal meals and gathered flowers for women who were not their mothers or wives—the work of kinship that many men normally do not perform.

Although Mother's Day may have been an exceptional holiday—as the one day of the year when women got to be first in line—Kato's photography of the occasion is representative of his broader contributions to affective kinship work that we see across decades of his album compilations. Kato photographed groups of close intimates, developed and selected snapshots, and then assembled them into scrapbooks and albums. Captioning each photograph with the names of men and women was further demonstration and dissemination of Kato's "kin knowledge."[54] His photographs recognize and account for relationships between non-biological kin, constituting a form of caregiving. Even as these Mother's Day images invoke normative patriarchal hierarchies, the labor Kato performed in his albums signals his eager participation in non-biological caregiving and a-filial kin work.

"THERE'S NOTHING LEFT FOR ME"

When Ed Kato died of cancer in 1998 at the age of eighty, his obituaries and remembrances described him as an "outstanding citizen" and someone "generous to a fault." One of his sisters said, "He was not the kind of person to talk about regrets." A Catholic priest recalled Kato smiling "even with his

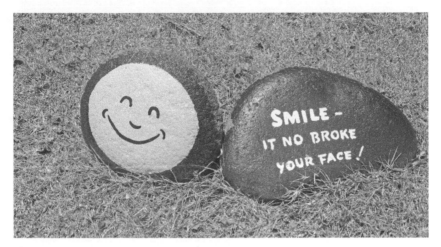

FIGURE 65. "Smile—It No Broke Your Face!" Smile rocks painted by Edward Kato, Kalaupapa settlement. Photograph by author.

own pains and hurts."[55] His public and private artistic work appears to hew to this self-presentation of cheery and selfless generosity. Kato painted rocks emblazoned with smiley faces and installed them in the settlement. These "smile rocks" exhorted residents and visitors alike, "Smile—It No Broke Your Face!" (figure 65). Kato filled his albums with similarly bright scenes of social gatherings, parties, and fishing expeditions. He and his subjects flash wide smiles for the camera, and he narrated these encounters with humorous and breezy captions like, "The beer was cold . . . the friendship warm," and "I'll be back, You can bet on it!"[56] So what might we make of one particular album whose title he carefully inscribed in cursive, "There's Nothing Left for Me . . . Among My Souvenirs" (figure 66)?

Although Kato does not make this explicit attribution, "Among My Souvenirs" is the name of a popular song recorded from the late 1920s to the 1970s by female and male singers alike. Its subject croons a sentimental reflection on the past: "There's nothing left for me/Of the days that used to be/They're just a memory among my souvenirs." As the ballad unfolds, the singer reveals his/her souvenirs as letters "sad and blue," a "photograph or two," a rose, and finally, a "broken heart."

The intertextual framing of snapshots by this song ruptures the optimism of Kato's images and announces a different structure of feeling. This structure of feeling shares something of a kinship with the "backward feelings" described by queer theorist Heather Love as the shame, depression, regret,

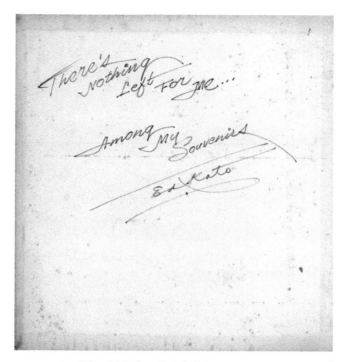

FIGURE 66. "There's Nothing Left for Me . . . Among My Souvenirs."
Inside cover, Edward Kato Album 13. Edward Kato Papers, KALA
17804. Courtesy of Kalaupapa National Historical Park.

and suffering prompted by social trauma. Spanning a two-year period in the
Kalaupapa settlement from December 1974 to December 1976, this "souvenir" album is largely a series of snapshots of visitors arriving, touring, and
leaving the settlement. Some appear to be friends, relatives, staff, and Catholic
pilgrims on tours. Kato poses in a few shots, smiling in front of identifiable
Kalawao and Kalaupapa landmarks. A recurring setting is the Kalaupapa
Airport and its white picket fence, where visitors are bedecked with floral lei
upon their departure. "Airport Farewell, Dec. 1974" reads one caption of an
older Hawaiian couple waiting to board the plane (figure 67).

Unlike several other albums of Kato's travels as a tourist, this album is
firmly grounded in the settlement. The resident experiences a constant flow
of visitors and enjoyable interactions, but page after page, the visitors leave.
The resident remains behind to experience "backward feelings"—souvenirs
of loneliness, regret, grief, even pain. We are not meant to know why the
album's compiler is left with a broken heart, but the album allows us to sense

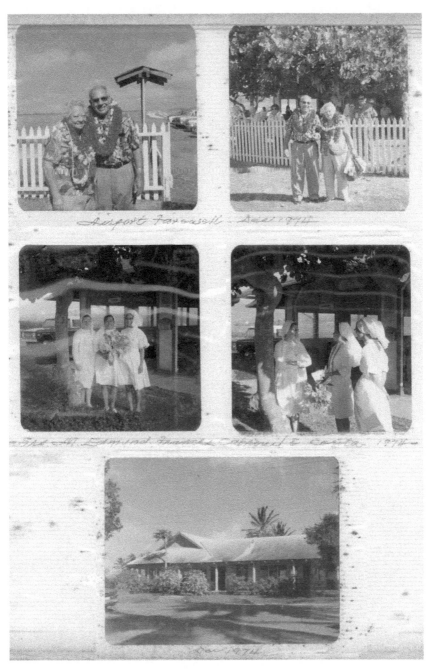

FIGURE 67. Pages 3-1 and 23-1, Edward Kato Album 13. Edward Kato Papers, KALA 17804. Courtesy of Kalaupapa National Historical Park.

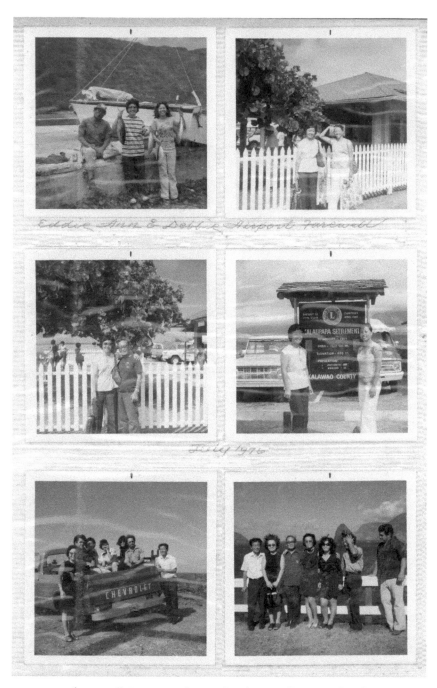

FIGURE 67 (continued). Pages 3-1 and 23-1, Edward Kato Album 13. Edward Kato Papers, KALA 17804. Courtesy of Kalaupapa National Historical Park.

his injuries. We may sit with these "negative affects" without having to rescue him from unresolved feelings.[57] Among the cheerful smiles, unfulfilled longings are also Kato's legacy.

Yet decades after Ed Kato compiled this melancholic souvenir album, it initiated unexpected encounters for new viewers. My graduate student Noah Dolim recognized his own family in Kato's album while reading a draft of this chapter. Dolim, who was raised primarily on Oʻahu, visits ʻohana (family) on topside Molokai frequently. The Hawaiian couple in the upper two farewell snapshots, shown bedecked in red carnation lei, were Elmer A. Wilson and his wife Abigail. Elmer Wilson was Dolim's great-great grandmother's brother. Wilson had been superintendent at Kalaupapa settlement. He was departing Kalaupapa upon retirement in 1974, after having worked in various capacities in the community for over thirty years.

Dolim responded with surprise and wonder at these heretofore unknown scenes of his family. Kato's album took on far less mournful interpretations in our seminar in California, as conversation shifted to our own wider relations in Hawaiʻi: Elmer Wilson's work as a minister in Hālawa Church; Dolim's cousins on topside Molokai; and Wilson's daughter, the singer Iwalani Wilson, who sang as a little girl in a Maui hula troupe, in a story shared with me by an endearing elder. While preoccupied with departures, Kato's album opened possibilities of future reunions across time and space: of astonishing, unforeseen kinship and reminiscences via the images within.

ANIMAL COMPANIONS AND CROSS-SPECIES KINSHIP

Ed Kato's photographs of some of his closest companions go back to the early 1950s. He placed a shot of a puppy named M.J. next to one of M.J. as a full-grown dog (figure 68). Another pet dog is dressed in a T-shirt and sits up on his hind legs. "M.J.," "Johnny," and at least two other of Kato's dogs grow older in snapshots, their ages and antics captured in handwritten captions: "M.J. couple months old," "Johnny and Oios," and "There's a fly on my nose, I've got to move!" Representing far more than pets, non-human kin became a recurring subject of patients' snapshots and paintings in the absence of human children, parents, and other intimate relations. Patients forged intense cross-species and queer kinship with domesticated and feral animals during exile. Whereas conventional family albums unfold onto pages of chil-

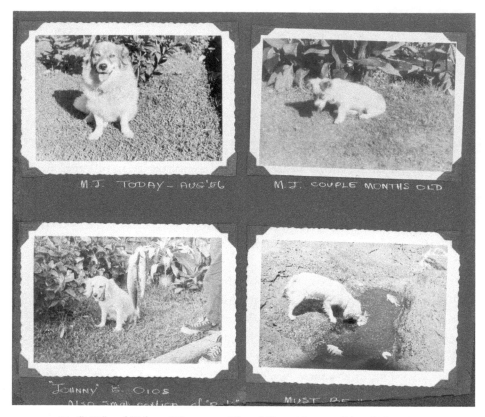

FIGURE 68. "M.J." and "Johnny." Page 22-1, Edward Kato Album 6. Edward Kato Papers, KALA 17804. Courtesy of Kalaupapa National Historical Park.

dren and multi-generational biological kin, exiled people enshrined "companion species" in two-dimensional works: kinship galleries of animals they adopted, fed, and loved.[58]

Physicians and health agents in Hawai'i enforced stringent prohibitions on co-habitation, caregiving, and touch between "clean" and "unclean" people, but did not police relationships between leprosy patients and non-human animals in the history of the settlement. In stark contrast to the removal of children from their care, patients were relatively free to adopt and lavish attention on non-human animals, caring for a range of domesticated, stray, and feral animals. In the early twentieth century, patient-residents chose to pose with their dogs in photographic portraits, as did a man named Naihe Pukai, from Kaua'i (figure 69). This dog may have been Pukai's companion during much recent loss. Pukai's wife died around the time of this portrait.

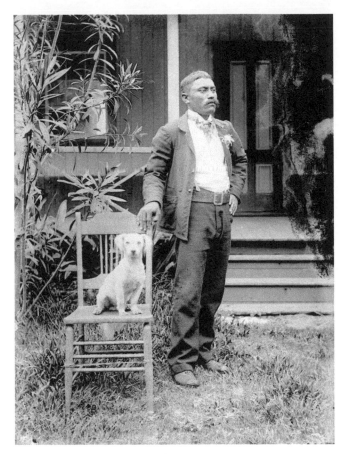

FIGURE 69. Naihe Pukai posing with his dog. Kalaupapa settlement, ca. 1910. Photograph likely taken by a brother or father of the Congregation of the Sacred Hearts. SG 086, Congregation of the Sacred Hearts of Jesus and Mary U.S.A. Province.

Three of their children had been born in the settlement, but one had died as a baby, while two others were taken to Oʻahu group homes for non-leprous children.[59] In the wake of such separations, people of all ages developed intimacy with animal kin, expanding their chosen families to diverse animals.

Kalaupapa patients expressed devotion by preparing special meals, creating portraits of pets, taking them riding in their cars, and making plans to be buried with them. They bestowed names like "Baybie," "Cupcake Akamai," "Candy Bar," and "Baby Pakalana."[60] Dogs and horses accompanied Franklin Mark and his friends on their 1930s adventures on the peninsula. One dog named Luckie Jr. was important enough to Mark to be

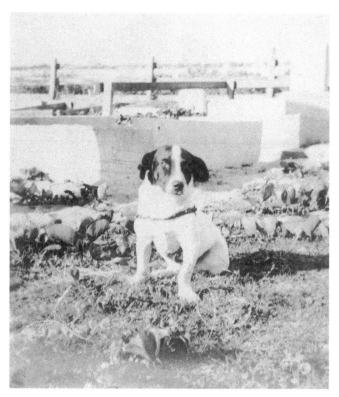

FIGURE 70. "Luckie Jr." Franklin Mark Album, KALA-00366.
Courtesy of Kalaupapa National Historical Park.

featured in solo portraits along the landscape (figure 70). As with Mark's
human "pals," dogs and horses were given individual recognition through
names he inscribed in his album: Luckie, Baybie, and Bunny. Beyond dogs,
cats, and horses, this companionship expanded to non-domesticated animals
like feral pigs and mongooses. However, this companionship did not mean
all animals were sacrosanct kin—patients and kōkua (non-patient workers)
alike took up deer hunting. They also slaughtered pigs, cows, and chickens
for food.

A cross-species intimacy between humans and some non-human species
echoes across institutional and carceral spaces. While prisoners deprived of
human contact in their cells were known to capture insects and mice for
company, Richard Stroud became one of the most famous in the twentieth
century. During a life sentence in solitary confinement at Leavenworth
Penitentiary in Kansas, Stroud found three baby sparrows in a nest in the

prison yard and raised them.[61] He crushed cockroaches and fed them to the sparrows using a toothpick. Stroud's interest in birds flourished, and he eventually published two books on ornithology. Stroud later became the subject of the 1962 film *Birdman of Alcatraz*.

Exiled patients' identification with animals under carceral conditions may have been based on analogous queerness and otherness. Kalaupapa patients' empathy with non-human life appears to have emerged from their awareness of having been marginalized as outcasts or having suffered injuries similar to animal companions. Gertrude "Gertie" Seabury Kaauwai, who became known as the "Cat Lady" of Kalaupapa, used a special knife to cut steak and meats while preparing twice-daily meals for a group of thirty or more cats at her home and others around the settlement.[62] She had names for all of them and could tell them apart. Recalling her painful childhood, Kaauwai said, "My stepmother used to starve me a lot. And I was so hungry, that I used to eat with the pigs. That was my first experience with animals. So when I came here [to Kalaupapa] and I saw cats and rabbits . . . I see a lot of them starving, and then I think back when I was young, that made me feed those animals." As an adult at Kalaupapa, Kaauwai felt unable to control her fertility due to the Catholic prohibition against sterilization. She gave birth to four girls, all of whom were taken from her. Kaauwai described the removal of her children as the "worst separation."[63]

Whereas some patients experienced estrangement from family members, did not have children, or found reunions with human kin fraught, animal companionship did not involve complicated negotiations. Animals anticipated regular feedings and seemingly bestowed affection on human caregivers; nor did they react pejoratively to non-normative human bodies. Edwin Lelepali treated his beloved dogs as surrogates for children and kin he and other patients did not have. Lelepali defied state groundskeepers who initially objected to him digging a plot for his three favorite dogs at Papaloa Cemetery. They told him the cemetery was for human beings, not animals. Lelepali explained to them, "I love those dogs. Those dogs just like our kids inside here. We no more children, see?"[64] When Lelepali died in 2016, these wishes were fulfilled; he was buried at Papaloa next to his many dogs and two predeceased wives.

Another woman patient, Katherine Costales, described the pure delight she received from her daily feedings of feral cats and wild mongooses: "When I see them, it gives me joy and I feel that life is wonderful . . . It brings joy to me, and I go inside and sit on my chair and think, I'm thanking God that all my animals are all being fed. . . . I make my rounds until I get home. And if I don't do it, I feel something is wrong."[65]

Patients pursued various aesthetic modes of capturing their kinship with animals. Elaine Kim Remigio painted large-format oil paintings of her cats and dogs (figure 71).[66] Representing only the animal's face rather than the entire body, her portraits rendered each animal distinct and recognizable. They represented not a type of "dog," or "cat," but an individual animal significant to the painter. In these anthropomorphic paintings, the animals offered a direct gaze and returned the look of the viewer. Other photographic efforts were meant to be seen, shared, and admired by others. Frank Mark photographed his dogs and placed them in an album with captions. Edward Kato placed snapshots of two of his dog companions in gold frames, presumably for display in his home.

If patients expressed ambivalence, if not a certain reserve, toward their own bodies and resisted becoming the object of stares, many enjoyed showing off their animals. They drove their pets in vehicles around the settlement. Dogs, cats, and pigs did not distinguish between people with "spoiled" and unspoiled bodies; similarly, exiled patients did not prize particular animals for their artful perfection.[67] A "poi dog" is a Hawai'i colloquialism for a mutt, and in a humorous inversion of the purebred pedigree dog show, the Kalaupapa poi dog contest pointedly celebrated the diversity of animal life. In a 1987 contest, one patient's dog named "Candy Bar" won the best in show trophy.[68] This practice of evaluating and viewing diverse kinds of living bodies also developed within the convention of the family albums.

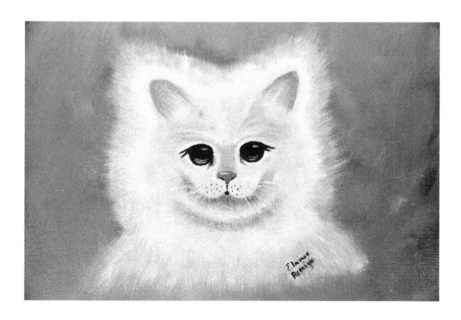

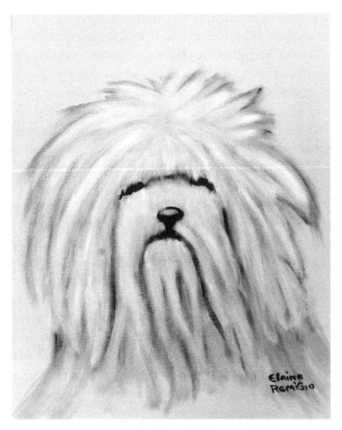

FIGURE 71. Oil paintings by Elaine Kim Remigio. KALA 21589 and KALA 21592. Courtesy of Kalaupapa National Historical Park.

ANTI-SPECTACULAR DISABILITY OPTICS

Young people detained as leprosy patients at Kalihi Hospital in the 1930s and 1940s were usually in the early stages of bacterial infection, displaying mild visual symptoms like raised hypopigmented (light-colored) patches of skin. Some did not appear sick or altered by leprosy.[69] However, once sent to Kalaupapa, they soon encountered "heavy," or more advanced, cases of people whose infections had manifested on their skin, eyes, and soft tissue.[70] Some patients were blind, had amputated limbs, and used wheelchairs, while others breathed through tracheostomy tubes that alleviated airway obstruction.

David Kalani Brede, a Hawaiian contemporary of Ed Kato's, arrived in Kalaupapa in 1942 as a young child. In Pidgin (Hawaiʻi Creole), Brede described the shock he experienced when he first saw patients with advanced cases at Kalaupapa: "When I first come I look the patients. Me, I patient myself, but I scared. You know the patients over here? You know the ear? All bandaged up. You no can see the ear. Was all covered with bandage. And then the thing drain through. You see all the gray or the pus or the blood. Scared, boy! I tell you! Me, I patient myself. That's why I tell plenty guys, even me I patient, I scared."[71] Children and young people entering leprosy institutions engaged in staring at leprous bodies. As a practice of "knowledge gathering," staring allowed new arrivals to make sense of unfamiliar bodies and create meaning out of chaos.[72]

John Kaona, a Hawaiian patient from 'Anini, Kaua'i, who was sentenced as a teenager, recalled how he had to reorient his way of looking when he arrived in the settlement in 1943. John's mother and brother warned him before he was sent to Molokai: "Boy, when you go up there, no *ho'a'a maka*" (Don't stare). "It means I look at you, no stare at you. And then, if they [the patients] talk to you, talk, but don't make fun. Just take them how they are."[73]

Young patients who initially found leprous bodies fascinating, horrifying, and frightening learned to control their staring. Knowing their own bodies were contingent and unstable, younger arrivals did not occupy positions as neutral observers of disability. They could not freely stare or participate in the stigmatization of older and often disabled patients. The question of when and if they themselves would become objects of stares was never far away. After regarding bandaged patients as Other, new residents learned how to manage the transition from Other to self: to see themselves in relation to this community of diverse bodies. John Kaona's visual reorientation therefore offers a significant vernacular theory of *observation without staring*, of accepting different bodies "as they are." What were these evolving observational practices and how did patients deploy them in photography? How did compilers of albums look at and represent diverse, disabled, and non-normative bodies, including their own?

If the clinical mode of looking at leprous bodies was to isolate and spectacularize disability and non-normative parts of the body,[74] disability in patient albums was represented via what I provisionally call the anti-spectacular. The anti-spectacular was produced visually in snapshots through an emphasis on bodily wholeness, the placement of the body in a wide, relational frame, and locating a person within a shared social environment. Catherine Zuromskis has theorized the snapshot as a particular amateur subset of the genre of vernacular photography and a "textbook example of banal conformity."[75] Pulling the snapshot into their own scenes of leisure, photographer-patients relied on the snapshot's cultural coding as "hopelessly ordinary and visually unremarkable" to resignify disabled bodies as anti-spectacular and banal.[76]

Photographer-patients from Kalaupapa avoided the visual disaggregation of bodies into parts. You will not find close-ups of spectacular hands, fingers, or faces in their albums. Instead, patients framed themselves and their bodies in wide shots and in social environments. Kato's tourist albums adopted this relational approach to the whole body. In his albums of a 1977 North American tour, his friend Kenso Seki is shown occupying avenues, a sidewalk, and an amusement park.

This ease in public space emerged over time as Seki and friends ventured out of the settlement. While at first uncomfortable with stares, Seki reflected on his growing nonchalance toward visibility. "We used to go to Honolulu quite a bit. When we went, we saw people turning around to look at us. Gee, that gives you a funny feeling. But then you notice quite a few handicapped people, and it's natural for everybody to look at what they're doing, how they manage. After that, I made up my mind that if they want to look at me, go ahead. Nothing's going to bother me."[77]

Capturing his friend as a fellow tourist, Kato does not focus on Seki's features, but he neither covers up nor exposes Seki's body. As outsiders to the albums, we may notice Seki's face and body appearing somewhat different from those of others, but Kato does not place Seki's face or fingers in tight focus. Nor is Kato concealing his friend's "extraordinary body," to use disability studies scholar Rosemarie Garland Thomson's term for bodies that perform a range of corporeal otherness.[78] Kenso Seki and other disabled patients from Kalaupapa are in plain view, but framed in social settings that made sense of them as tourists, consumers, and friends.

These tourist snapshots represent a mode distinct from the medical model of visualizing disability as pathology, as well as activist models of disability photography. The U.K.-based photographer David Hevey employed direct "camera-to-gaze" in his workshops and photographic portraits of disability in order to move from the victimhood of oppressive "charity advertising." His work aimed to show people's impairment and wounded-ness without representing them as victims. While Kato and Seki were not activist-oriented photographers, they eschewed self-representations as victims, objects of pity, or dignified heroes.[79]

Like any tourist in a wide shot, Seki is placed strategically in relation to a legible landmark to authenticate his presence at that site. The genre of the

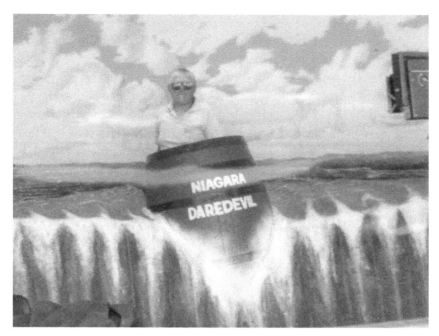

FIGURE 72. Kenso Seki as Niagara Daredevil, ca. 1977. Page 2-1, Kodak Folder, Box 11. Edward Kato Papers, KALA 17804. Courtesy of Kalaupapa National Historical Park.

banal tourist snapshot greatly aids in the de-spectacularization of disability and disease: within the quotidian scenario of leisure, Seki's body becomes relatively minor and incidental. In a spoof shot of a Niagara Falls barrel, Seki steps into a spot in which thousands of other middle-class travelers have been photographed, becoming Every tourist, not a disabled patient (figure 72). Within outdoor wide shots, the monument or natural wonder is meant to be legible as spectacular; Seki is not.

On a forty-five-day tour of Europe in 1972, Kato captured a woman and fellow traveler he called "Lei" in an obligatory en plein air tourist snapshot of Paris (figure 73). Lei stands full length in the foreground with the Eiffel Tower behind her. In two separate photographs placed on the same page, Ed Kato stands in almost the same location for his turn in front of the Eiffel Tower. Kato captioned this shot, "Me, too!" Another man, captioned in Kato's handwriting as "Sidney," also poses for a solo shot in front of the tower. I recognized Lei as a Hawaiian patient from Kalaupapa, while Sidney was a non-patient from Hawai'i, but it would be nearly impossible to parse patients and non-patients from a quick glance.

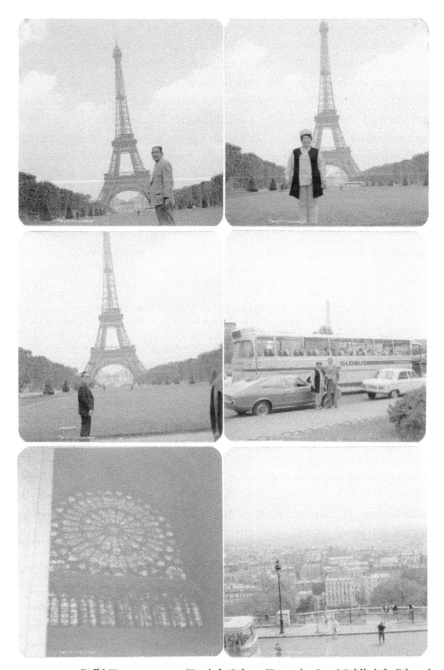

FIGURE 73. Eiffel Tower, ca. 1972. Top left: Sidney. Top right: Lei. Middle left: Edward Kato. Page 18-1, Edward Kato Album 14. Edward Kato Papers, KALA 17804. Courtesy of Kalaupapa National Historical Park.

As Kato photographed his self-described "Aloha Gang" on a tour that mingled patients and non-patients, we do not get a clear look at their bodies; each was dominated by the architectural wonders behind them.[80] The iconic family vacation snapshot, as Zuromskis has discussed, acts as a "passport to cultural normativity," a visual convention linking a family to a broader cultural ritual.[81] The "Aloha Gang" took this tour three years after the leprosy segregation law was terminated in Hawai'i in 1969. Patients had gained the formal and legal right to leave, making the snapshot an especially powerful signifier of cultural belonging and individual persistence for patients like Ed Kato and Lei. The square format of the Eiffel Tower shots repeated and assembled on one page performs both an authenticating and normalizing function: offering evidence of participation in the cultural ritual of tourism and rendering these potentially extraordinary bodies prosaic in public space.

CONCLUSION: ALBUMS ON THE PORCH

Can we call these family albums, or were they merely accidental collections of friends and fellow travelers? They are family albums in their deliberate construction of subjects and the social settings of their reception and sharing. With the abrupt interruption of other sustaining relationships, exiled youth imagined and constructed subjectivities and futures in these life-making albums. These were carefully crafted albums of chosen, a-filial kin: those with whom young people were sentenced to spend their lives in close proximity by happenstance of bacterial infection.

Recall the child Pete who sat protected by Kato in one of Ed Kato's first albums (figure 61). Pete and Ed Kato met at Kalihi Hospital in 1936 as newly diagnosed leprosy suspects. Like the majority of leprosy patients, Pete was Kanaka 'Ōiwi.[82] He was also one of Kalaupapa's lifelong bachelors. In his retirement years, Pete could no longer travel as far as his friends. His legs had been amputated; he used a wheelchair and lived in the Bay View Home, the settlement's dormitory for blind and disabled patients. However, at two p.m. every afternoon in the 1990s, Ed Kato and Kenso Seki joined Pete at Bay View Home to have a beer and "talk story." Ed Kato had no lineal descendants, the normative intended future viewers of family albums, so he did not create these albums for intergenerational transmission. However, I speculate that these albums were like slide shows, compiled to facilitate oral and social performances between kin.[83]

As intimate and sentimental artifacts, snapshots have the power to act as affective touchstones.[84] Carrying these portable albums to the shaded porch, Ed Kato would have been able to include his beloved bachelor gang in far-ranging adventures. In contrast to most heteropatriarchal families, the transmission of social knowledge through Kato's albums was lateral and a-filial. When Kato died in 1998, he had shared over sixty years of exile at Kalaupapa with Pete. These are family albums not only in what and whom they imaged, but how they were used to assemble and maintain kinship between men.

Biological families became frayed during exile, but patients remade and re-imagined kinship in subaltern albums, creating joyful and melancholic visions outside the mandates of curative time. Initially brought together by what was visible on the surface of their skin and what may have been hidden beneath, exiled patients forged affinities that exceeded reproductive, biological, and institutional hierarchies. Skin may have been what brought them to exile, but they chose to organize and represent themselves as chosen kin. These albums offer much for us to learn about the intimate and tender collectivities of people in institutions as they looked beyond skin.

Epilogue

HEALING ENCOUNTERS AT THE SETTLEMENT

IN A PHOTOGRAPH PASTED IN ONE of Edward Kato's albums, young men on the Kalaupapa Dodgers baseball team clasp hands and smile (figure 74). One player drapes his hand over a teammate's shoulder. In this season, the Dodgers won the championship. The Dodgers played against kōkua (non-patient staff) teams and teams from topside Molokai. The winning team photographed here included not only players like Kato, but also their friend Kenso Seki. Seki did not have fingers and did not play on the field, but he took on the vital job of scorekeeping and managing. The group's camaraderie and affection are palpable, and Kato captioned the photo with a ribbing, "Meet the Champs. Tho' They're 'Bums.'" Sports and recreation historically have been an important part of social life at the Molokai settlement since the early twentieth century. Men and women patients participated in organized sports, including volleyball, tennis, and baseball, though not on mixed-gender teams. As these men and women grew older, fewer patients participated in sports.

One of these Kalaupapa Dodger players, Edwin Lelepali, was a lifelong sports aficionado. When he no longer played on the field, Lelepali, or "Pali," as many called him, refereed volleyball games in the settlement. These pickup volleyball matches, played in mixed teams of "callers" (short-term visitors) and staff residents, became known affectionately as "Pali Ball." I met Uncle Pali, by way of an accident, at one of these games at Kalaupapa settlement.

Hawai'i's leprosy segregation law was officially rescinded in 1969, but a small cohort of people who were previously exiled chose to remain at Kalaupapa, the leeward village of the former leprosy settlement. Kalaupapa is no longer the carceral institution it was in the early 1900s, when thousands of patients populated the settlement. Since sulfone antibiotics were introduced

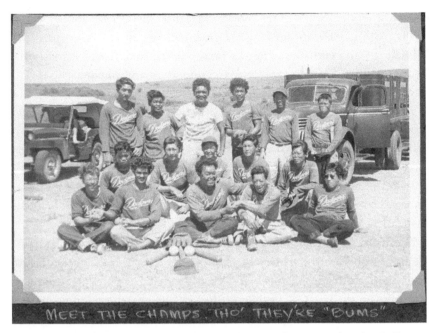

MEET THE CHAMPS THO' THEY'RE "BUMS"

FIGURE 74. "Meet the Champs. Tho' They're 'Bums.'" Kalaupapa Dodgers baseball team, ca. 1952. Edwin Lelepali is far right in middle row. Edward Kato is third from left in middle row. Kenso Seki is far right in third row. Page 18, Edward Kato Album 6. Edward Kato Papers, KALA 17804. Courtesy of Kalaupapa National Historical Park.

in the 1940s, patients have been able to obtain medical release, and enter and exit the community freely.[1] Although they were originally exiled there, Kalaupapa has become their home of choice and a sanctuary. Patients protested and led campaigns to protect Kalaupapa from possible closure and development. With their agitation, Kalaupapa was designated a National Historical Park by the U.S. Congress in 1980 with protection for its natural, cultural, and historical resources.

Kalaupapa National Historical Park (KNHP) manages the peninsula under the National Park Service, while the Hawai'i Department of Health (DOH) provides medical and social care for patients.[2] By state law, former patient-residents are guaranteed lifelong services in Kalaupapa from the DOH for the rest of their natural lives. As of mid-2015, there were nine former Hansen's disease patients and about one hundred state and federal staff residing full-time in Kalaupapa.[3]

"Patient" is the colloquialism preferred by Kalaupapa patients and resident workers. Patients are residents who were exiled under territorial or state law, while resident workers are known today as kokuas.[4] Even though cases of Hansen's disease are no longer active, patients and kokuas alike use "patient" to differentiate the former from workers and short-term visitors. Today, "patient" has a less segregative connotation and implies special elevated and honorific status.

In the spring and summer of 2015, debate about the future of the settlement was in full swing, prompted by public hearings held by the National Park Service (NPS) on management plans for the Makanalua peninsula after there are no patients.[5] Media attention and local chatter focused on diffusion, death, and dissipation of life. For instance, a feature article in the *Atlantic* about the future of Kalaupapa stated the issue plainly, "When the Last Patient Dies."[6]

Yet the focus on impending death misses ongoing struggles to maintain life and a future for the settlement. On research trips to Kalaupapa, I felt it replete with a different kind of biopolitics: life-giving gestures and practices that animate the space. If feelings of shame, fear, regret, and guilt underwrote the past century's experience of separation, what kinds of healing will the future bring? Communal acts of aloha, laughter, song, and reconnection are complementing and supplanting loss. The Kalaupapa hospital, as a necessary anchor of an aging community, provides medical and nursing personnel, hospital beds, I.V.s, heart monitors, dialysis machines, and medicine. However, healing encounters also take place beyond in the natural, social, and built environments of the settlement: at the bar, community halls, visitors' quarters, volleyball court, oceans, beaches, and cemeteries.

In Hawaiian, maʻi is a sickness or the state of being ill. Maʻi became shorthand for disease, as epidemics like smallpox, influenza, and cholera introduced to the islands decimated Kānaka ʻŌiwi in the eighteenth and nineteenth centuries. However, being sick in a Hawaiian context is not limited to the somatic body. Conflicts and breakdowns within the larger social body and environment also cause illness and distress, and these effects are distributed broadly.[7] Maʻi thus encompasses the social disorder and suffering caused by biopolitical responses to leprosy, including intense visual surveillance, stigma, racialized quarantine, exile, incarceration, and removal from loved ones.

As a meditation on history's stake in the present and future, this epilogue considers a series of life-making activities at the contemporary Molokai settlement that decenter the primacy of sight in favor of other sensory modalities and experiences. How are relationships being regenerated in informal and formal practices of community-oriented education, sports, recreation, and grave visitation? If exiled people were made to fear their own bodies and the way others looked at them, what ongoing acts, sounds, and encounters are reintegrating diverse forms of kinship?

SIGNS OF LIFE

The island of Molokai lies less than thirty miles southeast of Oʻahu, the main island, but it is a world apart. Visitors can enter Kalaupapa via one of two routes: by propeller plane or a daunting 3.5-mile hike down from topside Molokai.[8] Those arriving by air then drive into the settlement. On the side of the road, they are greeted by a large red painted sign, "Welcome to Kalaupapa." Those who choose to hike down the steep switchbacks face a far more hostile warning at the trailhead: "Hawaii Law forbids anyone beyond this point without written permit. Violators subject to citation and $500.00 fine." Both signs communicate the settlement's simultaneous warmth and wariness: residents are friendly, but have special cause to be cautious of outsiders. As a former medical institution under the jurisdiction of the NPS and the Hawaiʻi State DOH, Kalaupapa forms a protective cordon around its surviving patient-residents.

The second sign serves as an important reminder of the strict settlement rules established and maintained by the DOH. A maximum of one hundred visitors per day is set. All visitors must be sponsored by a current resident; register at the settlement administration office with a valid form of identification; stay within established settlement boundaries; wear a tag at all times; may not visit more than thirteen calendar days per quarter; may not be under sixteen years of age; and may not take photographs of residents or their private residences.

Officially, the settlement's mayor is the DOH director based on Oʻahu; she or he is the highest-ranking appointed health official. Despite retaining aspects of colonial hierarchical governance, Kalaupapa is, in key ways, a unique, patient-centric community in practice. The DOH settlement administrator consults with the Kalaupapa Patient Advisory Council, and patients exert a strong voice in regulations. Once a prison built to isolate patients, the settlement is, by patient design and intent, meant to keep gawkers from coming in. Access is limited largely because patients want to feel safe and not made the objects of stares. "Callers," or short-term sponsored guests, are marked off from authorized workers and patients functionally and symbolically by a tag that must be visible and clipped to one's clothing during the entire visit.

Yet the signage that I found most revealing of the tone, character, and pitch of Kalaupapa was far more informal and unofficial. It was posted somewhere unexpected: at the patient-owned community bar. The wooden sign at Fuesaina's Bar declared with idiosyncratic spelling and syntax: "Business Hours: We're Open most days about 9 or 10. Occasionally as early as 7, but Some Days as late as 12 or 1. WE'RE CLOSED about 5:30 or 6. Occasionally about 4 or 5, but Sometimes as late as 11 or 12. *Some days or afternoons we aren't here at all and lately I've been here just about all the time, except when I'm someplace else, but I should be here then too." Indeed, I soon discovered the bar might be open for a cold beer, talking story at a shady table, or catching a Wi-Fi signal, though at highly variable hours.

As in this sign, people at Kalaupapa have deployed humor in ways that disrupted the solemnity, sanctimony, and seriousness of its history. At the Lions Club annual Christmas party in 2013, wit, hilarity, and exuberance were prized over piety and pity. The patient-entrepreneur who owned the bar greeted the group heartily, "Aloha 'oukou! I figure after so many years of living here, I gotta learn some Hawaiian." This prompted cheers and applause from the hall. This aunty proceeded to admonish fellow residents to take more risks while decking their homes and yards with new and improved Christmas décor. She passed out small envelopes of cash, finally awarding best in show to the NPS worker who had festooned her front yard with brightly colored "Yo Gabba Gabba" inflatable figures and lights. With incongruous cartoon robot monsters flopping in the Molokai wind, this house also earned my private vote. Having experienced much loss, people here have reason to be somber, but they are also funny and irreverent. Longtime patient Pete (discussed in chapter 4) was known to offer this toast consistently with his afternoon beer: "Here's to those who wish us well. And those that don't can go to hell."[9] People cry, but they may laugh even louder.

LEARNING EXCURSIONS

I called Dr. S. Kalani Brady a few months after I began looking at public records on Hansen's disease (HD) in the Hawai'i archives. During a rare break at his Honolulu clinic, Dr. Brady lent his interpretations of historical

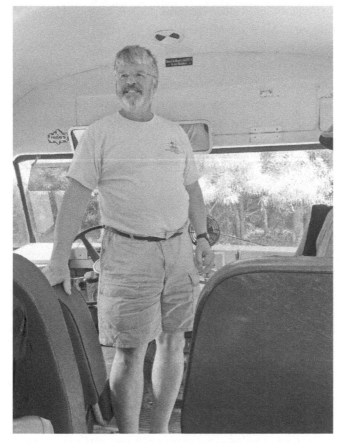

FIGURE 75. Dr. S. Kalani Brady, leading huakaʻi at Kalaupapa, Molokai settlement, July 2015. Photograph by author.

clinical photographs and answered my questions about HD treatment. Brady told me at our first meeting that he thought it would be important for me to experience Kalaupapa firsthand if I were going to pursue this research. He invited me to accompany him and his student interns on a huakaʻi (learning excursion) to the settlement. My first trip there was in 2013.

Dr. Brady is Kalaupapa settlement's physician, one of only a few Native Hawaiian doctors who have treated patients there in its 150-year history.[10] Now over the age of sixty, he has been the lead general practitioner for this group of HD patients since late 2003 (figure 75).[11] These residents, similar to other aging, Native Hawaiian, and Indigenous communities, require medical care for chronic conditions like heart disease, diabetes, and depression. They also may experience additional complications related to Hansen's disease, including amputations and peripheral nerve damage.

As with diabetes patients, HD patients who are cured may have little feeling in their peripheral nervous system and thus are at risk of developing gangrene from sores, infections, and wounds on their feet and hands. A simple activity like cooking on a hot stove can lead to severe burns that they may not notice; such injuries can lead to bone infections and amputations. Even small cuts need to be carefully monitored by nurses to ensure infection does not set in. If a bone does become infected, Brady must oversee the patient's transfer by air to Hale Mōhalu, the wing of Lē'ahi Hospital in Honolulu where patients can receive more intensive care and surgery. In these cases, patients are reluctant to leave their homes at Kalaupapa for the six-week administration of antibiotics.

Though Brady hates to fly, he takes a small propeller plane from Honolulu to Kalaupapa twice a month and stays overnight to treat his patients. At the time of my research, he also saw patients at the Lau Ola Clinic, an outpatient practice in Honolulu affiliated with the University of Hawai'i John A. Burns School of Medicine's Department of Native Hawaiian Health.[12] He also appears, as an unpaid public service, on the *Ask a Doctor* television segment broadcast locally on KHON-2 morning news. For over twenty years, Brady has answered medical questions sent in by viewers. Many of his Kalaupapa patients had seen him on the local news years before he became their physician. Through their TV sets, men and women at Kalaupapa enjoyed ample visual access to their physician in ways earlier generations of leprosy patients had not.

Soon after he began treating patients at Kalaupapa, Brady brought the first group of pre-medical and medical students on huaka'i to the settlement. The trip is voluntary for the students. Meaning "journey" in Hawaiian, huaka'i in contemporary Hawai'i often encompasses service learning at significant historical or spiritual sites, where participants are immersed in Hawaiian values and practices. Huaka'i for members of hālau hula (hula troupes), for instance, visit places honored in their mele (songs) and oli (chants). Regular huaka'i also are made to the island of Kaho'olawe, the district of Wai'anae, and the ancient fishpond Waikalua Loko. Participation is not usually limited to Hawaiians or locals (Hawai'i-born people), but Kānaka 'Ōiwi predominate.[13]

The students in the summer 2015 huaka'i were a mix of undergraduate interns interested in pursuing medicine or medical research as a career, and pharmacy students embarking on clinical rotations. The undergraduate students were interning with one of two summer medicine programs in Honolulu related to medicine: the Department of Native Hawaiian Health at the John A. Burns School of Medicine (JABSOM) and the Queen's Medical Center summer research group. Another small group of graduate students joined from the University of Hawai'i–Hilo Pharmacy School; they had completed their third year Pharm.D coursework and were doing rotations on O'ahu. None of the students received course credit for participating in the huaka'i. Four faculty and clinicians from University of Hawai'i–Mānoa medical and pharmacy schools accompanied the group. Other than one full-time staff coordinator from the Department of Native Hawaiian Health, all were voluntary participants.

The students were students of color or Indigenous students. Most were Kānaka 'Ōiwi, Pacific Islander, Asian American, or multi-racial. They had been raised in Hawai'i, except one Nigerian American born in California who was attending the University of Hawai'i pharmacy school. Of the 'Ōiwi students, three had attended the Kapālama campus of Kamehameha Schools, the private academy for students of Native Hawaiian ancestry. One young woman sported a tattoo on her wrist—"He Hawai'i Au" (I am Hawaiian) adorned with a heart. She professed, "I'm all about being Hawaiian."

Many of the undergraduates were attending elite colleges on the U.S. continent—Dartmouth, Emory, Claremont McKenna, and Amherst—and intended to apply to medical or professional schools after graduation. Brook's* dream was to practice medicine back home in Hawai'i; Mirai* wanted to become a cardiologist; Reese* hoped to become a trauma surgeon; and Michael* wanted to work as an ambulatory care pharmacist. Their summer projects with clinicians included research on health disparities, public health, and racialized access, as well as research focused on Native Hawaiians, Pacific Islanders, and Asian Americans. Harper,* for instance, was analyzing statistical and narrative data on the relationship between historical trauma, substance abuse, and health outcomes for residents of Papakōlea, a Hawaiian homestead on O'ahu.[14]

Despite having been raised and schooled in Hawai'i, they had not had any significant exposure to Kalaupapa settlement or its history before the excursion. They had not recalled learning about Kalaupapa, leprosy, or medical segregation in their public and private high schools. A few days before the trip, Brady gave a short introductory lecture on clinical aspects of HD transmission and treatment. The students also watched a video documentary about settlement life featuring resident-patient interviews.

Students stayed on the outskirts of the Kalaupapa community without specific programmatic goals. They toured significant historical sites and participated in informal social events. Notably, they were not allowed to treat or observe the treatment of patients. Patients and the community understood these annual trips as part of their doctor's larger kuleana (responsibility or mission).

The day before the students' arrival, a patient and I chatted at the bookstore. This man, whom I'll call Uncle Daniel, knew me as part of Dr. Brady's group, and he asked me when Dr. Brady was coming down. I reminded him that Dr. Brady's regular schedule at the hospital might be a little different since he was bringing in his students the next day. Uncle Daniel nodded, "Oh, yeah, the haumāna [students] coming down."[15] What would these haumāna see and experience during their trip to the settlement?

VOLLEYBALL AND RE-CREATION

The students' formal journey to Kalaupapa began on an uncomfortably humid Friday afternoon, with a short half-hour flight from Honolulu to topside Molokai. They rode a bus to the trailhead and then hiked their way down the sheer pali (cliff) to the settlement. Over the next hour, they descended a muddy, precipitous trail; at two thousand feet, the pali are some of the steepest in the world. The journey actually began earlier in the week with food shopping, packing, and the shipping of food and luggage by cargo plane into the settlement. There are no shops or grocery stores for visitors in the settlement, and all the foodstuffs for meals would have to be measured carefully in advance. Their approach by foot allowed them to appreciate how removed the settlement is. They would enter from above as outsiders, with slippery footholds on the trail.

As they carefully walked over three miles of switchbacks, the small town of about fifty homes and structures stretching along the ocean shore came into view from above. This lofty view would be replaced with close-up encounters in the settlement. What and whom did they expect to see? Kalaupapa is the one of the most intentionally undeveloped, rural, and ecologically pristine areas of Hawai'i, largely because it was established and maintained as a separate area in order to isolate patient-residents. Though I had grown up spending time with relatives in rural towns outside of the main island of O'ahu, Kalaupapa is easily the sleepiest Hawai'i village I have experienced. It has no restaurants, schools, or traffic lights.

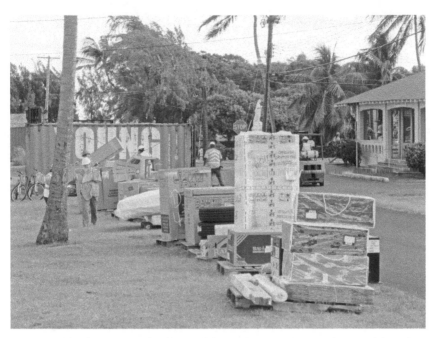

FIGURE 76. Barge Day at Kalaupapa, Molokai settlement, July 2015. Photograph by author.

One does not usually see many people walking or driving in the settlement, but this mid-July weekend was unusually busy and packed with visitors, likely edging close to, if not over, the hundred-person daily maximum set by the DOH. The usual soundscape of the settlement is an occasional car going by or the rattling of a window air conditioner, but the Kalaupapa pier on this Saturday was alive with the chatter and the buzzing of walkie-talkies, forklifts, and trucks.

Barge Day, also known as "Kalaupapa Christmas," is the only time of year patients and residents can ship large and heavy items that sustain the community: washers, cars, beer for the bar, lumber, and carpets.[16] The summer waters are calm enough to enable a large commercial barge to land at the pier. Community members gathered early Saturday morning down by the pier to watch the barge towed in by tugboats. Those who know how to operate forklifts donned hard hats and orange safety vests, off-loading and organizing the pallets and goods on the pier (figure 76). Residents drove over to inspect their pallets and admire their neighbors' haul. However, each year smaller loads come off the barge in a more subdued atmosphere, as the number of residents dwindles. During the previous Barge Day, the street from the pier was blocked off for safety; patients were not allowed to watch from the store, which caused some consternation.

Barge weekend was festive this year, however, with three outside groups visiting: haumāna (students) from Dr. Brady's group; the St. Vianney choir from Oʻahu, holding its annual concert and dinner at St. Francis Catholic Church; and Hoʻolohe Pono, a Protestant fellowship group from Oʻahu holding a service at Kanaʻana Hou Congregational Church. With youth from these groups, surely a volleyball match would be possible?

With patients growing older and dying in the twentieth century, fewer were able to participate in organized sports. Card games and cable television became favored forms of entertainment for older residents. Volleyball seems to have continued longer in the settlement, since unlike baseball it allows a more flexible number of players. Usually on Wednesdays, a pick-up volleyball match begins in the cleared field in front of the bar when enough kokuas and callers can be assembled in the settlement. Cheerleaders sit in the bleachers or under nearby trees in the shade with their dogs.

That Barge Saturday, everyone seemed to know that the longtime patient Edwin Lelepali was pulling the strings for a volleyball match. Sure enough, on our way to Barge Day earlier, Uncle Pali drove his pickup truck next to our school bus. He waved his arm out an open window at Dr. Brady, calling, "Volleyball later?" Dr. Brady smiled and told the students to get ready for a match, but said little more. Around five p.m., after swimming off the pier and purchasing ice cream and soda at Fuesaina's Bar, the twelve students assembled on the bleachers. Uncle Pali was already waiting for the game in the open grass field, sitting in a battered yellow Volkswagen van with no door—his refereeing throne. The van was purposely set next to the net, the best position to see and call plays (figure 77).

I had taken a bad fall the day before on rocky ground outside the village. Dr. Brady taped and wrapped my swollen ankle at Kalaupapa Hospital and scared up a pair of crutches previously used by a patient. When I hobbled onto the volleyball field on crutches, Uncle Pali took notice and felt sorry for me. He waved for me to come sit next to him in the van.

I did not know it then, but I would spend much of the next year in chronic pain, in and out of physical therapy and orthopedic surgery practices in Southern California. Ironically, or perhaps serendipitously, the one surgeon who had encountered my kind of injury and offered a clearer path forward was a foot surgeon who had operated on HD patients with nerve damage and foot wounds. He had done research at the Gillis W. Long Hansen's Disease

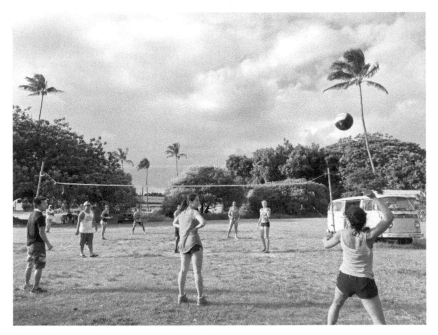

FIGURE 77. Volleyball match. Kalaupapa, Molokai settlement, July 2015. Photograph by author.

Center, formerly the National Leprosarium of the United States, in Louisiana. I eventually had surgery to remove a bone, shorten ligaments, and reconstruct my ankle, not unlike the procedures some people with Hansen's disease or diabetes may undergo, but that day, my injury appeared merely as a bad sprain.

It would have been rude to decline an invitation from an elder, so I settled next to Uncle Pali in his van on a zabuton (flat Japanese cushion). In the open door frame of the van, Pali sat on his faded cushion like an imperious emperor, propped up by his cane. Pali blew the whistle hanging around his neck and called for play to begin: "Game on!" Following each rally, he yelled the score. The set usually ended when one team's score hit eleven points. But when Pali was enjoying a long rally and wanted play to continue, he often ignored his previous score and called a second or third "deuce," prompting the players to reassemble for a new serve. After Pali reversed a score mid-play, one young man grimaced and laughed in front of the van, "That's 'Pali Ball' for you!" Some players pointed to the line to dispute whether a ball was in or out, but Pali's whistle was final. Many joked about the arbitrary calls. After I watched Pali call a couple of sets, he turned to me and said, "OK, you call score." I frequently miscounted, but Uncle Pali patiently confirmed the scoring till I reached eleven points. With relief, I turned the next game back to him.

Volleyball has been enjoyed for decades in the settlement, but instead of patients, new participants are filling these positions. Pali, pictured in the 1952 Dodgers team photograph with many of his friends, was the last surviving patient from that group. Besides patients dying, there is a painful reason why few young people live in the settlement today. Children were believed to be more susceptible to infection, and some data supports that hypothesis today. As part of the leprosy containment policy, patients who had children were forced to send their young children out of the settlement for adoption, fostering, or institutional care. Some patients may have been encouraged to submit to sterilization. Furthermore, to erase the stigma of having been born to leprosy patients, birth records were sealed or altered, making it difficult for adoptees to trace their lineage back to Kalaupapa. Many children grew up not knowing their relationship to the settlement. Parents and children alike lost track of each other.

One DOH official estimated that nearly every woman on Kalaupapa had given birth on the settlement, which could mean thousands of patients had a child or children removed.[17] However, even when reunions do occur, reconnections can become fraught. The respective parties may hold different expectations of intimacy. Adopted children have grown up with different kin, while patients may have reduced or heightened expectations of their relations with grown children. At least one patient couple made a conscious decision not to have children because separation would have been unbearable. Although this issue has been revisited many times, children under the age of sixteen may not come into the settlement by current rules. Children remain a contentious issue in the patient community, with some patient-residents supporting the return of children and others staunchly opposed.[18]

With biological ties strained, lateral social networks formed a vibrant community in the twentieth century. Patients built kinship through baseball teams, fishing clubs, crafting, and social clubs, as explored in chapter 4. On teams like the 1950s Kalaupapa Dodgers, some players became as close as brothers. In today's settlement, impromptu volleyball matches remake these social collectivities and communal spaces of exchange and conviviality between staff, patients, and temporary visitors.

On this afternoon, men and women of diverse abilities, ages, and personal connections to the settlement joined the volleyball match or stopped by to cheer. Benjamin,* a Hawaiian man who works for NPS, is himself a cousin of patients, similar to other kokuas. Benjamin swiveled his baseball cap backward and jumped in to play energetically. No one had to be a good or even minimally competent player, but Pali delighted in each skilled or fumbled pass, spike, and serve. He murmured about one player with college-level experience in our group, "Oh, she's good. Good server!" Pali directed all traffic on the field, blowing his whistle enthusiastically after each set. Pointing to the players, he choreographed new teams.

Between the action, Pali noticed people and animals coming to socialize on the margins of the field. He mentioned to me, "Oh, I like that dog!" about the well-behaved young pit bull someone had brought under the shade. Uncle Pali then reminisced about how he used to have a dog just like that one. "My pets are buried in the graveyard next to my wife," he remarked. As with many patients who cared for feral and adopted animals in the settlement, Pali's eleven dogs were his beloved children. Our conversation about the pit bull was an elliptical exchange about his own losses and connections. What Pali left unspoken, but implied, was his expectation to be buried somewhere in that space with his two deceased wives and pets. Uncle Pali died about six months after this volleyball game, and he was buried in that cemetery spot.

The sun was setting far faster than I had expected, and we knew the match would have to conclude soon. With no street lighting in the settlement, natural light ultimately would determine the duration of play. When the light had almost faded, Pali blew his whistle for the last time and called, "OK, good game. Shake hands." Pali directed the players to demonstrate good sportsmanship. Players from opposing teams high-fived each other in a line, saying, "Good game, good game" to each other. As darkness fell, the socializing finished, and "Pali Ball" was over. Uncle Pali climbed into his pickup truck on the field and drove back to his home about two blocks away.

The next day, when our group exited Catholic services, the haumāna found a piece of paper taped to the door of the school bus. It was a note handwritten on recycled notepaper with the letterhead crossed out. At first, they thought it was a parking ticket. But it was a message from Uncle Pali, who did not pass it to us at the Kanaʻana Hou Protestant Church services we had attended earlier. His note read: "This is not a citation. Thank you all for your participation [in] 'volleyball.' You all brought us so much joy and happiness." The note was signed, "C I Cheat Pali," a jocular reference to his arbitrary scorekeeping. The students read and passed the note on our bus ride back to our cottage. After returning to Oʻahu from the huakaʻi, the Department of Native Hawaiian Health interns pasted Uncle Paliʼs note of appreciation into their summer scrapbook.

Choreographing and participating in volleyball were integral parts of Uncle Paliʼs own health. Pali and other elderly patients are not able to jump or spike the volleyball, but volleyball was Uncle Paliʼs social and somatic compass. When Kekoa* worked as a clerk at Kalaupapa Hospital and became close to several patients, he did his best to schedule Paliʼs visits to Hale Mōhalu clinic on Oʻahu so Pali would not be out of the settlement on Wednesdays. Wednesday was when most of the volleyball matches between residents and callers were held. This scheduling often proved difficult, as the DOH expected Pali and other patients to fly out according to efficient and economical rationales. But Kekoa knew that volleyball made Pali feel the most well, motivating him to get out of bed in the morning. His care and concern for Paliʼs welfare and happiness included seemingly small acts like extra phone calls to reschedule flights and medical appointments.

Such regard for patients blurs established medical boundaries into respect for kūpuna (elders), ancestors, land, ocean, and iwi kūpuna (ancestral bones, where mana, or spiritual power, resides). The bar facing the volleyball field also forged communal life in the settlement (figure 78). It was the only place where people could buy beer, potato chips, and ice cream, or access a public Wi-Fi signal (with a five-dollar purchase).[19] The bar was and continues to be patient-owned. Passed down from patient to patient, it was owned by Mariano Rea in the 1960s, when it was called "Reaʼs Store." Rea was an immigrant from Ilocos Sur, Philippines, who had been exiled to Kalaupapa since 1937. After Rea died in 1994, fellow patient Elaine Kim Remigio bought the business and operated it as "Elaineʼs Place" until 2003. The most recent owner, Gloria Marks, renamed the establishment Fuesainaʼs Bar. "Fuesaina" is Marksʼs Samoan name. When the bar celebrated its tenth year of business in 2013, Marks held a block party with free Happy Hour drinks. The bar was decorated with photographs of Marksʼs late husband, Richard Marks, as well as droll signs. One sign read: "Bar rules: 1) If Youʼre Still Standing, You Need Another Beer."

Before its closing in 2018, the bar had been a central site of sociality where patients met their friends, talked story, played card games, and hung out. During a previous Christmas season, Uncle Pali ignored us carolers, preferring to watch YouTube videos with Kekoa on a laptop. Some women patients liked to play cribbage, while men tended to enjoy beer. Kenso Seki, a patient

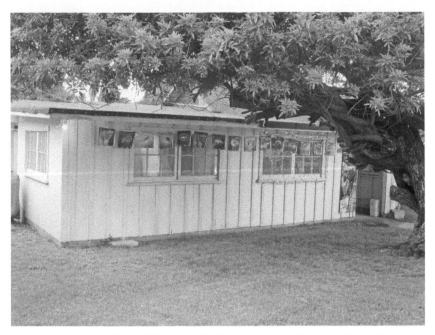

FIGURE 78. Fuesaina's Bar. Kalaupapa, Molokai settlement. Photograph by author.

who did not have fingers, designed and welded his own can openers so he could pop open aluminum beer cans and drink without having to ask for assistance (figure 79). Seki passed these freely out to friends, those with or without disabled hands. Assistive devices like can openers and modified pencils were as much social as they were pragmatic and material. As these tools were distributed and utilized, they strengthened social intimacies without subordination or dependence.

At the bar and McVeigh Hall (a former dormitory converted to a large community space), patients socialized and mingled with visitors and kokuas as interdependent entities outside of group homes and assigned residences. Through the early 2000s, groups of men and women patients and kokuas gathered to play cards on a near nightly basis.[20] Sizable sums of money could be wagered at cribbage, poker, and paiute (a card game rumored to have origins in Kalaupapa). Some women excelled at Scrabble and forged tight-knit friendships during these matches. Other patients preferred social drinking. During weekends, the patient-owned beach homes outside of settlement boundary lines also knew their fair share of carousing and drinking. If the surveillance optics of leprosy management excluded patients from civil

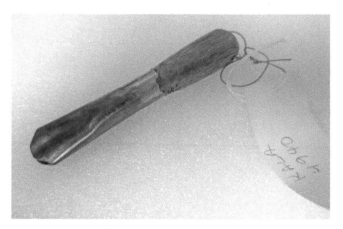

FIGURE 79. Metal beer can opener made by Kenso Seki. KALA 4940, Kalaupapa National Historical Park collection. Photograph by author.

society, then the volleyball field, social halls, and community bar were literal sites of recreation and re-creation; that is, it is where intimate bonds, social relations and civic rituals could be re-created.

ON SEEING AND NOT SEEING

Although medical students and residents touring the settlement over the past century had been able to inspect, and even photograph, living bodies in diverse stages of Hansen's disease, students today do not obtain access to patient-residents. To protect patient confidentiality, the haumāna do not spend time in the settlement hospital, nor are they allowed to treat or observe the treatment of patients. The excursions avoid medical or "dark" tourism, such as clinicians entering the settlement to catch a glimpse of disfigured and disabled HD patients, as they often did for decades. Dr. Brady is careful not to point out his patients to the group. Nor does Brady discuss specific experiences of his current patients or confidential medical information. The moʻolelo (historical stories) on his tour are composites of past patients from the early twentieth century. He maintains careful boundaries between his duties as the resident physician and huakaʻi leader, slipping away to the hospital to see patients while students are occupied with swimming at the pier.

Although the students loved meeting Uncle Pali and delighting him with a volleyball game, the objective of these excursions is not to learn directly from living patients. The haumāna only stopped briefly at the unpopulated side entry of the hospital to access restrooms before our bus ride to Kalawao on the eastern side of the peninsula. They did not see any patients there for treatment. It was only because an accident brought me to the hospital as a patient that I happened to see Dr. Brady interact with one of his longtime patients.

Dr. Brady and a nurse bound my leg in athletic tape on the chair where patients once sat to have daily dressings for their sores. Dr. Brady asked a woman in a wheelchair, a patient I'll call Aunty Ellen, if she minded sitting with me while he took care of some work at the hospital.[21] Aunty smiled, "Yes," so we sat and watched the local KHON-2 news without speaking until I left with a "mahalo" and "good-bye." With obvious mutual affection, Aunty Ellen beamed at Dr. Brady, while he called her "Tita" (sister). He joked with her, "Don't go dancing without me, OK?" He and Aunty Ellen laughed together.

The haumāna may have started off wanting to see the patients, perhaps like other medical tourists over the past century: doctors, nurses, scientists who came to Kalaupapa, documented patients, and exposed their bodies through photographs. Outsiders from the North American mainland and Europe take short bus tours through the settlement via Damien Tours, the patient-owned tour company. Even today, I have been told by residents that some of these tourists arrive with the hope of catching a glimpse of leprous bodies.

Hawai'i statutes on the books since 1923 specifically prohibit photography of patients in the settlement.[22] Today, a version of this law precludes videotaping and filming in the settlement without written permission of patients. By limiting photography and having strict guidelines like advance visitor registration, permits, and sponsorship of a full-time resident, the settlement attempts to limit the fetishizing of patients—the staring by curious outsiders at HD survivors.

At a past community event, NPS cultural anthropologist Ka'ohulani McGuire, who is herself 'ohana (family) of a patient, noticed a visitor shooting photographs of her aunt's hands as she clasped a beverage cup. An accomplished professional photographer, this man had found her aunt's fingerless hands interesting and wanted to take artistic close-ups of them. Ka'ohulani asked her aunt if she realized she was being photographed. When her aunt said, "No," she did not want to be photographed, Ka'ohulani blocked the camera lens.

The medical huakaʻi follows a similar ethos and practice of short-circuiting expectations of contact with patients. If the students harbored curiosity about leprosy in living bodies, they were soon thwarted by the fact that no one pointed out which residents were patients. Without prior knowledge, it is not apparent who the patients are in the settlement; they easily blended in with weekend visitors from the St. John Vianney Catholic parish on Oʻahu. The haumāna couldn't tell the difference between NPS workers, patients, and other callers during the weekend. One told me, "I couldn't tell them apart." Another said the patients were just like their "uncles and aunties." They had very few face-to-face interactions with patients.[23] Uncle Pali did not speak one on one with the haumāna, even on the morning following our volleyball match. We filed into church services at Kanaʻana Hou, the Protestant church of which he was the only remaining patient steward. Pali sat in the front while other guests from Oʻahu led the services. By leaving a thank-you note on the school bus, Uncle Pali did not need to be seen again by any of us.[24]

What might students on future huakaʻi learn from a settlement without patients? The huakaʻi does not depend on access to the presence of living patients. At mixed social engagements like church services and Barge Day, Dr. Brady does not introduce his haumāna to patients. There was one exception, when the group presented a thank-you card and an oli mahalo (chant of gratitude) for Mrs. Gloria Marks at her bar. Mrs. Marks was the official resident sponsor for the student group.

Without direct interaction with patients, the students visually documented their experiences. Never without smartphone cameras, they snapped hundreds of photographs and videos that they shared with each other later via Google Drive. Notably, not one of these images is of a patient. Their photographs instead focus on the landscape, their group, and communal activities: kanikapila (informal musical performances); an endangered monk seal sunning itself on a sandy beach; playing ʻukulele at night; performing hula at the cottage; hurling themselves into cannonballs off the Kalaupapa pier; Dr. Brady driving the bus; and meditating at gravesites.

GRAVESITES AND RECONNECTIONS

Medicine is far from the only site of learning and healing in the settlement. Healing takes place in suturing the living with the past, whether in the form of memorials or personal histories. A woman with a big operatic voice whom I'll call Debra has been visiting Kalaupapa as part of the Oʻahu-based St. John Vianney Parish choir for five years or more. Debra's operatic voice soared through St. Francis Catholic Church effortlessly during her solos. As happens frequently with outside callers, Debra realized only after visiting the settlement that she had family at Kalaupapa. Debra is Samoan and Hawaiian and had been adopted. She recently learned that her birth mother's family, her maternal great-grandparents, had been exiled at Kalaupapa. She contacted Kaʻohulani McGuire, a friend she had made during her past visits. Kaʻohulani, NPS cultural anthropologist, had been living in the settlement for nine years. Though Debra had been to Kalaupapa at least six times before, this was the first time she approached the settlement from the perspective and subjectivity of a family member. She asked, could my ʻohana possibly be buried somewhere at Kalaupapa? She knew some of their names.

While not immediately visible, graves dominate the landscape of the peninsula. Unmarked graves, cemeteries, scattered markers, and grassy expanses suggest the presence of thousands of once living people.[25] Kaʻohulani and I made a trip to Papaloa Cemetery over the weekend. It is an expansive strip of graves lining the road from the airport to the settlement. Papaloa, which means flat long area in Hawaiian, is dotted with twentieth-century gravestones written in Chinese, Japanese, Hawaiian, and English (figure 80). Church of Latter-Day Saints (LDS), Catholic, Buddhist, Americans of Japanese Ancestry (AJA), Hawaiian, and Protestant sections suggest the religious and ethnic affiliations of patients. Papaloa remains an active burial site—it is where Uncle Pali himself planned to be buried with his dogs and spouses. Some recent graves were marked by gleaming headstones and numerous offerings of lei.[26]

On this Saturday afternoon, Kaʻohulani leafed through thick binders of cemetery maps and indexes, searching for Debra's great-grandmother and great-grandfather. Kaʻohulani has been researching and caring for gravesites at KNHP; some descendants looking for exiled family members have found their way to her. Originally this was not part of her NPS work, but she now researches patient genealogies and helps to reconnect people to the gravesites and histories of their ʻohana. In the past two years, she has helped over three hundred people and continues to receive requests for information.

Kaʻohulani is, in a sense, similar to the people she is helping with reconnection. She earned a B.A. in anthropology at University of Hawaiʻi–Hilo in the early 2000s, when two professors hired her to do research as part of an

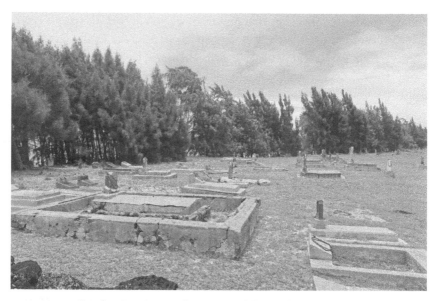

FIGURE 80. Papaloa Cemetery. Kalaupapa, Molokai settlement. Photograph by Noah Dolim, Hui Mālama Makanalua.

NPS-funded ethnographic study. Raised on a ranch on topside Molokai, she has extensive genealogical ties to Molokai, as well as training in a well-known hālau hula (hula troupe). She was aware her mother had a cousin who had been exiled and died at Kalaupapa. However, soon after arriving at Kalaupapa, she inquired about the cousin's gravesite and was shocked to learn from a patient that her mother had more relatives there, including a woman still living in the settlement. After Ka'ohulani found out, she ran to a payphone to call her mother on O'ahu. Her mother was unaware that she had younger cousins who had been exiled.

This cousin was named Cathrine Puahala. In island kinship terms, Cathrine effectively was Ka'ohulani's "aunty" because of their generational and age difference. They grew close. Over the next several years, Ka'ohulani's relationship to the patients shifted from anthropologist to the subjectivity of a patient descendant, and she retains this sensitivity and sense of protectiveness toward the patients. Her closest friends in the settlement, where she continues to live full-time, are patients.

On this afternoon, we were lucky. Ka'ohulani found Debra's ancestor's name in a cemetery binder. We crisscrossed overlapping sections of Papaloa Cemetery on foot, squinting to make out faded names on the stones. Though many gravestones had disintegrated or toppled over from exposure to saltwater air (some literally had exploded), the gravestones had been inscribed with great care and thought. Sometimes etched by hand, these graves were marked with names, affective relationships, dates, villages of origin, and sentiments: "Kia Hoomanao No Mrs. Helen Nauahi, Make Dec. 16, 1924, R.I.P." (Remembrance Stone for Mrs. Helen Nauahi. Died Dec. 16, 1924); "Hoapili, Me Ke Aloha" (Close Friend, with Love); "Beloved Son, David Keawe," "My Beloved Mother, Mrs. Mary Hatori, at Rest," and "In Memory of My Pal Lookie, 1904–1935, Rest in Peace." The Japanese head-stones were especially detailed, with dates, villages, towns, and prefectures of origin, such as one inscribed in Japanese and English, "Remembrance for Arakura Inohe, Died March 1, 1924, Sono, Shimizumura, Kikuchigun, Kumamoto." Some more recent markers had photographs set into the stone.

Despite our cross-referencing different maps, the graves were not often where they had been designated. Remains and markers had been moved, some by purposeful human design and some by natural events like the 1946 tsunami. After walking back and forth, we eventually located Debra's great-grandmother's grave, that of a "Mary M." Her name on the marker was barely visible. We then drove back to visitors' quarters and brought Debra to Papaloa. She walked gingerly between the graves until we came to Mary M.'s marker. Debra snapped a few photographs in silence with her camera phone. We asked her if she wanted one of herself next to the grave; she shook her head no. But a few minutes later, she changed her mind and handed her phone to Ka'ohulani. She thanked us and said she would share these photos with other family members.

What does it mean to find out that you're a descendant and related to people who have long passed? As with Debra, some of the students participating in Dr. Brady's huaka'i have discovered they have 'ohana in the settlement, either living or already passed. If you are Kanaka 'Ōiwi, chances are extremely high that you have 'ohana who were exiled between 1866 and 1969. Earlier in the twentieth century, when Hansen's disease was criminalized, it may have been shameful to discover such relations. However, today's responses suggest pride and reclamation are more common.

On this huaka'i, two young women began learning their own family histories in Kalaupapa. This was Harper's second time participating in the huaka'i. Since her first trip, she had learned that one of her Japanese grandparents had a sibling who lived in Kalaupapa. Her grandparents had spent time here on visits with their incarcerated relatives. These family members were now deceased, but Harper was spurred to come back to Kalaupapa and ask more questions about her family.

A Samoan-Hawaiian student on the trip learned recently from her grand-father that he was the cousin of two patients at Kalaupapa. Liane* wanted to be able to meet these two "aunties," and she shyly mentioned to Dr. Brady that she had these ties. She was hoping she would have a chance to introduce herself before hiking out of the settlement. He told her that the church services would be a good place to meet them. Liane met and hugged one aunty at the bar, but she did not know how she would recognize her second aunt. Later, at Catholic services, I was sitting next to Liane and whispered to her when I saw this aunt making her way up the aisle. Liane shyly approached her aunty after the service and explained their connection.

BIRTHING SANDS

Life and death are twin companions at Kalaupapa. Immediately behind Papaloa Cemetery lies a stretch of white sand beach. Nestled near rows of buried human remains, Papaloa Beach has become an active birthing and pupping area for a critically endangered species, the Hawaiian monk seal (figure 81). Hawaiian monk seals (Monachus schauinslandi) are indigenous and endemic to the Hawaiian Islands. There are only about 1,100 seals in the wild, and their population has been declining about 4 percent per year. While there have been no human births at Kalaupapa in many decades, two of its beaches have harbored over one hundred monk seal births since 1997, making the settlement a regenerative sanctuary for non-human life.[27]

Northern Molokai was not a frequent landing locale for monk seals in the twentieth century, and exiled patients did not recall seeing monk seals on settlement beaches prior to the 1990s. However, the very inaccessibility that transformed the peninsula into a prison has made it an unexpected, yet ideal, location for monk seals to birth and nurse their pups in the last two decades. With a small human population of one hundred residents and a tightly restricted visitor count, the sands and waters of Kalaupapa are life-giving for these endangered marine animals. New pups learn to swim and feed from their mothers in Kalaupapa's shallow reefs, protected from large waves, human disturbance, commercial fishing, and sharks.

Kalaupapa residents have become stakeholders in the protection of monk seals, developing a tentative guardianship of, if not a kinship with, these marine animals. Ecologists working for KNHP facilitate community aware-ness of the vulnerability of endangered seals. The community chalkboard in

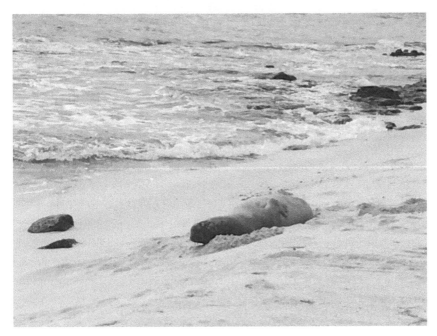

FIGURE 81. Hawaiian monk seal, Papaloa Beach. Kalaupapa, Molokai settlement. Photograph by author.

the village apprises residents of the number of seals born in settlement waters. By early summer of 2015, Monk Seal Pup #3 had arrived.

Native Hawaiian and non-Hawaiian communities in the main Hawaiian Islands have treated monk seals as an invasive species that competes for fish. Some have even killed seals, although they are a protected endangered species under state and federal laws.[28] By contrast, Kalaupapa patients and residents have grown supportive of monk seal conservation, taking pride in their relationship with the seals and their pupping colony. They agreed to the relocation of a captive monk seal to Kalaupapa from another island, while some in main Hawaiian Islands communities voiced opposition to similar proposals.[29] Patients have named new pups born on its beaches. In summer 2018, they suggested the Samoan name "Sole" for a male pup. When Sole was weaned too early from its mother and became malnourished, a marine agency rescued it after consulting with the patient community.[30]

As female seals often return to their birthing sands to give birth to their own pups, multiple generations of seals have made their way back to Kalaupapa beaches in recent years. "Mama Eve"—one of the first female seals in modern history to give birth at Kalaupapa in 1997—has had daughters and granddaughters returning to birth. At least fifty of Mama Eve's descendants have been born at Kalaupapa.[31] In the midst of these seal births, the patients have been unable to arrive at a compromise about the status of human children in their community. They remain deeply divided about whether to allow children into the settlement.

Children under the age of sixteen are not permitted in Kalaupapa. Some patients advocate change to current policy, expressing a desire to have their own mo'opuna (grandchildren) and other children of Hawai'i visit during their lifetimes. Clarence "Boogie" Kahilihiwa, a patient-resident of Kalaupapa since 1959, urged in a news interview, "Come when we [patients] alive . . . No come when we all dead." He affirmed, "I'd like to see the children and if they like hear our story, I can tell them personally."[32] Other patients continue to resist proposals for children to visit. Yet all seem to agree that the presence of baby seals is a common good. In future years, we may continue to see this shift from human-freighted activity toward non-human life on the peninsula.

CONCLUSION: SONIC PERFORMANCES

As endangered seals shelter at Kalaupapa, social activities are increasingly initiated by entities from outside the settlement. That July weekend, the community bulletin posted a notice written in colored chalk: "Summer concert and dinner—5:00-ish, Visitors Quarter. Italian Food—ono [delicious]." The small church choir making its annual visit from O'ahu invited the entire settlement to socialize and eat together.

An elderly Hawaiian man and his two younger family members attended the choir concert at St. Francis Catholic Church. I had taken the nine-seat propeller plane from Honolulu to Kalaupapa with them earlier that day. The oldest man, whom I'll call Uncle Leonard, appeared to be in his eighties and used a walker. He was accompanied by two younger family members. At the airline waiting area in Honolulu, they had greeted a patient. But I did not recognize the elderly Uncle Leonard as a former patient, and it was not immediately apparent how he was attached to anyone in the settlement. After the concert, the choir prepared a spaghetti dinner at Visitors' Quarters. Uncle Leonard rolled slowly up the ramp with his walker and sat on the bench.

A diverse group came to the visitor-hosted party: a former patient who lives "out" (outside the settlement on another island) drove another

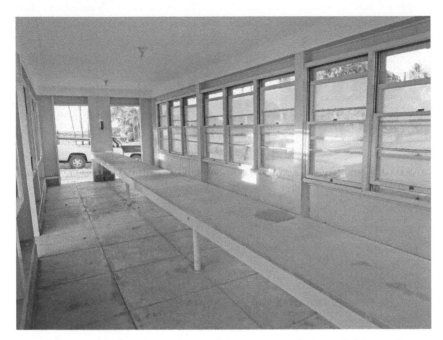

FIGURE 82. Longhouse, where visitors and patients met. Kalaupapa, Molokai settlement. Photograph by author.

patient-resident to the pāʻina (social meal); some NPS workers dropped by, and younger choir members poured drinks and boxed wine. We sat eating and talking story on benches outside the Quarters. This free mingling between staff, visitors, and patients would not have been possible for much of the twentieth century. A wire fence had been erected around the visitors' building to separate patients physically and symbolically from loved ones. The fence was removed only in 1947. Only a few steps away from the party was the reception building called the Longhouse, where patients once met their visitors. They sat face to face, but a physical barrier prevented them from touching (figure 82). Still intact, the Longhouse is a reminder of the enforced separation of patients and their kin, among other parts of the settlement's purposeful built environments.[33]

The al fresco dinner on paper plates led into kanikapila (informal performances) of ʻukulele and song for the next couple of hours. Songbooks were passed around, and residents and choir members strummed ʻukulele. Uncle Leonard's face brightened when he asked the musicians for the mele "Wailele ʻo ʻAkaka" (ʻAkaka Falls), a canonized Hawaiian love song celebrated for its falsetto vocals. The choir leader struck the first chords on the keyboard, and Uncle Leonard, his eyes closed, soared into a stunning falsetto. The clear notes of the chorus, "Kau maila i luna, Lele hunehune maila i nā pali," floated from the group, out past the lapping waves, and everyone fell quiet.

Uncle Leonard, as I later heard, was not a patient, but had been born in the settlement to patients. He, like many other hundreds of children, had been out-adopted as a baby and raised outside of the settlement; this was his first time back to Kalaupapa since he had been separated from his family over eighty years prior. Uncle Leonard's leo kiʻekiʻe singing an informal, unceremonial love song was the most sacred and memorable performance I heard that weekend. I cannot recall any of the Catholic or Protestant hymns performed in church services, but I can still feel the falsetto break Uncle Leonard held aloft for us that humid night, when he reached into his naʻau (guts) to carry that note.

Listening to Uncle Leonard that night, I was reminded of a story I was told about patients who used to sit out by the Kalaupapa lighthouse just to hear the laughter of children. The lighthouse lies outside the formal boundary of Kalaupapa settlement and is not subject to DOH jurisdiction. Children of patients were allowed to stay there, as long as patients did not touch them. Women who gave birth at Kalaupapa in the twentieth century were not allowed to hold their babies. They could only peer at them through a nursery window before the babies were removed from the settlement.[34] At the lighthouse, years after their own children had been taken from them, patients would gather and listen to the sounds of laughter carrying forth. Hearing children at play made life bearable *and* made them suffer, reminding them of the children they had lost.

I heard Uncle Leonard's voice that evening as a kāhea (calling) toward his family who had lost him as a child. Instead of patients furtively and lovingly listening to children who did not know they were being heard, his was an auditory beckoning back through time and space. Here was an elderly man singing, once a child mourned by those forced to give him up. His voice carried his aloha to Papaloa Cemetery to greet the bones of his parents and brothers buried there, the ones that were not allowed to raise him, as if to call to them, "I am back. I have returned. I have not forgotten you." The child once grieved was now performing a love song of reconnection and reunion. That night Uncle Leonard created a new memory for those of us listening.

Over the past one hundred and fifty years, there has been an intense focus on sight and struggles over the authority to control the optics of leprosy and the politics of touch in leprosy institutions. Yet sound travels even when touch is prohibited and sight is limited or overdetermined.[35] I favor contemplating what Kalaupapa will sound like as much as what will be seen there in the future. Whose laughter, songs, and cries might we hear? The soundtrack for Kalaupapa's next century will include the vocalizations of young monk seals and mele performed by the kin of Uncle Leonard and many others. Such is my hope.

ACKNOWLEDGMENTS

Through the uncertainty of hyperemesis gravidarum, childbirth, complicated orthopedic surgery, physical therapy, and the COVID-19 pandemic, many relationships, collaborations, grants, and conversations enabled this book to come to completion, albeit at an unpredictable pace.

The University of California Center for New Racial Studies, UC President's Faculty Fellowship in the Humanities, American Council of Learned Societies' Frederick Burkhardt Residential Fellowship and the National Institutes of Health/National Library of Medicine Scholarly Works in Biomedicine Grant no. G13LM011898-03 provided crucial support. In the early stages of this project, I received generous encouragement from Warwick Anderson, Cathy Gere, Philippa Levine, George Lipsitz, David Serlin, Alexandra Minna Stern, Elizabeth Watkins, and Katrine Whiteson. The University of California, Irvine Humanities Center provided publication support.

Presentations at the University of California Center for New Racial Studies, Huntington Library residential fellows seminar, University of Southern California American Studies and Ethnicity, Toronto Photography Seminar's Reframing Family Photography conference, University of California, Los Angeles Information Studies symposium, University of California, Santa Barbara Asian American Studies, Southern California Asian American/Pacific Islander History group, Princeton University American Studies, Washington State University-Vancouver gender and colonialism symposium, Pacific Coast Branch of the American Historical Association, UCLA Disability as Spectacle Conference, and meetings of the American Studies Association, American Association for the History of Medicine, and Native American and Indigenous Studies Association generated valuable feedback.

More personally, Susan Burch, Ryan-Lee Cartwright, Gordon Chang, Constance Chen, Anne Cheng, Rachael De Lue, Rayna Green, Judith Hamera, Jack Halberstam, Kerri Inglis, Lon Kurashige, Jim Lee, Julie Livingston, Valerie

Matsumoto, Aimee Medeiros, David Pellow, Thy Phu, Josh Reid, Shawn Michelle Smith, Jenny Thigpen, Paul Nadal, Linda Waggoner, John Troutman, Thuy Linh Nguyen Tu, Laura Wexler, Susie Woo, and Judy Wu enriched this work with sharp questions and scholarly engagement.

As a descendant of immigrant settlers to Hawaiʻi, I recognize the long, entangled histories of imperialism and immigration that have enabled me to settle, teach, and write on the ancestral lands of the Acjachemen and Tongva peoples. At the University of California, Irvine, I've benefited from the intellectual energy and generosity of Sharon Block, Andrew Highsmith, Rachel O'Toole, Allison Perlman, Kaaryn Gustafson, and Michelle B. Goodwin. The Medical Humanities program and center at UCI, spearheaded by Douglas Haynes, Johanna Shapiro, and James Kyung-Jin Lee, developed serendipitously as I worked on this book, providing a vibrant interdisciplinary outlet in which to teach and collaborate. The UCI Medical Center Ethics Committee enabled me to think through my research in relation to enduring bioethical issues in a hospital setting. My Ph.D. advisees Noah Dolim, Makanani Salā, and Ayuko Takeda, as well as students in Medical Humanities and Disability History, raised lively and generative questions which I've tried to answer within.

Julie Livingston read drafts of two early chapters and provided important feedback on modern quarantine regimes. Bob Moeller offered expert guidance in modern German history for chapter one. Adrienne L. Kaeppler of the Smithsonian National Museum of Natural History, Ruthard von Frankenberg of Cologne, Germany, and Omer P. Steeno of Leuven, Belgium shared insights and research on Eduard Arning. Dermatologist Melinda Longacker channeled her interest in the study of skin, and art historian Stacey Pierson lent her keen eye. I cannot thank Susan Schweik, Regina Kunzel, Lisa Sun-Hee Park, Kim Nielsen, Phil Deloria, Noelani Arista, Kaʻohulani McGuire, and John Ioane Hoomanawanui enough for reading full drafts of the manuscript, lending their wide-ranging expertise, and improving the book immeasurably. Vicki L. Ruiz remains an inimitable model of mentorship and wisdom. She continues to remind me of the centrality of people's stories in our work. I've made it this far in the profession because of her refreshing humor and steadfast support. Some of the ideas in this book were planted years ago when I was an undergraduate in Laura Wexler's "Photography and the Body" seminar at Yale. Little did I anticipate I would write a book on photography, but Laura's elegant and moving words continue to resonate as if it were yesterday. I'm further grateful to readers for University of California Press who helped me refine many arguments. At UC Press, Robin Manley, Kate Hoffman, and Niels Hooper brought this book to fruition.

I also owe archivists and curators a special debt for making their collections accessible: Kalani Kaanaana at Queen's Hospital; Julia Aleszczyk and T. Scott Williams at Kalaupapa National Historical Park; Helen Wong Smith at Kauaʻi

Historical Society; Stuart Ching at the Congregation of the Sacred Hearts of Jesus and Mary U.S.A Province; Jennifer Higa and Elizabeth Seaton at the Hawaiian Historical Society; Elizabeth Schexnyder at the National Hansen's Disease Museum in Carville, LA; and Eric Boyle at the National Museum of Health and Medicine in Silver Spring, MD. Patricia Lai and Melissa Shimonishi at the Hawai'i State Archives went above and beyond with their assistance and guidance. They made each research trip an extraordinary experience, as did fellow researchers like David Forbes who offered additional resources and leads.

In Hawai'i, Mona-Ann Cardejon of the University of Hawai'i-Mānoa's Department of Native Hawaiian Health, made participation in a Kalaupapa huaka'i possible, as did fellow students and faculty who welcomed me on this excursion. I warmly mahalo Catherine 'Īmaikalani Ulep for her meticulous research assistance. Lynn Davis, foremost scholar of Hawai'i photography, pointed me to little seen resources. Isaac Moriwake, while litigating on behalf of 'āina and waterways, lent his acumen to interpret Hawai'i territorial and state statutes.

While I'm unable to name every person at Kalaupapa settlement whose imprint reverberates in this book, I am especially grateful to Kalani Brady, Jun Look, Ben Young, Kerri Inglis, and Ka'ohulani McGuire for sharing situated knowledge that guided my interpretations. Kalani, in the earliest days of this research, breathed life into ancestors. Simply put, without Ka'ohulani's friendship, writing this book would have been a listless experience. She guided me through obscured records, sponsored my settlement visit, and offered numerous suggestions. As we made journeys to Louisiana, Wai'alae, and downtown Honolulu together, she made this work even more meaningful and personal.

As this book concerns kinship and care, I cannot emphasize enough how my own a-filial and filial kin keep me afloat. The Pierson-Pan clan—Patty, Arnold, Phoebe, and Penelope—delivered meals and endless treats when I couldn't walk, arranged celebrations, and shared latte strolls. Catherine Sameh pitched in with my kids, cooked, and poured wine. Kim Gilmore, Julie Chu, Jen Sung, Grace Wang, and Julie Sze kept checking in, and Emily Thuma commiserated. The humor and musicality of Aaron Salā and 'ohana enlarged my world. Cindy I-Fen Cheng, regardless of time zone, has been a fount of enthusiastic support and intellectual rigor; I continue to learn from her compassion and integrity. Along the way, Eleana Kim read every fragment and paragraph I've written and helped untangle frustrating knots; I owe arriving at the finish line to her brilliance, constancy, and friendship.

My relations near and far—Warren and Dorothy Imada, Jeanette Yamanaka, Lori Arakawa, and sweet cousins Sheldon, Brandon, and Jenn—enriched each trip back home with favorite meals, treats, music, and laughter. Marcy Imada and Stacy Toyama, Rae Yamanaka, the Mimura and Oak families, as well as Shari Smith and family, shared time, nourishment, playdates, and care packages. Glen Mimura, who cleared so many pathways to make this book possible, will recognize his acute insights woven throughout, I hope. Our children Naia and Saku learned to walk, read, and play catch as I was researching and writing. I trust they will come to understand their mother chose to write this story of love and connection because of them.

NOTES

ARCHIVAL ABBREVIATIONS

260 Box 30, HSA   260 Box 30, Folder (Kalihi Boys' Home, Non-Leprous Children Sent to Kalihi, 1890–1929); Bureau of Leprosy, 1866–1930, Kakaako and Kalihi Receiving Stations and Kalihi Hospital; Records Related to Hansen's Disease 1866–1981, Series 260; HSA.

331 Vol. 115, HSA   331 Volume 115 (Visits to Kalihi Station, November 23, 1904–September 17, 1917); Board of Health Letterbooks (Other Agents and Officers); Outgoing Letters of the Board of Health, 1865–1981, Series 331; HSA.

334-14, HSA   Folder, Letters 1889, A–C; Box 334-14; Incoming Letters of the Board of Health, 1850–1904, Series 334; HSA.

334-34, HSA   Folder, Reports by Physicians on Leperous [sic] Persons, 1880–1886 (Hansen's Disease, 1867–1941); Box 334-34; Incoming Letters of the Board of Health, 1850–1904, Series 334; HSA.

334-35 Arning, HSA   Folder, Records re: Dr. Edward Arning, 1883–1888 (Hansen's Disease, 1867–1941); Box 334-35; Incoming Letters of the Board of Health 1850–1904, Series 334; HSA.

334-35 Kalihi, HSA   Folder, Records re: Kalihi Receiving Station, 1887–1893 (Hansen's Disease, 1867–1941); Box 334-35; Incoming Letters of the Board of Health, 1850–1904, Series 334; HSA.

334-37, HSA   Folder, Newspaper clippings, 1907–1929 (Hansen's Disease, 1867–1941); Box 334-37; Incoming Letters of the Board of Health 1850–1904, Series 334; HSA.

335-11, HSA	Folder: House of Representatives re: Lepers 1907–1911; Box 335-11; Correspondence of the Board of Health, 1905–1917, Series 335; HSA.
335-12 (1907), HSA	Folder, Kalaupapa Settlement, July–December 1907; Box 335-12; Correspondence of the Board of Health, 1905–1917, Series 335; HSA.
335-12 (1909), HSA	Folder, Kalaupapa Settlement, January–June 1909; Box 335-12; Correspondence of the Board of Health, 1905–1917, Series 335; HSA.
335-13, HSA	Folder, Kalihi Hospital, 1905–1909; Box 335-13; Correspondence of the Board of Health, 1905–1917, Series 335; HSA.
335-16, HSA	Folder, Mrs. Emma Nakuina, 1905–1910; Box 335-16; Correspondence of the Board of Health, 1905–1917, Series 335; HSA.
AEA	Arning Ethnographic Album, Eduard Arning Albums and Research Material, Arnsteiner Patres, Werne, Germany.
ALA	Arning Leprosy Album, Eduard Arning Albums and Research Material, Arnsteiner Patres, Werne, Germany.
Box 5, NBE	Box 5, Medical Papers; Series One: Emerson's Research Material; Nathaniel Bright Emerson Papers, 1766–1944; The Huntington Library, San Marino, California.
Box 6, NBE	Box 6, Research Material (Mele); Nathaniel Bright Emerson Papers, 1766–1944; The Huntington Library, San Marino, California.
CBC-HSA	C. B. Cooper Collection, Hawai‘i State Archives, Honolulu, Hawai‘i.
CBC-Q	Charles Bryant Cooper, M.D., Collection, Queen's Hospital Historical Room, Honolulu, Hawai‘i.
CMR	Caroline M. Reader Collection, 1978–1998, KALA 12364; Kalaupapa National Historical Park, Kalaupapa, Hawai‘i.
CPNP	Catalog Photograph/Negativ Platten, Eduard Arning Collection, Hawaiian Historical Society, Honolulu, Hawai‘i.
CSH	Congregation of the Sacred Hearts of Jesus and Mary U.S.A. Province, Honolulu, Hawai‘i.
EK	Edward Kato Papers, KALA 17804, Kalaupapa National Historical Park, Kalaupapa, Hawai‘i.

ER	Elaine Remigio Collection; Kalaupapa National Historical Park, Kalaupapa, Hawai'i.
FM	Franklin Mark Album, KALA-00366; Kalaupapa National Historical Park, Kalaupapa, Hawai'i.
GMC	George McCoy Collection/Lantern Slide Set, ca. 1948; Otis Historical Archives 225; National Museum of Health and Medicine, Silver Spring, Maryland.
HD-3, HSA	Volume HD-3 (Records of Deaths in Leper Settlement [Monthly], 1889–1923); Patient Registers and Indexes; Bureau of Leprosy, 1866–1930, Kalaupapa Leprosarium; Records Relating to Hansen's Disease, 1866–1981, Series 260; HSA.
HD-4, HSA	Volume HD-4 (Kalawao Deaths, January 3, 1909–October 4, 1912); Kalawao County Vital Statistics Registrar's Records; Bureau of Leprosy, 1866–1930, Kalaupapa Leprosarium; Records Relating to Hansen's Disease, 1866–1981, Series 260; HSA.
HD-5, HSA	Volume HD-5 (Kalawao Deaths, September 1, 1914–October 5, 1917); Kalawao County Vital Statistics Registrar's Records; Bureau of Leprosy, 1866–1930, Kalaupapa Leprosarium; Records Relating to Hansen's Disease, 1866–1981, Series 260; HSA.
HD-6, HSA	Volume HD-6 (Kalawao Deaths, July 19, 1927–November 24, 1931); Kalawao County Vital Statistics Registrar's Records; Bureau of Leprosy, 1866–1930, Kalaupapa Leprosarium; Records Relating to Hansen's Disease, 1866–1981, Series 260; HSA.
HD-7, HSA	Volume HD-7 (Persons Apprehended and Examined for Leprosy, 1874–1932); Patient Registers; Bureau of Leprosy, 1866–1930, Kakaako and Kalihi Receiving Stations and Kalihi Hospital; Records Relating to Hansen's Disease, 1866–1981, Series 260; HSA.
HD-A, HSA	Volume HD-A (map) (Children Residing in the Settlement, 1880–1925); Registers of Non-Leprous Children; Bureau of Leprosy, 1866–1930, Kalaupapa Leprosarium; Records Related to Hansen's Disease 1866–1981, Series 260; HSA.
HD-B, HSA	Volume HD-B (Boys' Home, Honolulu, 1908–1935); Registers of Non-Leprous Children; Bureau of Leprosy, 1866–1930, Kalaupapa Leprosarium; Records Related to Hansen's Disease 1866–1981, Series 260; HSA.

HD-C, HSA	Volume HD-C (map) (Girls' Home, Honolulu, 1885–1935); Registers of Non-Leprous Children; Bureau of Leprosy, 1866–1930, Kalaupapa Leprosarium; Records Related to Hansen's Disease 1866–1981, Series 260; HSA.
HHS	Eduard Arning Collection, Hawaiian Historical Society, Honolulu, Hawai'i.
HSA	Hawai'i State Archives, Honolulu, Hawai'i.
JL	Papers of Jack London, Photograph Albums and Large Albums; The Huntington Library, San Marino, California.
KNHP	Kalaupapa National Historical Park, Kalaupapa, Hawai'i.
Leprosy Cases, NBE	Leprosy Cases 1 to 184; 1879–1883; EMR 1314; Series Five: Ephemera and Bound Volumes; Nathaniel Bright Emerson Papers, 1766–1944; The Huntington Library, San Marino, California.
MER, HSA	Medical Examination Records, 1896–1910; Bureau of Leprosy, 1866–1930, Kakaako and Kalihi Receiving Stations and Kalihi Hospital; Records Relating to Hansen's Disease, 1866–1981, Series 260; HSA.
NBE	Nathaniel Bright Emerson Papers, 1766–1944; The Huntington Library, San Marino, California.
NPS	U.S. National Park Service.
SSC	Stanley Stein Collection, NHDM-19578.12; National Hansen's Disease Museum, Carville, Louisiana.
Vol. 2, Box 1, HSA	Volume 2, Box 1 (Honolulu—Persons Examined—No. 1 [Bk. I]—1881–1885); Patient Registers; Bureau of Leprosy, 1866–1930, Kakaako and Kalihi Receiving Stations and Kalihi Hospital; Records Relating to Hansen's Disease, 1866–1981, Series 260; HSA.
Vol. 3 Folio, HSA	Volume 3 Folio (Bureau of Leprosy, 1866–1930, Kalaupapa Leprosarium); Patient Registers; Honolulu—Persons Examined—No. 2 [Bk. II], 1881–1900; Records Relating to Hansen's Disease, 1866–1981, Series 260; HSA.
Vol. 5, Box 3, HSA	Volume 5, Box 3 (Clinical Records, 1896–1897); Medical Examination Records; Bureau of Leprosy, 1866–1930, Kakaako and Kalihi Receiving Stations and Kalihi Hospital; Records Relating to Hansen's Disease, 1866–1981, Series 260; Hawai'i State Archives.

Vol. 7 Folio, HSA	Volume 7 Folio (Kalihi Boys' Home, 1908 to [1934]); Bureau of Leprosy, 1866–1930, Kakaako and Kalihi Receiving Stations and Kalihi Hospital; Records Related to Hansen's Disease 1866–1981, Series 260; HSA.
Vol. 7 Minutes, HSA	Volume 7 (January 15, 1897–December 31, 1898); Minutes of the Board of Health, 1858–1983, Series 259; HSA.
Vol. 15 Minutes, HSA	Volume 15 (January 16, 1907–June 17, 1908); Minutes of the Board of Health, 1858–1983, Series 259; HSA.
Vol. 16 Minutes, HSA	Volume 16 Folio (July 9, 1908–December 22, 1910); Minutes of the Board of Health, 1858–1983, Series 259; HSA.

PREFACE: ENCOUNTERING THE PHOTOGRAPHS

1. Campt, *Listening to Images,* 24–26.
2. Iwi kūpuna (ancestral bones) are protected and treasured by Native Hawaiians, and grave desecration is considered an act of spiritual defilement.
3. Armitage, *Healers,* 107, 121.

NOTE ON LANGUAGE

1. *Oral Histories of the Native Hawaiian Elderly,* 276.

INTRODUCTION: AN ARCHIVE OF SKIN, AN ARCHIVE OF KIN

1. The exact number is not known, but between seven and eight thousand people were sentenced and removed to a settlement on Molokai between 1866 and ca. 1949. The number of suspected people apprehended was much larger. In the last two decades of the leprosy removal policy (1949–1969), sulfone drugs became accepted as a cure, and people newly diagnosed with leprosy were confined and treated at a new facility, Hale Mōhalu, on Oʻahu. By the 1969 rescindment of the policy, more people were treated as out-patients without the need for confinement. While there is considerable debate about the correct spelling and pronunciation of Molokai, I have chosen to spell it without the ʻokina, or glottal stop. Pukui, Elbert, and Mookini's *Place Names of Hawaii* writes "Molokaʻi" with an ʻokina, but Molokai elder Harriet Ne pronounced and spelled it without an ʻokina. Edward Halealoha Ayau, Ne's grandson, was told by Ne that the name shifted to "Molokaʻi" in the 1930s because musicians began pronouncing it this way. Mary Kawena Pukui called Ne to correct

the island's spelling to Molokai; Pukui also determined Molokai means "the gathering of the ocean waters." Pukui, Elbert, and Mookini, *Place Names,* 20; Ne, *Tales of Molokai,* vi.

2. Keliiahonui entered Kalihi Hospital and Detention Station on September 10, 1903, and died in the settlement April 10, 1914, at the age of seventeen. Although his place of origin was noted as Hilo, Hawaiʻi, he had been born in the Molokai settlement to exiled patients around 1897. According to the 1910 U.S. census, he was living with other boys and single men in Baldwin Home in the Kalawao settlement. Keliiahonui's record is case 336, Box 18 (Medical Examination Records 1903); MER. His death is in HD-3, HSA.

3. The earliest appearances of an illness that may have been leprosy in Hawaiʻi were recorded in 1823 through the 1830s. Mouritz, *Path of the Destroyer,* 29–30.

4. Section 3 of the 1865 Act to Prevent the Spread of Leprosy read: "The Board of Health or its agents are authorized and empowered to cause to be isolated and confined, in some place or places for that purpose provided, all leprous patients who shall we deemed capable of spreading the disease of Leprosy . . . and it shall be the duty of every Police and District Justice to cause to be arrested and delivered to the Board of Health or its agents, any person alleged to be a leper . . . and it shall be the duty of the Marshal of the Hawaiian Islands and his Deputies, and of the Police Officers, to assist in securing the conveyance of any person so arrested, to such place as the Board of Health or its agents may direct, in order that such person may be subjected to medical inspection, and thereafter to assist in removing such person to place of treatment, or isolation . . ." Section 4 granted the power to send to "a place of isolation . . . all such patients as shall be considered incurable or capable of spreading disease of Leprosy." *Laws of His Majesty Kamehameha V, 1864–1865,* 63–64.

5. For a rich pre-and post-leprosy settlement history of Makanalua and the sustaining interactions between residents and exiled patients, see Inglis, "Nā Hoa."

6. Francis N. Frazier translated "luakupapaʻu kanu ola" as "the grave of living corpses" in her foreword to "True Story of Kaluaikoʻolau," 2. I have benefited from conversations with scholar Noelani Arista about reinterpretation of these Hawaiian-language descriptions. In contrast to "grave of living corpses," a "grave where the living are buried" diminishes horror in favor of pathos toward Kānaka who were cut from society. The original account of Koʻolau was written and published in Hawaiian by Kahikina Kelekona (John Sheldon) in 1906. The latter two terms are among many notated from Hawaiian-language newspapers in Clark, *Kalaupapa Place Names,* 141.

7. Chapter XVI, An Act Relating to Divorce, in *Laws of His Majesty Kamehameha V, 1870,* 18.

8. The first people exiled to the Molokai settlement in 1866 all were Kānaka ʻŌiwi. As more foreigners arrived in the islands, their numbers increased in the settlement. Between 1901 and 1920, for example, between 79 and 94 percent of those exiled were Kānaka ʻŌiwi, with the largest foreign, immigrant, and non-Indigenous populations usually represented by Portuguese, Chinese, Japanese, Koreans, and Filipinos. Those categorized "English" and "American" or from Western European

countries (e.g., "Belgian," "German") constituted the smallest groups. With increased racial mixing in nineteenth- and twentieth-century Hawaiʻi, the Board of Health disaggregated "Hawaiians" and "Part Hawaiians," but I include both in the category of "Hawaiian," as was the preferred practice of Kānaka ʻŌiwi. For a sample of these racialized national statistics, see *Report... Ending December 31, 1902*, 268; *Report...Ended June 30, 1915*, 42; and U.S. Department of the Interior, *Report of the Governor of Hawaii, 633*.

9. The term "mai Pake" ("maʻi Pākē" in contemporary orthography) suggests some association between Chinese and this new disease, but it does not constitute evidence that Chinese introduced leprosy to Hawaiʻi. While leprosy may have been transmitted to Hawaiians from Chinese contract laborers, physician Arthur Mouritz suggested other plausible theories about the origins of leprosy in Hawaiʻi, including crews from whaling ships recruited from places with endemic leprosy like Cape Verde, the West Indies, Malaysia, India, and Mozambique. *Path of the Destroyer*, 28. Transnational interactions in the nineteenth century likely introduced leprosy to Hawaiʻi, whether Hawaiians traveling and returning to the Islands, or the arrival of diverse foreigners to Hawaiʻi's shores. Yet BOH use of the English-language translation "Chinese leprosy" during its proceedings indicates how physicians and settlers racialized the disease as Asian in origin, while debating methods to quarantine Native Hawaiians with the disease. By 1870, "Chinese leprosy" was codified in Kingdom of Hawaiʻi law; a spouse contracting this disease could be divorced by the non-leprous party. *Supplement*, 4–7; *Laws of His Majesty Kamehameha V, 1870*, 18.

10. In the United States, Australia, and New Zealand, Chinese immigrants and their descendants were targeted as pestilent people in the nineteenth and twentieth centuries. Fears of Chinese spreading leprosy, syphilis, and plague in the United States fueled immigration restriction, including the 1882 Chinese Exclusion Act. Gussow stresses, in contrast, that even if Chinese were named as the origin of leprosy in Hawaiʻi, this association was not harnessed as an argument to restrict their immigration to the islands. Rather, Hawaiians were detained and exiled. Gussow, *Leprosy*, 95–96, 125–26. On Australia's exclusion of Chinese from the national body, see Bashford, *Imperial Hygiene*, 88, 142, 143.

11. For example, statistician and health reformer Frederick Hoffman, testifying in 1916 before a U.S. Senate committee vetting a federal leprosy facility, offered a characterization of the "excessive" representation of "native and oriental" people in the Molokai leprosy settlement. *Care and Treatment of Persons*, 135.

12. Mouritz, *Path of the Destroyer*, 165; Gussow, *Leprosy*, 85. Bashford refers to the rigid practice of leprosy isolation in the British Empire as "spatial exclusion." *Imperial Hygiene*, 88. In comparison to Hawaiʻi, Japan's official period of leprosy isolation lasted from 1931 until 1996.

13. Gussow and Tracy argue that three main events in the 1860s and 1870s brought leprosy into Western prominence in the modern period: 1) the outbreak of leprosy in Hawaiʻi; 2) the discovery of *M. leprae* in 1873; and 3) the news that Father Damien had contracted the disease and later died in 1889. "Stigma," 432.

14. Bloombaum and Gugelyk, "Attitudes," 69; Bashford, *Imperial Hygiene,* 88. Victor Heiser, the U.S. Director of Health in the Philippines, searched for an island similar to Molokai to establish the Culion leprosy colony. Anderson, "Leprosy and Citizenship," 712. Leprosy policy in the Cook Islands, a British protectorate in the late nineteenth century, was loosely based on the Molokai isolation model, and one of the islets where people were segregated was named Molokai. Lange, "Leprosy in the Cook Islands," 310–11.

15. Although there is recent research suggesting some individuals may have a genetic susceptibility to infection, about 95 percent of people exposed to the bacteria will not develop the disease because their immune system will fight the infection; www.cdc.gov/leprosy/world-leprosy-day/index.html. On the shift from "leprosy" to "Hansen's disease" in the 1960s, refer to note on language.

16. Medical classifications of leprosy have shifted significantly over time. Lepromatous and tuberculoid leprosy had become two major diagnostic categories by the 1940s. Lepromatous was the more severe and contagious type, characterized by nodules, while tuberculoid was less contagious and characterized by skin lesions. To add to the confusion, "tubercular" was the term formerly used to refer to the severe form that became known as lepromatous. By the early 1900s, Hawai'i-based medical officers classified leprosy cases as tubercular, anesthetic, and mixed. The tubercular type later became known as lepromatous, and the anesthetic type as tuberculoid. Muir, *Manual;* U.S. Treasury, *Transactions,* 88; U.S. Treasury, Public Health and Marine-Hospital Service, *Report upon Treatment,* 10. It is a common myth that fingers of leprosy patients "fall off." When fingers and toes suffer nerve damage, people may lose feeling and injure these areas, developing infections that result in tissue loss and cartilage absorption. Hence, some experienced shortened bones and fingers. S. Kalani Brady, interview, December 18, 2013.

17. Sontag, *Illness as Metaphor,* 128–31.

18. Tuberculosis, in stark contrast to leprosy and HIV/AIDS, did not attach sexualized stigma to its sufferers. Rather, tubercular people retained associations with heightened creativity, romantic genius, and sexual desirability.

19. The field of tropical medicine that studied infection emanating from "tropical" people and places was prompted by Western fears of the corporeal and moral corruption of colonial populations. Worboys, "Tropical Diseases," 512–26; Bashford, *Imperial Hygiene,* 81, 83–89. Bashford observes how leprosy became conceptualized as a tropical disease, even though leprosy public health programs were initiated in "untropical" places like New Brunswick, British Columbia, and Robben Island in Cape Colony. The term "imperial danger" comes from H. P. Writers, *Leprosy: An Imperial Danger* (J. & A. Churchill, London, 1889). See also Edmond, *Leprosy and Empire,* 7–8, 44–45, 96, on the rediscovery of leprosy in Norway in the 1840s and the hysteria prompted by leprosy cases in England in the 1880s after leprosy became re-associated as a foreign disease.

20. Gussow and Tracy argue the racial stigma of leprosy and ensuing public health model of mandatory confinement arose in specific relationship to colonial expansion. Gussow and Tracy, "Stigma," 425–49. Bashford discusses "racial cordons

sanitaires" in settler colonial Australia that closely tied the disease management of leprosy with racial conduct and contact. *Imperial Hygiene*, 82.

21. People with leprosy relocated to leprosaria outside of towns and cities were still connected to religious charity and care. Brenner, "Recent Perspectives," 397.

22. Alison Bashford argues this shift to a cordon sanitaire model of prevention and protection marked leprosy management in the age of empire. *Imperial Hygiene*, 87.

23. Osorio, *Dismembering Lāhui*, 224. Mark Rifkin also analyzes the subordination of Hawai'i to global imperial powers as "debt sovereignty." "Debt and Transnationalization of Hawai'i."

24. J. Kēhaulani Kauanui argues that the Hawaiian Kingdom exercised a "colonial biopolitics of governmentality" as a "protective measure against Western imperialism." Chiefly elites attempted to protect the lives of their people by adopting Western monarchical forms and law. In the process, the monarchy criminalized domestic and sexual arrangements; she names these practices "Hawaiian state racism." *Paradoxes of Hawaiian Sovereignty*, 23–24.

25. Merry, *Colonizing Hawaii*, 89.

26. By the time of the 1893 U.S.-backed overthrow of the Hawaiian Kingdom, BOH membership was composed of equal numbers of physicians and lay members.

27. Hawaiians pushed back against the sanctioning of Western biomedicine at the expense of Native medicine. The legislature established a Papa Ola Hawaii (Native Hawaiian Board of Health) in 1868. This Native board licensed some kāhuna to practice legally in the kingdom. Bushnell, "Hawaii's First Medical School," 110; Chun, *Kāhuna*, 59.

28. Foucault, *Society Must Be Defended*, 243–45, 247; Foucault, *History of Sexuality*, 139.

29. Moblo, "Blessed Damien," 698–99; Gussow, *Leprosy*, 90–96. These economic concerns continued through the 1920s, with BOH leaders tracking the representation of leprosy in Hawai'i by business leaders in the United States. These compiled news clippings are in 334-37, HSA.

30. Blaisdell, "Historical and Cultural Aspects," 8; Herman, "Out of Sight," 276. By the time leprosy isolation was enacted in 1865, the Native people of Hawai'i had declined to an estimated 59,000 from 300,000 since Western contact in 1778. Bushnell, "Hawaii's First Medical School," 109.

31. Moblo, "Blessed Damien," 697. Moblo says that tuberculosis was responsible for four times as many deaths as leprosy in Hawai'i.

32. Influenza killed 202,000 and tuberculosis killed 194,000 people in 1900; they were the number one and number two causes of death in the United States. Jones, Podolsky, and Greene, "Burden of Disease," 2336. The estimated figure of 278 people with leprosy is in *Letter from the Surgeon-General*.

33. The relationship between colonial expansion and racialized phobia of leprosy, particularly in the Pacific, has been well established. Gussow and Tracy, "Stigma." David Arnold has observed that it "would not be hard to construct" a "definitive colonial history of leprosy," while Luker, Buckingham, Inglis, and other contribu-

tors to a special issue on leprosy in the Pacific have demarcated the colonial history of leprosy in the Pacific's "Commonwealth zone." Arnold notes how leprosy "rapidly became in a perceptual, if not in an epidemiological, sense naturalized in the Pacific, reinforcing the perception that it was, or had become, a largely 'tropical' disease." Arnold, "Leprosy: From 'Imperial Danger,'" 407, 411; Luker and Buckingham, "Histories of Leprosy," 266.

34. Gussow and Tracy, "Stigma," 440. The authors do not name Indigenous Pacific Islanders, but inhabitants of the Western, North, and Central Pacific are specified in Anglophone reports from the turn of the century.

35. Arning, "Appendix E," lxi. Arning's letter to BOH President Gibson was dated April 10, 1884.

36. Entry dated March 11, 1880; Leprosy Cases, NBE.

37. Fitch, "Appendix E," 120.

38. Hagan, "Leprosy on the Hawaiian Islands." Hagan offered little proof for this assertion, nor do BOH records validate the claim of European and American settlers becoming infected at higher rates. Yet this leitmotif and anxiety repeated itself in the writings of white settler physicians like American George Fitch, who documented white men's sexual transgressions with women who became leprous. See Fitch, "Appendix E."

39. The biopolitical regulation of colonial prisoners was connected through institutions like plantations, detention hospitals, jails, insane asylums, and reform schools. Leprosy suspects were surveilled and caught in these spaces. Within a short span of four years, three kingdom laws were passed that moved people into state-sponsored custodial institutions. An act establishing an insane asylum was passed in 1862, an act establishing an industrial and reform school for neglected children and juvenile offenders in 1864, and a year later, in 1865, an act to control leprosy. By 1866, all institutions had opened and were housing offenders. People with psychiatric disabilities, dementia, and unsightly cases of leprosy were institutionalized, along with the poor and juveniles who had committed truancy or petty crimes. For the 1862 insane asylum act, see *Na Kanawai o Ka Moi Kamehameha*, 33, *Compiled Laws of the Hawaiian Kingdom;* and *Pacific Commercial Advertiser,* October 16, 1862, 4. For the 1864 reform school and 1865 leprosy acts, see *Laws of His Majesty Kamehameha V, 1864–65*, 32, 62–64.

40. Fanon, *Dying Colonialism,* 122–24.

41. I use "regime" to suggest how the medical prison operated as more than a discrete institution. As Dylan Rodriguez argues, the prison is not an institution or apparatus, but a "state-mediated practice of domination and control." *Forced Passages,* 40. Sarah Haley usefully discusses the role of physicians in the Jim Crow South's carceral regime. "Carceral physicians" kept prisoners in shape so they could labor in the service of neoslave convict camps. *No Mercy Here,* 75. Warwick Anderson links public health-oriented discipline and therapeutic responsibility to the production of "carceral citizenship" at the overlapping site of Culion leprosy colony in the Philippines. "Leprosy and Citizenship," 721.

42. While the BOH was dominated by Western medical practitioners, prominent Hawaiians responded in a number of ways to epidemics and Hawaiian depopu-

lation. A group of Hawaiian educators, lawyers, and legislators founded the ʻAhahui Lāʻau Lapaʻau of Wailuku (Association of Hawaiian Healing and Medicine) in December 1866. Its members, all men except for one woman, undertook an intensive series of interviews with kāhuna (trained traditional healers) to investigate whether Native Hawaiian medicines were appropriate treatments for diseases in the kingdom. The ʻAhahui's findings were discussed in the 1868 Legislative Assembly, and later that year, the legislature created the Papa Ola Hawaii, a Hawaiian Board of Health, that went on to license some practitioners of Native medicine. These activities indicate the intense interest Hawaiians had in maintaining their own paradigms of healing within and outside of the authority of the Western settler-dominated Board of Health. Chun, *Kāhuna*, 125, 141, 154, 159.

43. McDonald, "Diagnostic Examination," 1567. J. T. McDonald was a Canadian-born doctor who became a naturalized U.S. citizen. He was a pathologist at Kalihi Hospital and Detention Station from 1901 to 1910. Although McDonald was describing the territorial period that began in 1900, the system of dividing the islands into public health districts was established under the Hawaiian Kingdom.

44. The Kakaʻako Branch Hospital and Receiving Station opened in 1881 and closed in 1888. A similar detention facility, the Kalihi Hospital and Detention Station, operated from 1865 to 1875 and from 1889 to 1949. Both located on the Honolulu waterfront, these facilities admitted and examined people suspected of having leprosy.

45. Kunzel, *Criminal Intimacy*, 8.

46. Kaeppler, *Old Hawaii*, 51.

47. On German anthropology and photography, see Edwards, "Photographic 'Types.'" On Bertillon, see Anderson, "Case of the Archive," 542; and Cole, *Suspect Identities*, 43, 47–48.

48. On Lombroso, see Gould, *Mismeasure of Man*, 156–65; Gibson, *Born to Crime;* Lombroso, *Criminal Man;* and Lombroso and Ferrero, *Criminal Woman.*

49. "Patients Must Obey the Rules," *Hawaiian Gazette*, July 30, 1909; 334–37, HSA. BOH agents borrowed from these circulating technologies that attempted to find root causes and symptoms of criminality, but also departed from these, as I discuss in chapter 2.

50. U.S. census records, which began in Hawaiʻi in 1900 with U.S. territorial status, referred to settlement patients as "institutional inmates."

51. For example, *Report . . . Ended June 30, 1923*, 144.

52. This slide is not reprinted here. George McCoy was director of the Leprosy Investigation Station in Hawaiʻi (1911–1915), then went on to lead the two national entities that preceded today's National Institutes of Health: the Hygienic Laboratory and the National Institute of Health, between 1915 and 1937.

53. The slide was captioned "leper boy" and was manufactured by A. D. Handy Company in Boston, Massachusetts. It was originally in the lantern slide collection of USA-East Lantern Slide Collection, Congregation of the Sacred Hearts of Jesus and Mary U.S.A. Province, and is now in CSH. The latter also holds another slide of Keliiahonui. Slide LS8-48; Box 8 (Oahu and Molokai views); Ss 1d.2 (Glass

negatives [lantern slides]); Series I (Photographic Forms); Special Collection, RG IX; CSH. The same image of Keliiahonui was published originally in Jourdan, *Le Père Damien*, 176.

54. Sekula, "Body and the Archive," 6.

55. Ann Stoler has called archives "commitments to paper" in *Archival Grain*, 1. The U.S. army inserted bodies in its archive in the 1890s, basing its identification system on Alphonse Bertillon's criminal identification system from the 1880s. However, it was too complicated and time-consuming for the army to include photographs. Anderson, "Case of the Archive," 542. Bertillon's system used photographs, but preferred narrativized physical description. Cole, *Suspect Identities*, 43, 47–48. The U.S. federal government utilized photographs to regulate Chinese immigration from 1875 to the 1920s, as Anna Pegler-Gordon has analyzed in *In Sight of America*.

56. Stanley Burns observed that photographs were used for patient consultation in the United States in the late 1850s. American doctors made and used daguerreotypes for clinical purposes beginning in the late 1840s. *Early Medical Photography*, 1263, 1267.

57. Stoler, *Archival Grain*, 20.

58. Pinney, "Parallel Histories," 77.

59. Sontag, *On Photography*, 154.

60. Foucault, *Birth of the Clinic*, 122.

61. Albert Londe, director of photography at Salpêtrière Hospital in the 1880s, quoted in Didi-Huberman, *Invention of Hysteria*, 32.

62. While not specifying its application for the study of leprosy, physician Boardman Reed advocated the camera's optic truth in 1889. He argued photographs provided the "best of all records" for medical cases, such as facial paralysis, spinal curvature, hip-joint disease, and marked skin disease. They would be useful for "future reference" and diagnosis. Reed, "Why Physicians Should Cultivate Photography," 514–15.

63. Epidemics: Bubonic Plague, 1900; Folders PP 19-1; PP 19-2; PP 19-3; Photograph Collection; HSA.

64. Heinrich, *Afterlife of Images*, 74.

65. Mouritz, *Path of the Destroyer*, 21.

66. Entry dated July 30, 1906, p. 84; 331 Vol. 115, HSA.

67. For example, four photographs of patients taken in 1898 in Honolulu were included in a U.S. Senate Committee on Public Health and National Quarantine report. *Letter from the Surgeon-General*, at 8.

68. Images do not appear in Bashford, *Imperial Hygiene*, or Gussow, *Leprosy*. Mouritz's *Path of the Destroyer* (1916), one of the earliest books on "Hawaiian leprosy," included color plates of Hawaiian patients with no attribution. More recently, Inglis's *Maʻi Lepera* and Tayman's *Colony* include photographs of patients as illustrations. Sander A. Gilman's *Disease and Representation* remains a pioneering model for making visual culture central to histories of medicine. Stepan's *Picturing Tropical Nature* and Heinrich's *Afterlife of Images* also rely on visual culture for historical analysis.

69. Here I take a cue from disability studies scholar Rosemarie Garland Thomson, who uses "extraordinary" to reference bodily diversity in a non-pejorative way. *Extraordinary Bodies*.

70. Immigrants from Puerto Rico and Portugal were also photographed, but with far less frequency. In transnational media, images of Native Hawaiians and Asian immigrants to Hawai'i represented the scourge of leprosy emanating from Hawai'i. Stepan has shown how photographic "tropical-disease portraits" in medical atlases conflated tropical disease with the bodies of colonized people. *Picturing Tropical Nature,* 171–72. Neel Ahuja argues that the circulation of disabled and racialized Hansen's disease narratives and images justified medical segregation on Molokai by heightening the "interspecies" merging of patients and animals. *Biosecurities,* 19, 31.

71. Mulvey, "Visual Pleasure."

72. As discussed in chapter 1, Ponepake Lapilio was one of a group of twelve boys who were returned to Kalihi Hospital for experimental treatments in 1895. His record and photographs are in Vol. 5, Box 3, HSA. A boy named Joseph William Lapilio was born on November 14, 1903, and he may have been Ponepake and Louisa Lui Lapilio's first child. Their other children were Bernardo (Benenato) Lapilio, born February 1905; Leilehua Lapilio, born March 1908; Fred Lui Lapilio, born June 1909; Anastasia (Annie) Lapilio, born May 1912; and Mary Ann Louisa Lapilio, born August 1913. After petitioning for re-examination with 160 other inmates from the settlement, Ponepake Lapilio was medically discharged as non-leprous in 1909, according to BOH meeting minutes from November 11, 1909. Of the fifty-six people declared non-leprous, fourteen applied to remain in the settlement as kōkua (unpaid caregivers). Lapilio was granted permission to serve as a kōkua for his wife Louisa, along with three others discharged. Later known as William Bonaface Lapilio, he returned to Honolulu after her death and cared for his grandchildren in Kaka'ako. Vol. 16 Minutes, HSA. The children's records are in 260 Box 30, HSA; HD-A, HSA; and HD-C; HSA.

73. Bernard Palikapu was born in 1870 and was from Hanalei, Kaua'i. He was admitted to leprosy detention in December 1897. He died at Molokai on October 23, 1919. Nathaniel B. Emerson took his case history on December 10, 1897, and recorded his name as Polikapu Keakuahanai. He was married and had no children. Case 05146, Box 5 (Medical Examination Records 1896–1898); MER, HSA. While his name is recorded variously as Palikapu and Polikapu in U.S. census and BOH records, his gravestone at St. Philomena Church in Kalawao reads "B. Palikapu." As of 1900, Palikapu and Ponepake Lapilio were living in Baldwin Home, the Catholic home for boys and men, in Kalawao. In addition to sharing a dormitory, Lapilio likely was Palikapu's pupil; the latter is listed as a schoolteacher and Lapilio "at school" in the 1900 U.S. census.

74. Pukui, Haertig, and Lee, *Nānā i Ke Kumu* 1:95, 98.

75. Joseph and Bernardo Lapilio were admitted to Kalihi Boys' Home on May 2, 1908. The brothers were released later from the Boys' Home and married women in Honolulu. 260 Box 30, HSA and HD-B, HSA.

76. Walter Johnson has offered an important caution against the romantic notion of "recovery" and the trope of agency in the writing of history of slavery. "On Agency."

77. Imada, *Aloha America,* 18, 63–64.

78. Wexler, "State of the Album."

79. Hagan, "Leprosy on the Hawaiian Islands." See Imada, *Aloha America,* on the valences of aloha during imperial expansion.

80. Povinelli, "Notes on Gridlock," 217. Bringing their interests in ethnography to bear, physicians George Fitch, Eduard Arning, Nathaniel B. Emerson, and Sidney Bourne Swift produced such genealogical grids to track the possible relationship between leprosy and biological relatedness. See Leprosy Cases, NBE; Fitch's record of Kaka'ako and Molokai cases in *Supplement,* 161–83; Swift, "Case of Keanu"; and Arning, "Eine Lepra-Impfung beim Menschen," 12. That leprosy appeared to run in some families, but not in others, troubled doctors. They debated theories of inheritance in which leprosy was passed from parent to child and discussed whether spouses transmitted leprosy through intercourse or cohabitation.

81. Leprosy Cases, NBE.

82. Agamben, *Homo Sacer,* 139. The existing literature on leprosy has tended to treat the modern practice of leprosy exile as the exertion of "total institutions" that consigned people to social death. See Goffman, *Asylums.* Bashford's *Imperial Hygiene* and Edmond's *Leprosy and Empire* focus on the rationale and ideological practices of institutionalization in colonial sites, while Anderson demonstrates the production of "biomedical citizenship" and inculcation of bodily and civilizational reform in the Culion, Philippines, leprosy colony. *Colonial Pathologies,* 168–71, 177–78.

83. Povinelli, "Notes on Gridlock." While the field of anthropology was built on the bedrock of genealogical and biological kinship, contemporary anthropologists theorize and track political-economic and social kinship in institutions, transnational adoption, gay and lesbian reproduction, and assisted reproductive technologies. Cartsen, *Cultures of Relatedness;* Kim, *Adopted Territory;* Strathern, "Displacing Knowledge"; Weston, *Families We Choose;* Yanagisako, *Producing Culture and Capital.*

84. Hawaiian genealogical and kinship connections are produced and defined through deeds, actions, and character, not blood, as J. Kēhaulani Kauanui has argued. Inclusive genealogical and kinship practices of Kānaka Maoli rely on principles of common descent, rather than blood quantum. Yet, the federal Hawaiian Homes Commission Act of 1921 designated homesteads only to those "native Hawaiians" who could prove 50 percent blood quantum. *Hawaiian Blood.* In a parallel arena, kinship in leprosy institutions during the territorial period was also defined narrowly through blood, marriage, and descent.

85. Here I am borrowing from scholars of family photography. Phu, Brown, and Dewan, "Family Camera Network"; Fleetwood, "Posing in Prison."

86. See Law, *Kalaupapa;* Inglis, *Ma'i Lepera;* Silva and Fernandez, "Mai Ka 'Āina." John R. K. Clark has republished numerous Hawaiian-language newspaper articles written about and by patients. Clark, *Kalaupapa Place Names.* Fred E. Woods discusses the history of Mormon patients in Kalaupapa, as well as short oral

histories with contemporary patients and stakeholders in the settlement. *Kalaupapa; Reflections of Kalaupapa.*

87. Baynton, "Disability," 33, 41.

88. In a contemporary context, Nirmalla Erevelles has analyzed the simultaneous racialization and disablement of students of color via the school-to-prison pipeline in *Disability and Difference.* Julie Livingston, Jasbir Puar, and Eunjung Kim have marked critical distinctions between debility and disability in their respective works. Livingston offers debility as supplement to disability that incorporates an ethos of communal care beyond a rights-based understanding of personhood. Debility, as sharpened by Puar, suggests an aggregate or population-based subordination, injury, or disability in which some bodies are made more vulnerable to incapacity by political, economic, military, and neoliberal capitalist forces. Kim has analyzed the debility produced in South Korea through an embrace of able-bodied heteronationalism in the wake of colonialism, war, and neoliberal economic regimes. I have chosen to rely on disability as a concept that incorporates an aggregate sense of incapacity and debility, as disability was mobilized by settlers in this particular way in Hawai'i. Livingston, *Improvising Medicine;* Puar, *Right to Maim,* xv–xvii; Kim, *Curative Violence,* 18–19.

89. Imada, "Decolonial Disability Studies?"; Bishop, *Why Are the Hawaiians Dying Out?*

90. Baynton, "Disability," 33.

91. Schweik, "Kicked to the Curb" and *Ugly Laws.* While not using the language of disability per se, Gussow and Tracy in an earlier assessment suggest that the deformity and helplessness associated with the disease produced the Western stigma of leprosy. Gussow and Tracy, "Stigma," 444.

92. Letter from E. Cook Webb, MD, June 12, 1886; 334-34, HSA. In general, when the disease had progressed or was deemed incurable, patients were shipped out of sight to Kalawao and Kalaupapa settlements on Molokai. Otherwise they were detained at Kalihi Hospital in waterfront Honolulu, where they were more accessible to family members, friends, and business associates.

93. Sharon L. Snyder and David T. Mitchell have described disability as "systems of anticipatory classification . . . based on bodily aesthetics rather than literal abilities." *Cultural Locations,* 41.

94. Fitch, "Leprosy," 544.

95. Fitch, "Appendix E," xxxiv.

96. Segregation of Lepers, 5 Haw. 162 (1884).

97. Physician Nathaniel Emerson, lamenting the care and devotion Hawaiians bestowed on leprous loved ones, wrote, ". . . [C]all it what you will it is a blindness that not less severely leads to death." Emerson, Report to President of the Board of Health (1879); EMR 188; Box 5, NBE.

98. Nakamura, "Spectacle of Disability (Studies) in the Age of Trump."

99. The 'ō'ō is a forest bird endemic to Hawai'i, likely now extinct, and valued for its beautiful yellow feathers. Kealakai, "He Hoomanao Kanikau." An English-language translation of the kanikau is in Clark, *Kalaupapa Place Names,* 337–38. Kealakai also

may have composed an ardent love song, "Nuuanu Waipunu a Kealoha" (Nuuanu's spring waters), for his first wife, Akiu Haupu, as the 1894 kanikau describes Akiu as his "beloved wife from the cliffs of Nuuanu." Akiu Haupu's clinical record notes that she entered detention in 1891, escaped from the settlement in September 1892, was recaptured in September 1893, and died in August 1894. Mekia's younger brother, Charles Nakipi, was also exiled in 1891 and died in Kalaupapa in May 1898. Mekia Kealakai was not a leprosy patient. A talented musician, he became a well-known troubadour with the anticolonial Hawaiian National Band in 1895–1896 and on Hawaiian music circuits in the early 1900s. HD-3, HSA; Imada, *Aloha America,* 114, 115, 149–50.

100. Imada, *Aloha America,* analyzes how the staging of gendered hula performance encouraged and eased the incorporation of Hawai'i into an American insular empire.

101. Musick, *Hawaii, Our New Possessions,* 91.

102. Imada, *Aloha America,* 11, 67–68, 154. Hula had become the dominant imagery of Hawai'i by the 1930s, eclipsing leprosy.

103. Browne, *Paradise of the Pacific,* 196.

104. "Series of Gross Misstatements," *Hawaiian Gazette,* November 9, 1909; 334-37, HSA. The article protested the "brand of misinformation being published in a section of the Northwest from which Honolulu hopes to attract tourists and settlers."

105. This woman's mother was Frances Nahinu, who died in 1936.

106. Decades later, at the age of eighty-one, this woman found her mother's gravesite at Kalaupapa. Other performers, such as Mekia Kealakai (see note 99), had kin incarcerated in the settlement, while others had ancestral ties to Molokai lands that were expropriated for use by the Board of Health. These were Kini Kapahukulaokamāmalu and Jennie Napua Woodd. Leprosy incarceration was perhaps one of the harshest instantiations of settler colonialism, pushing Native Hawaiians to seek opportunity structures outside of Hawai'i, including in commercial entertainment circuits.

107. Love, *Feeling Backward,* 4. My use of queerness signifies disqualified non-normativity, rather than same-sex desire or practices.

108. Hoppe, *Punishing Disease.* Hoppe does not draw this explicit connection between leprosy and HIV.

109. Henry Nalaielua described the feeling of "degrading, humiliating, shaming . . . where I was stared at, poked and prodded, like a bug you then step on." Nalaielua, *No Footprints,* 19.

110. A vocal cohort of Hawaiian patients wrote letters to newspapers, submitted petitions to Papa Ola, and signed petitions against the U.S. annexation of Hawai'i in the late 1800s. See Silva and Fernandez, "Mai Ka 'Āina." On 1970s self-determination, see Trask, "Birth."

111. To save money, the state of Hawai'i wanted to centralize HD care at another hospital, against the express desire of patients. On this patient movement, see *Hale Mohalu* and "Save Hale Mohalu News" 2, no. 2 (March 1979); Folder 1; CMR.

112. For example, the United Nations campaign and its traveling exhibits on ending Hansen's disease stigma was entitled "Quest for Dignity." Likewise, July

1998, featuring the display at Honolulu Hale, was designated "Quest for Dignity Month." Law, *Collective History*, 485–87. Current commemorative efforts include erecting a plaque of approximately eight thousand names of exiled patients in the Makanalua peninsula.

113. Regina Kunzel astutely analyzes how gay activist efforts in the 1970s to disavow stigma, claim pride, and align homosexuality with health also functioned as a "project in normativity and exclusion." "Queer History," 316, 318. See also Halperin and Traub, "Beyond Gay Pride," 3–8.

114. Anne White, "Isle of Exile," *Beacon Magazine of Hawaii,* February 1968; Folder NHDM-19576.9; SSC. In January 1969, *Beacon* put Marks on its cover again as "Man of the Year." Marks railed against the hypocrisy of being treated as an outcast while being told it was against state law to name a person a "leper," himself included.

115. Noelani Goodyear-Kaʻōpua has outlined useful principles of engagement for "ethical Hawaiian studies research." "Reproducing Ropes," 14.

116. Smith, *Decolonizing Methodologies.*

117. Three patients I met at the Molokai settlement have since passed away.

118. Simpson, "On Ethnographic Refusal." Taking up Simpson, Tuck and Yang have urged active forms of refusal toward settler colonial social science research that voices only the pain of subaltern people. Tuck and Yang, "R Words."

119. "Topside" is a colloquial term for the rest of Molokai, excluding the Makanalua peninsula. Kalawao and Kalaupapa rest two thousand feet below mountainous cliffs; hence "topside" for the portion of Molokai above it.

120. Descendants of two enslaved people of African descent named Renty and Delia, among seven men and women photographed for a series of medical daguerreotypes in 1850, filed a lawsuit against Harvard University, which owns the photographs. The plaintiffs argue that the photographs are stolen property. Schuessler, "Your Ancestors Were Slaves."

121. Dolmage, *Disabled upon Arrival;* Livingston, *Improvising Medicine;* Sharpe, *In the Wake,* 118–19; and Caswell, *Archiving the Unspeakable,* 163. I have also benefited greatly from conversations with Susan Burch and Regina Kunzel about their ethical use of medical records and names in historical research on the psychiatric incarceration of Native American women and queer histories of psychiatry, respectively.

122. Caswell, *Archiving the Unspeakable,* 163.

123. Feminist disability scholars Ellen Samuels and Izetta Autumn Mobley, in their respective discussions of performers Millie and Christine McCoy, include self-reflexive discussions of how they are using images of disability in their scholarly work. Samuels chose to crop commercial portraits of the McCoy sisters. Samuels, "Examining Millie and Christine McKoy," 70–71, 74–75; Mobley, "Troublesome Properties."

124. Prosser, *Light in the Dark Room.*

125. Hattori, "Re-membering the Past," 317.

126. Susan C. Lawrence discusses how privacy protections for the living, such as the provisions in the Health Insurance Portability and Accountability Act

(HIPAA), are complicating preservation of and access to materials about deceased individuals. *Privacy and the Past*, 17. Relying on interviews with scholars who have accessed and analyzed medical records for historical research and confronted ethical, legal, and pragmatic conundrums, Lawrence argues that historians "need to make deeply contextual decisions" about weighing medical disclosure and the protection of individual privacy. On related challenges posed for archives holding medical information, see Novak Gustainis and Letocha, "Practice of Privacy."

127. Motivated by similar concerns about privacy, memory, and the uneven exposure of Indigenous people, women, and people with disabilities in historical works, scholars have deployed different naming and disclosure tactics. Alice Wexler began using pseudonyms in her research on the history of Huntington's disease, a fatal genetic disease, but shifted to the real names of deceased people in order to lessen stigma. Susan Reverby used select pseudonyms to protect the memories of some family members of African American survivors of Tuskegee syphilis experiments. Susan Burch included actual names of American Indian women incarcerated in South Dakota's Canton Asylum (though the names were available in archives) only when the women's families granted permission. See Lawrence, *Privacy and the Past*, 108–10; Wexler, *Woman Who Walked into the Sea;* Reverby; *Examining Tuskegee;* and Burch, "Dislocated Histories," 143.

128. S. K. M. Nahauowaileia's letters from Kalawao dated August 27, 1909, were published as "Papa Inoa o Na Mai Lepera" in *Ka Nupepa Kuokoa,* September 3, 1909, and "Na Mea Hou o Kalaupapa" in *Kuokoa Home Rula,* September 3, 1909. His letter dated October 19, 1909, was published as "Nanaia Na Ma'i o Molokai" in *Ka Nupepa Kuokoa,* October 29, 1909. S. K. Maialoha's letter dated August 2, 1909, was published as "Na Mea Hou o ke Kahua Ma'i," in *Ke Aloha Aina*, September 4, 1909. I gratefully acknowledge Sahoa Fukushima's blog, nupepa-hawaii.com, which alerted me to these articles. The writer used two poetic pen names, Nahauowaileia (the dews of Waileia) and Waikakulu (a freshwater pool). Marriage, 1910 U.S. census, and HSA BOH records suggest S. K. Maialoha was a man, possibly with the full name S. Maialoha Kapela. Clark; *Kalaupapa Place Names*, 297–98, 309. While writing as Nahauowaileia, Maialoha included his names "Maialoha" and "Kapela, Maialoha" in the list of patient-petitioners published in *Ka Nupepa Kuokoa,* September 3, 1909, and *Kuokoa Home Rula,* September 3, 1909.

129. For example, a woman patient named Mrs. H. P. Paniani wrote a moving tribute and mourning poem on October 5, 1912, to her deceased friend, a Mrs. Kalamau, who resided at Bishop Home with the writer. As memorialized by her friend, Mrs. Kalamau hailed from Pahala, Ka'ū, Hawai'i, and she was exiled from March 29, 1912, until her death on September 27, 1912. Paniani, "Hoomanao Ana i Ka Mea i Hala."

130. In some HD communities in Japan and Louisiana, patients were given a new name upon entering the leprosarium to protect their families from stigma, although this was not the case in Hawai'i.

131. Pukui, Haertig, and Lee, *Nānā i Ke Kumu* 2:290.

132. Pukui, Haertig, and Lee, *Nānā i Ke Kumu* 1:94–95, 100–101.

133. In the context of contemporary Inuit society, anthropologist Lisa Stevenson has discussed Inuit names as similarly outlasting the physical body, and their significance for individual and community survival. *Life Beside Itself,* 125–26.

CHAPTER 1. OCULAR EXPERIMENTS AND UNRULY TECHNOLOGIES OF THE BODY

Arning, "Appendix I," xliii.

1. Nathaniel B. Emerson was posted as resident physician at Kalawao from 1878 to 1880. He later served as president of the Board of Health, from October 1887 to January 1, 1890.

2. Pukui and Elbert defined pōhaka as splotches and spots in *Hawaiian Dictionary,* 334. Emerson described pohaka as patches of skin, irregular in shape or color in Leprosy Cases, NBE.

3. Leprosy Cases, NBE, 355.

4. Leprosy Cases, NBE, 111–13. Emerson described William Keliaka, kāne (male), age thirty-five, from Lāhainā, Maui, on October 25, 1879. His sketch is on p. 113.

5. Leprosy Cases, NBE, 120–22. Emerson described Iana Puhi, kāne (male), age forty-three, from Ka'ū, Hawai'i, October 29, 1879. His sketch is on p. 120.

6. Leprosy Cases, NBE, 361. The man Emerson described and sketched was Lolo Kuila, kāne (male), twenty-one years, Waikāne, Ko'olaupoko, O'ahu, July 19, 1880.

7. Leprosy Cases, NBE, 305. This woman was named Margaret Kahaulolio from Hilo, Hawai'i, and her case history spanned from 1879 to 1882.

8. Bushnell, "Dr. Edward Arning." Bushnell's article provides illuminating context as well as a lively read. Bushnell later created a character based on Arning for his historical novel *Molokai.* In addition to writing novels and medical history, Bushnell was a professional microbiologist in Hawai'i.

9. George Fitch, BOH physician at the Kaka'ako Branch Hospital and Molokai settlement, reported an average of 750 patients at Kalawao in 1884. Fitch also noted that the Kaka'ako Branch Hospital had received 531 patients, of which 365 were removed to Kalawao. Fitch, "General Report," 140, 142.

10. Arning photographed European settler families and the cultural activities of Japanese immigrant laborers and New Hebrideans, but his subjects were mainly Native Hawaiian people, landscapes, seascapes, and material culture.

11. Arning used terms like "anesthetica," "tuberosa," and "maculosa" to classify types of leprosy in patients. "Anesthetic" corresponds to a later twentieth-century classification of tuberculoid leprosy, which is less contagious, while "tuberosa" (tubercular) became known as lepromatous, the more severe contagious type of leprosy. Ester Kanepuu was likely a girl named Ekekela Kanepuu. She entered leprosy detention on March 16, 1884, along with Halakii Kanepuu, who may have been her sister or mother. They were from Iwilei, O'ahu. Vol. 2, Box 1, HSA. Ester Kanepuu's photograph is ALA, p. 12, and listed as negative no. 3.27.

12. Dermatologists in the nineteenth century experimented with photographic material and technologies to illustrate dermatological conditions and pathological types. Neuse et al., "History of Photography," 1494.

13. Arnsteiner Patres is known in English as the Congregation of the Sacred Hearts of Jesus and Mary, or by its acronym SS.CC. It relocated several times from Aachen to Lahnstein, and now is in Werne, Germany.

14. Many of these are the only known copies of Arning's photographs, which likely were shot on dry plate negatives.

15. The Congregation of the Sacred Hearts of Jesus and Mary were the first Roman Catholic missionaries to Hawai'i, arriving in 1827. Ching, "Portraits of Kalaupapa Residents," 146. Belgian priest Damien de Veuster was from this congregation. Arning diagnosed Damien with leprosy at Kalawao, Molokai, in 1884. Damien died of leprosy in 1889 and became world famous as the "martyr priest."

16. After suitably posing and lighting a subject, a photographer inserted the dry glass plate into a holder in the camera. He would slide the cover from the plate holder, thereby uncovering the plate, and then uncover and re-cover the camera lens. The exposure time was less than a second. After the cover was slid back over the dry plate, the plate was removed for processing in a darkroom. In the darkroom, the glass plate negative was developed by moistening the plate and covering it with developing fluid. After the image emerged, the fluid was washed off. The plate was placed in a bath of fixing solution, washed, and dried. The glass negative then could be used to print an image onto light-sensitive paper. The paper was fixed to the negative with a frame. The paper was exposed to natural or artificial light until the image appeared, then it was washed in water, toner, fixing solution, and finally dried. https://pastonglass.wordpress.com/2016/02/16/getting-the-picture-understanding-the-basics-of-glass-plate-negative-photography/.

17. To my knowledge, these albums are the only two extant that demonstrate Arning's process of category making. Anthropologist Adrienne L. Kaeppler located approximately 237 glass plate negatives of Arning's in the Hamburg Museum of Ethnology (Hamburgisches Museum für Völkerkunde), but these were not assembled in albums. Prints of these negatives are in the HHS and described in Kaeppler, "Eduard Arning's Hawaiian Collections."

18. Arning did not title this album of leprosy photographs. However, he categorized the latter images as "Lepra" (Leprosy) in his corresponding catalogue of negative plates, CPNP. The lepra album includes a few images of Europeans with eczema, psoriasis, and lupus in 1889 and 1890, taken in Germany upon his return.

19. Arning, "Lecture by Eduard Arning," 51.

20. Penny, *Objects of Culture,* 31. Bastian said natural people would "succumb to a quick physical decline and die out." Quoted in Zimmerman, "Adventures," 161.

21. Arning, "Lecture by Eduard Arning," 53.

22. Osorio, *Dismembering Lāhui.*

23. Nathaniel B. Emerson was one member of the "Hawaiian League," a group of haole (white foreigner) men that forced King David Kalākaua to sign the Bayonet

Constitution in 1887. The Bayonet Constitution severely limited the Hawaiian monarch's powers. Osorio, *Dismembering Lāhui,* 197.

24. Bishop, "Why Are the Hawaiians Dying Out?"

25. Fitch, "Etiology of Leprosy," 298, 302.

26. As historians of medicine and disability have pointed out, people with disabilities were used for experiments in the nineteenth and twentieth centuries, but Arning and his contemporaries operated with far less discretion outside of continental Europe and North America. See Lederer, *Subjected to Science,* 7–9, on experiments on institutionalized people. Arning's contemporary, British physician Arthur Mouritz, conducted experiments on non-leprous kin of leprosy patients at the Molokai settlement from 1884 to 1887; see chapter 3.

27. Historian H. Glenn Penny has discussed this collecting as the "relentless empiricism" of nineteenth-century German ethnology that produced the world's largest ethnographic museum, more than a decade before colonial territorial expansion. *Objects of Culture,* 3.

28. According to the 1865 Act to Prevent the Spread of Leprosy and subsequent laws in Hawai'i, people determined to have leprosy also were treated as living dead. George Fitch described them as those "civilly dead, while mortally living." Fitch, "Appendix A," vi.

29. Bergmann, "Tödliche Menschenexperimente," 144. This sourcing of bodies is not unique in the history of biomedicine. Enslaved African women, for instance, were an invaluable resource for pioneering gynecologists, as Laura Briggs has discussed. Zimmerman has analyzed the German "skin trade" of natural scientists, which relied on prisons, graveyards, and colonies to source bodies for nineteenth-century science. Briggs, "Race of Hysteria," 249–50; and Zimmerman, "Adventures."

30. George Fitch described the site of the Kaka'ako Branch Hospital as "most wretchedly chosen" and prone to flooding. "General Report," 142.

31. The seven men Arning named were Kaniu, C. Stillwell, W. Cook, T. Birch, Luhilea, C. Shawn, and Kalua. The four "females," both young girls and women, were Ester (Ekekela) Kanepuu, Halaki Kanepuu, Ellen Davis, and Emele. Letter from Eduard Arning to W. M. Gibson, December 20, 1884; 334-35, HSA.

32. Arning, "Appendix I," xlv.

33. Zimmerman, "Adventures," 157.

34. Lederer states, "At no time were American investigators free to do whatever they pleased with their human subjects. Neither their peers nor the public would have stood for reckless experimentation that endangered human lives." *Subjected to Science,* xv–xvi.

35. In a different locale in the Jim Crow South, carceral physicians at convict camps sometimes treated prisoners in order to enable the latter to labor, as Sarah Haley has discussed in *No Mercy Here,* 75.

36. On November 14, 1883, Fitch inoculated six leprous girls with syphilis; all were under the age of twelve. Fitch, "Leprosy," 544. Fitch also requested the use of death-row prisoner Mendosa for an experiment, but was turned down right before Arning's application for Keanu. Nicholas Turse has described the "experimental

ethos" that enabled physicians to gain access to colonized and subordinated bodies, including in the "neocolony" of Hawai'i. "Experimental Dreams," 139.

37. Arning, "Appendix I," liii.

38. The organism was often a human patient. Lederer, *Subjected to Science*, 3. Gerhard Armauer Hansen, who had discovered the leprosy microbe, was removed from his position as medical director of leprosy hospitals in Bergen, Norway, for attempting to inoculate a female patient's eye with leprosy in 1879.

39. Neisser discovered the bacteria *gonococcus* in 1879.

40. Arning, "Appendix I," xlii.

41. Arning, "Appendix E," lxi.

42. Arning, "Appendix I," lxii.

43. Arning, "Appendix I," xliii.

44. Latour, *Science in Action*, 4.

45. The murder trial was described in *Pacific Commercial Advertiser*, July 15, 1884; *Daily Bulletin*, August 1, 1884. Keanu's father Kuliaiou (possibly Kuliouou) was from Kohala and his mother, Keawe, from Makapala, both located in northern Hawai'i island. Arning, "Eine Lepra-Impfung beim Menschen," 11.

46. *Daily Bulletin*, September 22, 1884.

47. This claim of no family history of leprosy would be proven false. Sidney Bourne Swift, the resident physician at the Molokai settlement during this period, established a history of leprosy among Keanu's family members after Arning's experiment. These kin included Keanu's son Eokepa and his nephew David. Swift, "Case of Keanu."

48. Arning, "Eine Lepra-Impfung beim Menschen."

49. Parts of Arning's experiment on Keanu are described in Mouritz, *Path of the Destroyer*, 154, and Fitch, "Leprosy," 534. In 1919, a Hawaiian writer identified the girl in the experiment as a "Emale" (transliterated as "Emily" in English). A girl named "Emele," about age eleven, was apprehended at the Honolulu police station on June 28, 1884. The mid-1884 date makes the latter a possible match to the girl in Arning's September 1884 experiment. "He Ma'i Lele I'o Anei Ka Ma'i Lepera?" (Is Leprosy Truly a Contagious Disease?) *Ka Nupepa Kuokoa*, March 28, 1919, in Clark, *Kalaupapa Place Names*, 145. The police record is in 334-34, HSA. Arning also may have photographed this girl at Kaka'ako Hospital; she may be the subject of photographs labeled as negatives 3.29 and 3.30, in ALA.

50. Keanu would not develop symptoms of leprosy until after Arning had returned to Germany.

51. "Contagious Nature of Leprosy"; Morrow, "Personal Observations"; Swift, "Case of Keanu"; "Etiology of Leprosy"; "Alleged Communication of Leprosy"; Montgomery, "Report of Histological Examination"; and Tebb, *Recrudescence*.

52. Arning's contemporary Albert Neisser injected female prostitutes with syphilis in Germany ca. 1898. British leprologist Tebb called Arning's experiment "utterly unjustifiable." Tebb, *Recrudescence of Leprosy*, 125.

53. Articles that discuss Arning's medical experiments do not analyze his photographs, even if they reprint them. Turse, "Experimental Dreams"; Bushnell,

"Dr. Edward Arning"; and Bergmann, "Tödliche Menschenexperimente." Meanwhile, Arning's ethnographic photography has garnered separate attention. Kaeppler, "Eduard Arning."

54. Arning listed the series of glass plate negatives made of Keanu as 2.13, 2.14, 2.15, and 2.16 in his handwritten "Anthropologie" catalogue, CPNP. Photograph 2.13 of Keanu is at the Hamburg Museum of Ethnology and HHS. Photographs 2.14, 2.15, and 2.16 of Keanu were listed in CPNP, but the negatives are not in the Hamburg Museum of Ethnology. Their location is currently unknown.

55. Arning's original German for negative no. 2.13 reads, "Keanu. Hawaiian. Front. Ganze figur." HHS in Honolulu retains a copy of Arning's negative plate catalogue handwritten in German and a commissioned English-language translation. CPNP.

56. Arning, "Eine Lepra-Impfung beim Menschen," 12.

57. Arning, "Appendix I," xliv.

58. Arning, "Eine Lepra-Impfung beim Menschen," 15–16.

59. CPNP. Photographs of Kina and Kahalelau listed as 2.25a, 2.25b, 2.25c, and 2.26a, 2.26b, and 2.26c are not in the HHS, and their location is unknown. M.C.'s photograph 2.27a is in the collection, but 2.27b, 2.27c, and 2.27d are missing.

60. Arning's arrival in Hawai'i was noted in *Ko Hawaii Paeaina*, November 17, 1883, and posted on nupepa-hawaii.com on December 21, 2017. Sahoa Fukushima's nupepa-hawaii.com provides significant Hawaiian-language sources on Hansen's disease, Kalaupapa, and Kalawao. Over thirty years after Arning's departure, an exiled Hawaiian patient at Kalaupapa discussed Arning's leprosy experiments in detail. He cited it as proof that leprosy was not contagious, save "when the infected pus enters or is inserted into a body in good health." "He Ma'i Lele I'o Anei Ka Ma'i Lepera?," 145.

61. Hawaiians came dressed in their finest to sugar plantation engineer Christian Hedemann's home photography studio in Hāna, Maui, to have their portraits taken on Sunday in the early 1880s. Twenty years earlier, Hawaiians living in the remote district of Ka'ū wrote a newspaper to ask photographers to come to their communities. *Ka Hae Hawaii*, November 27, 1861; Davis, *Photographer in the Kingdom*, 55.

62. Anthropometric photography had been developed in Europe in the 1860s and 1870s, as exemplified by the influential racial projects of T. H. Huxley and John Lamprey. The British Huxley advised photographing individual nude subjects in full length using front and profile views, while Lamprey's method involved placing nude subjects against a mesh measuring grid, also in front and profile views. These methods were taken up in various European colonial and penal sites in the British Empire, including Australia. Edwards, "Photographic 'Types.'"

63. Arning, "Eine Lepra-Impfung beim Menschen," 12.

64. Pualokelani was listed as subject of negatives 2.18a, 2.18b, and 2.18c in CPNP. Prints of these negatives are in HHS. The skin color scale Arning used may correspond to the skin color table developed by his mentor, the anthropologist-pathologist Rudolf Virchow. Zimmerman, *Anthropology*, 21.

65. Arning's negatives of Kealoha are listed as 39.a, 39.b., and 39.c in CPNP, and include a photograph of her back and buttocks. Arning's caption describing Kealoha in ALA differs slightly from his fuller notation in CPNP. The latter three negatives of Kealoha, as translated from German, read, "3.39a. Kealoha, girl, 13 years old, in Kakaako. Leprosy papulocircinata. Full figure. Front. 3.39b. The same. Full Figure. Back. 3.39c. The same. Part of the back." Although Arning indicated Kealoha's age as sixteen in his ALA caption, his CPNP notes, as well as BOH and census records, indicate she was about thirteen years old in 1885.

66. Arning collected other wooden kiʻi (symbolic representations of Hawaiian deities) and photographed them. He described the origins of this particular figure: "When in March 1884, Chinese workers turned an old taro plantation near Wailuakai, Kauaʻi, into a rice field, Pukalu, a Hawaiian teacher, found a roughly carved ʻahakea wood sculpture. Together with the base, it is 92 cm high; the figure itself is 37.5 cm high. According to the Hawaiian Kahele in Lihue, it represents the god Luaalii, a guardian god to whom the Hawaiians prayed before going on a journey by sea or by land and before going to war." Arning, "Old Hawaiʻi," 215. Luaaliʻi's exhumation from Hawaiian land was tied to the kingdom's political economy, which was increasingly subject to Western economic development, trade, and treaties. Large-scale plantations like the rice plantation referred to in Arning's passage were operated by Euro-American businessmen and supported by cheap immigrant labor from Asia. To my knowledge, a deity named "Luaalii" is not discussed in extant Hawaiian-language historiography or newspapers. Nor was it referenced in contemporaneous chants or oratory.

67. Arning, "Appendix I," xliii.

68. Stoler, *Archival* Grain, 65–66.

69. Fatima Tobing Rony has theorized this taxidermic gaze. Writing of Edward Curtis, Rony believes that the taxidermic impulse of the filmmaker requires that Nanook be "always dead" in order to look alive. *Third Eye,* 116.

70. Arning, "Appendix I," xxxvii.

71. Arning, "Eine Lepra-Impfung beim Menschen," 12.

72. Arning, "Old Hawaiʻi," 81, 107, 109.

73. Letter from Eduard Arning to Nathaniel Emerson, May 10, 1888, p. 6; 334–35, HSA.

74. Arning, "Appendix I," liii. Arning probably exhumed this body in 1884.

75. These activities did not go unnoticed by Hawaiians. One newspaper reported that Arning had ordered bodies exhumed at Kalawao in order to study them. *Ke Ola o Hawaii,* March 22, 1884 (posted on nupepa-hawaii.com, December 22, 2017).

76. *Ka Nupepa Kuokoa,* June 13, 1885, 3 (posted on nupepa-hawaii.com, December 22, 2017).

77. Arning, "Old Hawaiʻi," 259.

78. The pathologist-anthropologist Rudolf Virchow, who was Arning's field research sponsor for Hawaiʻi, for instance, recommended that travelers bring back bones, hair, salted skin, and dried hands. These could be collected at public executions, prisons, hospitals, and battlefields. Zimmerman, *Anthropology,* 158–59.

79. Pukui, Haertig, and Lee, *Nānā i Ke Kumu* 1:108–9, 111–12. These sacred relationships between iwi, land, and ancestors are invoked in significant terms, such as kulāiwi (land of bones, or a homeland) and ʻōiwi (a person whose bones are the land, meaning a Native person). On iwi repatriation, see Abad, "Long Journey"; Wong, "Iwi Kūpuna"; Ayau, "Hui Mālama."

80. Sharp, along with the geographer William Libbey from Princeton University, took approximately sixteen human skulls from "superficial graves" along the coast at Kīpūkai, Kauaʻi. These skulls were deposited in the Academy of Natural Sciences in Philadelphia. Allen, "Study of Hawaiian Skulls."

81. "State Medical Society of Pennsylvania," 601. Benjamin Sharp's lantern slide collection is in Collection 349, Benjamin Sharp papers and glass lantern slides, 1844–1893, Academy of Natural Sciences, Philadelphia.

82. In 1889, the Board of Health reprimanded William T. Brigham for taking unauthorized photographs for Morrow. Brigham later became director of the Bernice Pauahi Bishop Museum of Polynesian Ethnology and Natural History in Honolulu. Letter from William Brigham, November 14, 1889; 334-14, HSA. Morrow later published some of these images in "Personal Observations; "Leprosy"; and *Leprosy*.

83. Morrow, "Personal Observations," 85.

84. Ibid. He gave this illustrated lecture on July 6, 1889.

85. Morrow, "Leprosy and Annexation," 587.

86. Arning, "Lecture by Eduard Arning," 53.

87. Steeno, "Eduard Arning."

88. Arning, "Eine Lepra-Impfung beim Menschen," 21.

89. Garland Thomson, "Seeing the Disabled," 348.

90. On the medical gaze, Foucault, *Birth of the Clinic*, 29.

91. Zimmerman, "Adventures," 158.

92. Arning, "Appendix I"; "Appendix O," xl and lvii–lviii.

93. Arning's proposed salary would have been donated by prominent white "gentlemen" residing in Hawaiʻi, including Charles R. Bishop and J. B. Atherton. "Appendix U," lxi. Arning remained a sore point decades later for some members of the BOH, including President Charles B. Cooper, who complained in 1904 that Arning had refused to leave his scientific research in Hawaiʻi. The board since learned to stipulate that research produced by physicians in its employ remain BOH property. U.S. Treasury Department, Public Health and Marine-Hospital Service, *Transactions*, 94.

94. Letter from Eduard Arning to Nathaniel Emerson, May 10, 1888; 334-35 Arning, HSA.

95. Letter from N. B. Emerson and "Committee on Treatment of Leprosy," May 9, 1885; EMR 208, Box 6, NBE.

96. Vol. 5, Box 3, HSA.

97. Vol. 5, Box 3, HSA. This report, dated January 1, 1895, was written by James T. Wayson, MD. Furthermore, lead bacteriologist Luis Alvarez did not care enough, it seems, to take any photographs of these experimental treatments to the 1897 Leprosy Congress in Berlin, where he served as Hawaiʻi's official delegate and

presented a report on the experiment. *Report . . . for the Biennial Period Ending December 31, 1897,* 92–94.

98. Vol. 7 Minutes, HSA. Also see chapter 2.

99. Sekula, "Body and the Archive," 6.

100. Buerger, "Art Photography," 1–2. Arning's artistic and professional pursuits are described in Steeno, "Eduard Arning." The Hamburg photograph society was the Gesellschaft zur Förderung der Amateur-Photographie (Society for the Promotion of Amateur Photography).

101. Arning's photograph *Sonnenschein,* which used his wife Helene Sophie as a subject, was published in the photo journal *Photographische Rundschau* (1896). See also 1898 and 1899 issues of *Die Kunst in der Photographie.* Examples of his other work are in *Kunstphotographie um 1900,* 66–71, 180–82.

102. Arning remained at St. Georg Hospital until his retirement in 1924, after achieving several promotions. Steeno, "Eduard Arning."

103. Ruthard von Frankenberg, email message to author, October 25, 2013.

104. Arning did not notate all of the names of his subjects in the lepra album (ALA) or negative catalogue (CPNP). Kahalemake was from Lahaina, Maui. He was born ca. 1870 and sent to Molokai in March 1884 at age fourteen. Arning photographed him at the Molokai settlement in May 1885; his photograph is ALA, p. 29, and negative no. 3.37, CPNP. He died February 9, 1890, at age twenty. Joseph Kulanui, identified by Arning as "Kulanui," was from Hāna, Maui, and entered leprosy detention on October 24, 1885, around the age of eight. His photographs are ALA, pp. 36–37, and nos. 3.45a and 3.45b, CPNP. Kulanui died February 23, 1894, at age seventeen. The woman Arning identified as Lahela, age sixty, Kakaako Hospital, in CPNP no. 3.31, and ALA p. 24, was likely Lahela Hookualana, who was from Kōloa, Kauaʻi. She entered leprosy detention on November 13, 1883, and died November 22, 1890, at age sixty-three. Arning also indicated he made a plaster mask of Lahela. HD-3, HSA.

105. Kealoha was born about 1872 and was from the ʻEwa district of Oʻahu. Kealoha and Lui Nailima had at least nine children between 1891 and 1908: Anna E. Nailima, born 1891; Kane Nailima, born 1892 or 1893; Joseph Hoaeae Nailima, born 1894; Kuheleloa Nailima, born 1896; [Louis] Kahalewai Nailima, born 1897; Benedicta Waialii, born 1902; Wahineaukai Nailima, born 1903; Kaka Nailima, born 1907; and Mileka Nailima, born 1908. HD-A; HD-C; HD-3; HD-5, HSA.

106. Stoler, *Carnal Knowledge.*

107. By my estimate, the portrait was taken around 1915. The photographer, probably a father or brother of the Catholic mission in the settlement, is unknown. Many patient portraits in the early 1900s appear to have been taken by Father Paul-Marie (Joseph) Julliotte, whose dates of residence in Kalaupapa were 1901 to 1907. Based on the sons' ages in the photograph, the Nailima portrait likely was taken after Julliotte's 1907 departure from the settlement.

108. Brilliant, *Portraiture,* 13–18. Portraits "concretize the individual portrayed," as Brilliant writes. The portrait, however, is not an inherently stable category separate from ethnographic science. In early twentieth-century Germany, the photogra-

pher August Sander would marshal the portrait-photograph for a comparative study of types, what Walter Benjamin would call "an atlas of instruction," leading from the peasant to the "highest representatives of civilization" and back down to "imbeciles." Benjamin, "Short History," 21, 22.

109. *Hawaiian Gazette,* June 4, 1909; 334-37, HSA; "Now 171 Lepers Knocking at the Door of Hope," *Hawaiian Star,* August 24, 1909. Nailima family members, including Kuheleloa Nailima, Kahalewai Nailima, and Hoaeae Nailima, were named as 3 of the 133 re-examination candidates in Nahauowaileia, "Na Mea Hou"; "Papa Inoa"; and "Nanaia Na Maʻi."

110. The infant Kuheleloa Nailima was born in August 1917 and died two months later. Louis Kahalewai Nailima and Keahi Humphreys Schutte married in 1919 and would have at least three more children: Claude, Margaret, and Elaine. Keahi Schutte was also known as Mary Keahi Schutte; her parents were from Hawaiʻi island. Upon being diagnosed with leprosy in 1913–1914, Keahi Schutte left behind a husband, a German-Hawaiian man named Claude Schutte, and their children in Honolulu. Despite legal and medical mandates that separated them, people continued to express and perform enduring connections. Claude Schutte died in an accident on Oʻahu in 1917. When Keahi Schutte and Kahalewai Nailima had a son in May 1923, they named him Claude, the same name as Keahi's first husband. HD-A; HD-B; HD-C; HD-3; HD-5; 260 Box 30, HSA.

CHAPTER 2. A CRIMINAL ARCHIVE OF SKIN

1. Daland, "Leprosy in the Hawaiian Islands."

2. Goodhue, "Surgical Cure," 267.

3. John (Keoni) Kapuahi's record is case 148, Box 14 (Medical Examination Records 1901–1902); MER, HSA. Kapuahi was unmarried and from Kalihi-waena in Honolulu. He was exiled to Molokai on March 18, 1902, and died December 14, 1910. HD-3, HSA.

4. The detention compound to which I refer is Kalihi Hospital and Detention Station, which operated from 1865 to 1875 and 1889 to 1949. A separate facility in nearby Kakaʻako, the Branch Hospital and Receiving Station, opened in 1881 and closed in 1888. Kalihi Hospital, as it was commonly known, was also called "Kalihi Receiving Station" until ca. 1908. Kalihi Hospital admitted and examined people suspected of having leprosy. Those deemed incurable were sent to Molokai settlement. By the early twentieth century, Kalihi Hospital had expanded to a compound that included a receiving building, separate men's and women's quarters, infirmary, and a keeper's cottage. By the 1930s, Kalihi had a social hall, school, chapel, and playground. After closing in 1949, Kalihi Hospital was replaced by Hale Mōhalu in Pearl City, Oʻahu, which provided rehabilitation services. Meaning "the edge" in Hawaiian, Kalihi was an ahupuaʻa (land division running from the uplands to the sea) in the moku (district) of Honolulu on the mokupuni (island) of Oʻahu. Kalihi Hospital was located in Kalihi Kai (the seaward area of Kalihi) at the makai

(seaward) end of Puʻuhale Road. Photographs and textual descriptions are in *Molokai Settlement* and Binford, "History and Study."

5. Photographs may have been incorporated into leprosy segregation practices in other global sites by the mid-twentieth century. A class-action lawsuit filed in 2016 by Hansen's disease patients against the Japanese government notes that photographs were part of some patient documentation and incarceration practices after World War II. McCurry, "Like Entering a Prison."

6. Stoler, *Archival Grain,* 20; Anderson, "Case of the Archive." See also Azoulay, "Archive."

7. See, for example, Moran, *Colonizing Leprosy;* Inglis, *Maʻi Lepera;* and Bashford, *Imperial Hygiene.* A notable exception is Stepan, *Picturing Tropical Nature,* which analyzes the terrifying optics of tropical diseases like elephantiasis for Western viewers as the field of tropical medicine became institutionalized. The forum "Beyond Illustrations" in *Bulletin of the History of Medicine* centers the visualization of anatomy and disease in historical analysis of medical science. Berkowitz, "Introduction: Beyond Illustrations."

8. Sekula, "Body and the Archive," 6.

9. Didi-Huberman, *Invention of Hysteria,* 30.

10. At an annual commemoration called Lei Haliʻa O Kalaupapa (Kalaupapa Garlands of Remembrance), community members from Hui Mālama Makanalua make, bless, and bring lei to the Makanalua peninsula and place them on known grave markers. It is one recent example of people from outside the settlement honoring patients and their caregivers who lived and died on the peninsula.

11. Much of the Board of Health's collection of clinical records is either missing or was never transferred to the state of Hawaiʻi archives.

12. The Papa Ola commissioned photographs of patients for its 1878 visit to Kalawao, Molokai; twelve patients were photographed by Honolulu photographer Henry L. Chase on this occasion. These wet glass plate negatives are in CBC-HSA. "Report of the Special Sanitary Committee" and "Expenses of Special Sanitary Committee." Photographs of leprosy patients also were taken at BOH detention facilities possibly as early as 1881, when American George Fitch became head of the Kakaʻako Branch Hospital. Clinical intake photographs of leprosy patients at Kakaʻako were produced as trial evidence in a libel trial initiated by Dr. Fitch in 1883, suggesting this photographic practice began as early as 1881 or 1882. The location of Fitch's photographs is currently unknown.

13. In the 1880s, approximately 10 percent of Hawaiian government revenue went to the Board of Health, and more than 50 percent of the board's budget was allocated to leprosy care and treatment. Inglis, *Maʻi Lepera,* 67, citing Daws, *Holy Man,* 126.

14. Ott, "Contagion," 86.

15. Danielssen and Boeck, *Om spedalskhed;* Ober, "Can the Leper Change His Spots?" 49. See also Ehring, "Leprosy Illustration," 872, discussing representations of leprosy through symbolic forms and its depiction of more medically accurate symptoms during the Renaissance. Neuse et al., "History of Photography," also

outlines dermatologists' experimentations with photographic technologies to illustrate pathological conditions.

16. Stanley Burns observes that photographs were used for patient consultation in the United States in the late 1850s. American doctors made and used daguerreotypes for clinical purposes beginning in the late 1840s. Burns, *Early Medical Photography*, 1263, 1267. While not specifying its application for the study of leprosy, physician Boardman Reed advocated the optic truth of the camera in 1889. He wrote that photographs provided the "best of all records" for medical cases, such as facial paralysis, spinal curvature, hip-joint disease, and marked skin disease. They would be useful for "future reference" and diagnosis. "Why Physicians Should Cultivate Photography."

17. *Biennial Report . . . 1890*, 9.

18. In the 1920s, quarantine at Kalihi Hospital was usually six months long, according to James T. Wayson, a medical superintendent from this period. In the early 1900s, some people with milder cases were allowed to stay at Kalihi for treatment. For instance, the child Nailima Lishman, discussed later in this chapter, was kept at Kalihi for four years, from 1907 until exile in 1911. However, detention was often much shorter before shipment to Molokai, at times only a matter of a few weeks. For example, people examined and confirmed as leprous at Kalihi Hospital in early to mid-May 1900 were shipped to Molokai on May 22, 1900. Cases 5291–300, Box 7 (Medical Examination Records 1897–1900); MER, HSA. Wayson, "Notes on Kalahi [*sic*] Hospital," 45.

19. "Report of Insane Asylum Affairs," *Hawaiian Gazette*, January 15, 1901.

20. Vol. 7 Minutes, HSA. Dr. Clifford Wood initiated the photography motion at a BOH meeting on May 5, 1898. Along with other Euro-American scientists with keen interests in amateur photography, Wood belonged to the Hawaiian Camera Club, founded in 1889. Wood had arrived in Hawai'i in 1886 and was appointed a member of the BOH by settler businessman Sanford B. Dole. Dole had become the first president of the pro-American republic of Hawai'i, after he, Nathaniel Emerson, and other influential haole overthrew the Hawaiian Kingdom and proclaimed a republic in 1894. On the Hawaiian Camera Club, see Davis, *Photographer in the Kingdom*, 90, 98.

21. *Laws of His Majesty Kamehameha V, 1864–65*, 62–64; *Supplement*, 8–10.

22. *Biennial Report . . . 1892*, 29; *Molokai Settlement*, 13.

23. As of the 1920s and 1930s, a minority of suspects with "quiescent" cases could be released to their own communities, but remained subject to BOH examination and supervision. Wayson, "Leprosy," 15.

24. According to BOH reports and the statistical snapshot provided by officials, anyone rounded up for these health examinations was far likelier to be declared a "leper" than to be released as a "suspect" or "not a leper." *Biennial Report . . . 1888*, 9. For example, 368 people were examined in 1888, and of these, 304 were declared "lepers," 42 were suspects, and 22 were "not lepers." It is unclear whether 368 was the total number in 1888 or a shorter period. As of 1907, a suspect who later showed negative bacteriological readings had his or her photograph stamped "not a leper" and was discharged.

25. Maria Alexander's record is case 70, Box 13 (Medical Examination Records 1901); MER, HSA. Her clinical record lists Maria as Hawaiian, nineteen years old, and married. Alexander was her husband's surname. Before being admitted to Kalihi Hospital on August 19, 1901, she had been living with her husband, Solomon, in Kalihi, Hawaiʻi, and others in a boarding house. She arrived in Molokai on October 1, 1901. She died December 1907 at the age of twenty-eight. HD-3, HSA.

26. See for instance, *Biennial Report . . . 1888*, 9. The BOH passed a resolution in 1887 requiring the judgment of at least three competent physicians for someone to be sent to the leprosy settlement. In 1888, the BOH official physicians consisted of two physicians in active practice in Honolulu. These men had the authority to pronounce someone leprous and dispatch him/her to the settlement. By 1892, the medical group responsible for examining suspects increased to five men. *Biennial Report . . . 1892*, 29. By 1907, the Board of Health had adopted the language of rights and asserted that its examination rules protected the rights of the suspect. *Molokai Settlement,* 12.

27. Amirault, "Posing the Subject"; Maehle, "Search for Objective Communication," 572.

28. Meleana Pookalani's record is case 263, Box 17 (Medical Examination Records 1903); MER, HSA. She was from Waipiʻo, Hawaiʻi, and admitted to Kalihi Hospital on March 24, 1903. She was sent to Molokai on June 30, 1903. She gave birth to two sons in the settlement and died in November 1914 at age twenty-five. HD-3 and HD-5, HSA.

29. Gibson, *Born to Crime,* 17, 30.

30. Cole, *Suspect Identities,* 51.

31. On Lombroso, see Gibson, *Born to Crime,* 121, 123. On Galton's criminal composites, see Cole, *Suspect Identities,* 24–25. Elks, "Believing Is Seeing."

32. Didi-Huberman, *Invention of Hysteria,* 33.

33. Ibid.

34. *Biennial Report . . . 1890,* 8–9.

35. The board's procedures for monthly medical reinspections of suspects and deployment of sheriffs to apprehend leprous people were published in *Biennial Report . . . 1892,* 29, 31.

36. Mary Akim's record is case 05201a, Box 6 (Medical Examination Records 1898–1899); MER, HSA. Also known as Malia Keawe, she was from Kohala, Hawaiʻi. She was sent to Molokai on June 16, 1898, and died there on March 20, 1900, at around age thirty-three. HD-3, HSA, and Vol 3. Folio, HSA.

37. Didi-Huberman, *Invention of Hysteria,* 63.

38. The earliest extant clinical forms occasionally include bacteriological results in the final "Remarks" sections. Beginning around 1901, the blank forms were revised to include a more specific final section, "Bacteriological Findings."

39. These cases are known today as paucibacillary cases (leprosy cases with negative or few bacilli readings). This problem of false-negatives was discussed at the 1897 leprosy conference in Berlin. "Report of Dr. L. F. Alvarez, Delegate to the Leprosy Conference, Berlin, in *Report . . . Ending December 31, 1897,* 98–99.

40. McDonald, "Diagnostic Examination," 1568.

41. These articles are, respectively, "Discharged from Kalihi Station," *Hawaiian Gazette,* June 4, 1909, and "Victims of a Terrible Mistake," *Evening Bulletin,* June 3, 1909; 334-37, HSA. Two boys had been at the Kalihi Boys' Home (a Honolulu facility for non-leprous male children of Molokai patients) and nine were at Molokai. James Harvey, age seven, and John Ku, age six, were from Kalihi Boys' Home. Charles Wainui, Ioane Kaimu, J. W. Puiehaka, J. K. Alapai, John Kaapuni, Kahele Kana, Kealiiahonui, Naiwi, and Augusta Freitas were released from Molokai settlement. All were issued certificates clearing them of leprosy. Territorial resolutions supporting individual petitions are in 335-11.

42. See note 84, below, regarding paucibacillary cases as defined by the World Health Organization.

43. "Now 171 Lepers Knocking at the Door of Hope," *Hawaiian Star,* August 24, 1909.

44. U.S. Treasury, Public Health Service, "Statistical Report," 9.

45. Sekula, "Body and the Archive," 351.

46. Letters from Mrs. Emma Nakuina, June 8 and June 15, 1909; 335-13, HSA; Letter from Moses K. Nakuina and E. M. Nakuina, September 26, 1905; 335-16, HSA. Frank Carr's record is case 81, Box 13 (Medical Examination Records 1901); MER, HSA. Carr was from Hāmākua, Hawai'i, and had a German American father and Hawaiian mother. His father, also named Frank Carr, had been exiled to Molokai from 'Auwaiolimu, O'ahu, in 1895. The senior Frank Carr died in the settlement in 1906, his son in 1910. The widowed Emma Nakuina Carr remarried a fellow patient named Solomon Kamohoalii later in 1910. Kamohoalii and the younger Frank Carr may have become friends during detention and exile; they entered Kalihi Hospital days apart in 1901, were examined on the same day, and sent on the same ship to Molokai. They had consecutive case records, 81 and 82. Kamohoalii died in 1912, and Emma Nakuina Carr died in 1916. HD-3, HD-4, and HD-5, HSA.

47. Portuguese immigrants, while not considered "white" or "haole," occupied a middle stratum between haole and Asian settlers in Hawai'i, particularly within the racially stratified plantation labor economy. They were offered American citizenship after the United States annexed Hawai'i as a territory in 1898, while immigrants from Asia were not. Immigrants coming to Hawai'i from the Portuguese colony of Cape Verdes were Portuguese nationals of mixed African and European origin and, thus, may have been racialized as "black." Today Portuguese commonly are included in the category of "local"—people born and raised in Hawai'i, such as Chinese, Japanese, and Filipinos.

48. Thompson, "Leprosy," 289.

49. Moblo, "Institutionalising the Leper," 242–43. Japan repatriated some of its nationals before and after exile to Molokai, but Japanese immigrant laborers also were photographed and their images circulated. See case of Wari Goto, case 755, discussed later in this chapter. A royalist who criticized the 1893 overthrow, Georges Trousseau had far more complicated professional and personal dealings with leprosy. His longtime partner Makanoe's two children were eventually exiled in 1896 and died in 1906. Keoki (Hawaiian for George) Kaeepa, born around

1878, may have been Trousseau's namesake. Greenwell, "Doctor Georges Phillipe Trousseau."

50. Theories of Hawaiian predisposition were discussed at the 1897 Berlin International Leprosy Congress. *Mittheilungen und Verhandlungen,* 119. Physicians also speculated Chinese immigrants to the islands were the original source of leprosy, citing one of leprosy's names in Hawaiian, "maʻi Pākē" (Chinese disease).

51. Fitch, "Etiology of Leprosy," 301.

52. Daland, "Leprosy in the Hawaiian Islands," 1129.

53. Kaulili Kuula's and Makanui Kanehe's records are case 382, Box 19 (Medical Examination Records 1903–1904) and case 241, Box 16 (Medical Examination Records 1902–1903); MER, HSA. Kaulili Kuula was married and from Lahaina, Maui. She was admitted to Kalihi Hospital on March 12, 1904, and arrived in Molokai on April 21, 1904, when she was about fifty-five years old. She died there at the age of sixty-three in December 1912. Makanui Kanehe and her husband Haumea Kanehe (case 240) were ages twenty-one and twenty-six, respectively, when they were admitted to Kalihi Hospital on December 24, 1902. They were from Wainiha, Kauaʻi. During his exam, Haumea said he and Makanui had "been hiding in the bush for two years past" to evade detention. After their exile in February 1903, they petitioned the BOH to allow their daughter in Waimea, Kauaʻi, to join them at Molokai, but this was denied. The daughter was sent to Kapiʻolani Home for Girls in Honolulu. Three years later, in 1906, Haumea died at the settlement at age twenty-nine. Makanui Kanehe appears to have been discharged in November 1909. *Hawaiian Gazette,* June 5, 1903, p. 5. HD-7, HSA.

54. I have cropped nude photographs that draw or may draw scopophilic attention to these bodies, following the example of feminist disability scholar Ellen Samuels in "Examining Millie and Christine McKoy," 70–71, 74–75. Oliwaliilii and her mother Kinolau were admitted to Kalihi Hospital on August 28, 1903. They were from ʻAuwaiolimu, Honolulu. Both were exiled to Molokai on September 16, 1903. Kinolau died March 3, 1912, at age sixty-one, and Oliwaliilii on February 14, 1916, at age thirty-one. Cases 328 and 329, Box 18 (Medical Examination Records 1903); MER, HSA. HD-3 and HD-5, HSA.

55. A series of undated photographs in a separate box of Medical Examination Photographs, Series 260, HSA, feature predominantly nude patients, suggesting that images were culled from different files to form a separate erotic archive.

56. Heinrich has usefully observed how the medical gaze was conjoined with the erotic gaze in Western doctors' clinical photographs of Chinese patients during a contemporaneous period in China. Heinrich, *Afterlife of Images,* 100–107.

57. Didi-Huberman, *Invention of Hysteria,* 59.

58. Sarah Sunter's record is case 253, Box 17 (Medical Examination Records 1903); MER, HSA.

59. *Report . . . Ending December 31, 1902,* 268; *Report . . . Ending June 30, 1903,* 92. Sunter died in the settlement less than a year later, on January 8, 1904. HD-3, HSA.

60. McVeigh described the spacious home for "white foreigners" in *Report . . . Ended June 30, 1909*, 190. The building on which McVeigh had "set his heart" in 1908 was meant to house "twenty-three white lepers." "Board of Health Adopts Important Change in Policy," *Hawaiian Gazette*, August 14, 1908; 334-37, HSA.

61. *Friend* 41 (February 1904), 14.

62. Birth determined makaʻāinana (commoner) or aliʻi (chiefly) rank for Hawaiians. In 1,400 extant photographs in the archive, I have seen no other attempt to anonymize or shield the identity of a Hawaiian or Asian woman, man, or child.

63. Letter from Moses K. Nakuina and E. M. Nakuina, September 26, 1905; 333 16, HSA.

64. Emma K. Nakuina's record is case 548, Box 22 (Medical Examination Records 1905); MER, HSA.

65. Stoler, *Archival Grain*, 20.

66. As early as 1901, oil derived from the seeds of the Southeast Asian chaulmoogra nut (Hydnocarpus plant) was used as a treatment on patients in Hawaiʻi. Intravenous injections of chaulmoogra oil were painful. It seems to have had a palliative effect and reversed some symptoms in early cases, but it was not a cure.

67. U.S. Treasury, Public Health Service, "Statistical Report," 12.

68. U.S. Treasury, Public Health Service, "Treatment of Leprosy, with Especial," 1959.

69. During this time, 249 paroles were granted to 242 leprosy patients; seven of these were second-time paroles. To be released on parole, a patient submitted to a final examination by a board of three physicians. Parole meant at least four years' release, with periodic medical exams and inspections. U.S. Treasury, Public Health Service, "Statistical Report," 12, 13, 15.

70. U.S. Treasury, Public Health Service, "Statistical Report," 23.

71. Mikala Kaipu's writ of habeas corpus in 1904 is discussed below. On other court challenges, see Tayman, *Colony*, 205–6.

72. American penologist Zebulon Brockway pioneered parole and prison reform experiments throughout his career. He instituted a formal parole program at Elmira State Reformatory in New York State, which opened under Brockway's supervision in 1876. Brockway, *Fifty Years of Prison Service*. See also Bottomley, "Parole," 321–322. David Rothman historicizes the emergence of U.S. correctional institutions as a response to perceived social disorder. He suggests wardens in the 1830s to 1860s advocated conditional release to encourage prisoner compliance and more flexible prison administration. *Discovery of the Asylum*, 252.

73. In 1917, all prisoners convicted of felonies, except those sentenced for first-degree murder, were eligible for parole in the territory of Hawaiʻi. Lindsey, "Historical Sketch," 67.

74. U.S. Treasury, Public Health Service, "Statistical Report," 23.

75. The board used the language of "public menace." In a treatment experiment on injections of ethyl esters of chaulmoogra oil conducted between 1921 and 1923, 23 percent of patients were paroled as "no longer a menace to the public." U.S. Treasury, Public Health Service, "Treatment of Leprosy with Derivatives," 10. Hasseltine was

a U.S. Public Health Service surgeon and director of the U.S. Leprosy Investigation Station at Molokai when he published this article.

76. While photographs have been a part of biomedical experiments on leprosy patients in Hawai'i since at least the 1880s, they appear to have intensified when the federal investigation station opened in 1909 in Kalawao. Federal scientists began transferring from Kalawao to Kalihi Hospital between 1910 and 1914. Binford, "History and Study," 419.

77. U.S. Treasury, Public Health Service, "Treatment of Leprosy with Derivatives," 3.

78. The male and female patients under experimental treatment appear to have been Hawaiian, "Part Hawaiian," Filipino, Japanese, and Portuguese. Only one Portuguese patient in the group of twenty was listed. U.S. Treasury, Public Health Service, "Treatment of Leprosy with Derivatives," 5–7.

79. Hasseltine offered no data for how he measured "improvement" or "excellent progress," but his use of photographs and visual observation suggest that these constituted evidence for the cessation of "active leprosy." U.S. Treasury, Public Health Service, "Treatment of Leprosy with Derivatives," 7–10.

80. Broad interest in Hawai'i's leprosy experiments is indicated by physicians from Venezuela, South Africa, and the Philippines visiting and observing at Kalihi Hospital. Ester treatments supplied from Kalihi Hospital were adopted as well. *Report . . . Ended June 30, 1922*, 136; *Report Ended . . . June 30, 1923*, 148.

81. Parole meant discharge from Kalihi Hospital or Molokai settlement. U.S. Treasury, Public Health Service, "Statistical Report," 12.

82. *Report Ended . . . June 30, 1923*, 144.

83. Hasseltine discussed relapses in U.S. Treasury, Public Health Service, "Statistical Report," 13.

84. It is now believed that a negative bacteriological reading does not mean leprosy is arrested; bacterial counts may wane over time. S. Kalani Brady, interview, December 18, 2013. In paucibacillary leprosy cases, patients show negative bacteria in skin smears. "Classification of Leprosy," World Health Organization, accessed October 28, 2015; www.who.int/lep/classification/en/.

85. The more altered the skin, the less likely a person was to be paroled. More than half of patients with "anesthetic" leprosy, the milder form of the disease, were paroled, whereas only 25 percent of the more severe, nodular, cases were paroled. By the 1940s, these two types of leprosy were being classified as "tuberculoid" and "lepromatous," respectively. Furthermore, patients who had slight paralysis, such as of the eyelids, as first evidence of disease had a much greater proportion of parole. See U.S. Treasury, Public Health Service, "Statistical Report," 21–22.

86. McDonald and Dean, "Constituents of Chaulmoogra Oil," 1471. According to McDonald, Kalihi Hospital supervising physician, 50 percent of patients who entered the hospital recovered and were paroled between 1920 and 1921.

87. *Pacific Commercial Advertiser,* November 17, 1921, 2.

88. "Out of the Darkness into the Light," 35.

89. "Mrs. R. Blaisdell Gives Impressive Story of her Cure of Leprosy," *Pacific Commercial Advertiser,* September 9, 1920. Blaisdell relapsed and was sent to Kalaupapa in August 1928. She died March 1930. HD-6; HSA. Tayman, *Colony,* 216.

90. Letter from James Keao, December 2, 1912; 335-13, HSA.

91. The lawyer representing both Kaipu and Maunakea was former Kingdom of Hawai'i attorney general Clarence W. Ashford. After the writ's denial in U.S. District Court in 1905, Emma Kaipu appealed to the U.S. Supreme Court, but the case was dismissed on May 13, 1907, due to Mikala Kaipu's death. In the Matter of Kaipu, 2 D. Haw. 215 (1904); Kaipu v. Pinkham, 51 U.S. 1191 (1907). Mikala Kaipu was admitted to Kalihi Hospital on September 23, 1904, from Kaua'i. She was forty-seven years old and listed as "½ Hawaiian, ½ white." Case 450, Box 20 (Medical Examination Records 1904); MER, HSA. Anamalia Maunakea was admitted on November 10, 1907, from Kuamo'o, North Kona, Hawai'i; she was thirty-nine years old. Her record is case 740, Box 26 (Medical Examination Records 1907–1908); MER, HSA. In re: Maunakea, 19 Haw. 218 (1908). *Report . . . Ended June 30, 1909,* 10.

92. These attempts to see loved ones are palpable in a log of visits granted by the BOH president and sent to the keeper of the Kalihi Receiving Station. The keeper was the head jailer. Only one log remains, with the bulk of recorded visits in the years 1904–1908. 331 Vol. 115, HSA.

93. Letter from F. Wittrock to Dr. John Pratt, February 21, 1913; Letter from Dr. John Pratt to F. Wittrock, Februrary 24, 1913; 335-13, HSA.

94. The children to whom Frederick refers were likely Ella and Augusta. Augusta would have been nineteen years old in 1913; she had been married in Honolulu in 1911. Her sister Ella was about nine years old. Later, two of their brothers, George and Walter Wittrock, would be exiled to Molokai. Ella married a fellow patient named Manuel Borge (also spelled Borges) at Kalaupapa in July 1921 and had at least four children. One child named Manuel George was removed from Kalaupapa settlement to the Kalihi Boys' Home for non-leprous children and later readmitted to Kalihi Hospital. 260 Box 30, HSA; HD-A; HD-B, HD-C. Frederick Wittrock was deputy sheriff of Maui when he died on April 25, 1913. Although he and Kukonaalaa had seven children, a Honolulu obituary notes he was survived by "a widow and five children," suggesting his daughters with leprosy may have been considered socially dead. "Two Pioneer Citizens of Hawaii Pass to Beyond," *Honolulu Advertiser,* April 27, 1913.

95. Tayman, *Colony,* 214.

96. In 1889, the Board of Health reprimanded ethnologist William T. Brigham for taking photographs of patients on behalf of visiting American researcher Dr. Prince A. Morrow. During this visit, Brigham photographed Father Damien, other "pathological cases," and landscapes. Letter from William Brigham, November 14, 1889; 334-14, HSA.

97. "Board of Health," *Hawaiian Gazette,* August 8, 1893; R. W. Meyer, Letter, *Hawaiian Gazette,* August 22, 1893. After Hawai'i became an incorporated U.S.

territory in 1900, the BOH continued to restrict use of cameras in the "leper settlement." BOH president L. E. Pinkham issued a warning to the publisher of *Leslie's Weekly* not to publish photographs of inmates after one of its correspondents had been noticed taking unauthorized photographs. Letter to The Judge Company, July 15, 1907; 335-12, HSA.

98. Kauikeaouli (King Kamehameha III) first organized the BOH in 1850, and membership was a kingdom political appointment. After the 1893 overthrow, only occasionally did its ranks include a Hawaiian man. Shortly after the overthrow, three American doctors, three laymen (i.e., non-physicians), and the attorney general ex-officio constituted the BOH. The three lay members were influential merchants. Only one, John Ena, was Kanaka ʻŌiwi, and he was a wealthy investor in a shipping line affiliated with plantations. Several members in the 1890s participated in pro-U.S. annexationist groups, including Lorrin A. Thurston and Theodore F. Lansing.

99. Imada, *Aloha America,* 11, 154–57, 180; Imada, "Aloha ʻOe," 41.

100. Andrews, "Fine Island Views."

101. Fitch, "Appendix E," xxxiv.

102. Morrow, "Leprosy and Hawaiian Annexation."

103. The BOH's formal interdiction of unauthorized photography in August 1893 was issued seven months after the U.S.-backed overthrow of the Hawaiian Kingdom.

104. Bushnell, "United States Leprosy Investigation Station," 76.

105. The earliest extant clinical images of patients taken by photographer Henry L. Chase during the BOH's 1878 Kalawao, Molokai, visit were part of Dr. Charles B. Cooper's own collection when the territorial archives acquired them in 1930. CBC-HSA. This suggests Cooper created a personal archive of skin.

106. U.S. Treasury, Public Health and Marine-Hospital Service, *Transactions.*

107. No photographs were printed in the dry, eight-page pamphlet on leprosy that Cooper brought to the U.S. continent. "Leprosy in the Hawaiian Islands."

108. "Dr. Cooper at Capital," *Hawaiian Gazette,* June 21, 1904. Letter from Surgeon-General, at 8.

109. These four people's records are in Box 5 (Medical Examination Records 1896–1898); MER, HSA. Halauwai's record is case 05172. She was about twenty years old when she was admitted to leprosy detention in May 1898. She was from the Hāmākua district of Hawaiʻi. She was sent to Molokai on June 16, 1898. As of 1900, Halauwai was living in the settlement; she died March 26, 1903. HD-3, HSA. Kaupe's record is case 05191. She was about age fifty when she was incarcerated in June 1898. She was from Kohala, Hawaiʻi, and died September 29, 1905. HD-3, HSA. Juan de Freitas's record is case 05174. Also known as John Freitas, he was admitted to detention on June 16, 1898, from Wailuku, Maui, and died January 9, 1899, at around age fifty-four. HD-3, HSA. Henry K. Apolo was from Aliamanu, Kauaʻi. His record is case 05213; he was examined at Kalihi Hospital on June 25, 1898. He was sent to Molokai in August 1898. As of 1900, Apolo was living at Baldwin Home for Boys in Kalawao. He died February 11, 1906. HD-2, HSA.

110. Letter from Walter Wyman, Surgeon General of the United States of America, to Charles B. Cooper, July 20, 1904; and Letter from Charles B. Cooper to Walter Wyman, August 12, 1904; CBC-Q.

111. Act to Provide for Investigation of Leprosy (1905). Michael, "Leprosy Investigation Station," 204. There were two separate congressional bills for leprosy funding in 1905; the one funding the investigation station passed, while the one for national leprosarium appropriation did not. Moran, *Colonizing Leprosy*, 33–34.

112. Before, during, and after treatment shots of Hawaiian patients were an integral part of experiments conducted at federal leprosy investigation laboratories at Kalawao and Kalihi. See, for example, Brinkerhoff and Wayson's 1909 experiments with nastine, a bacterial fat. U.S. Treasury, Public Health and Marine-Hospital Service, "Report upon the Treatment." I have identified the three Hawaiian male patients whose images were in these reports as ten–year-old Louis Aloisa, twenty-year-old Vivian Holstein, and forty-one-year-old F. J. Cook. The chaulmoogra oil experiments between 1921 and 1923 that prompted parole also were conducted under the direction of U.S. federal scientists. See U.S. Treasury, Public Health Service, "Treatment of Leprosy with Derivatives."

113. O'Day delivered an illustrated lecture on leprosy in 1913, as reported in *Medical Century*, 349. His articles on Hawai'i include "Hawaii and Her Leprosy" and "Visit to the Leper Colony." O'Day may have received permission to use the photographs because he wrote favorably of the board's care of inmates and stated leprosy was not contagious.

114. O'Day, "Visit to the Leper Colony," 248.

115. Wari Goto and Puaiku Iokepa's records are cases 755 and 760, Box 27 (Medical Examination Records 1909–1910); MER, HSA, respectively. Goto had immigrated to Hawai'i from Japan in 1902. Although she had been exiled to Molokai, Goto was brought back from the settlement and repatriated to Japan "at request of the Japanese Consul." She was shipped to Japan on February 6, 1909, along with a child and a Korean named Chin Chun Yok. BOH records do not indicate whether the child was Goto's, but Goto had given birth to a girl named Shino in July 1908. This child was discharged on February 3, 1909. Vol. 16 Minutes, HSA, p. 90. HD-A, HSA. According to Japan's first leprosy prevention law in 1907, if Goto did not have family members to shelter her, she may have been placed in one of five public leprosaria opened in 1909. Puaiku Iokepa was from Kawaihae, Hawai'i. He was admitted to Kalihi Hospital on April 3, 1908, along with his father Konia and older brother Keahi (cases 758 and 759, Box 27). Keahi was discharged as non-leprous, but Konia and Puaiku were sent to Molokai on April 17, 1908. Puaiku died August 1909 at the age of sixteen, and Konia died December 1911 at age fifty-six. HD-3 and HD-4, HSA.

116. Edward S. Goodhue was the brother of William J. Goodhue, who served as medical superintendent of Molokai settlement from 1902 to 1925. William Goodhue eventually contracted leprosy himself and left the settlement. Quotations are from Goodhue, "Physician in Hawaii," 141, 143.

117. Chase agreed to the price of fifty dollars for the negatives and an additional six dollars per dozen of "impressions of said negatives." "Expenses of Special Sanitary Committee."

118. The person labeled "nerve leprosy" was a woman named Kalamau, fifty years old, from Honolulu, who had been at Kalawao five years. The person labeled "tubercular leprosy" was a man named Naluaai, fifty-six years old, from Kalihi, Oʻahu, who had also been at Kalawao five years. "Report of Special Sanitary Committee." Chase's original wet glass plate negatives, 772A-772L, are in CBC-HSA, Box PNLPC26.

119. For example, better papers to print photographs had become available by the 1880s, including silver-print gelatin papers and non-silver papers, replacing albumen prints. Burns, *Early Medical Photography*, 1251.

120. Daland, "Leprosy in Hawaiian Islands"; Goodhue, "Surgical Cure"; Goodhue, "Cure of Leprosy"; Cottle, "Photographs of Lepers"; U.S. Treasury, Public Health Service, "Treatment of Leprosy with Derivatives."

121. GMC, ca. 1948.

122. William Eli Hodge's record is case 211, Box 16 (Medical Examination Records 1902); MER, HSA. He was Hawaiian and from Waihina, Hanalei, Kauaʻi. Hodge was examined on September 25, 1902, sent to Molokai on October 6, 1902, and died August 30, 1915, at age twenty-one. HD-3 and HD-5, HSA.

123. Forrester, "Strange Case"; Kalisch, "Strange Case."

124. *Care and Treatment of Persons,* at 145–47.

125. Moran, *Colonizing Leprosy,* 41.

126. For example, "Carville, U.S.A.," Folder 3 (Booklets, Pamphlets, Guides, 1945–1960); Box 11; Public Health Service Hospitals Historical Collection, 1895–1982; MS C 471; National Library of Medicine, Bethesda, Maryland, ca. 1950–1953. Despite Carville's emphasis on rehabilitation and medical reform rather than incarceration, the racialization of its patients did not end. Carville practiced racial segregation in the form of separate living quarters for whites, African Americans, and Asians. Moran, *Colonizing Leprosy,* 128. Furthermore, physicians took clinical photographs of Carville patients, but Dr. George McCoy's lantern slide collection selected African American patients from Carville as his clinical examples, not white patients. McCoy's scientific career spanned Hawaiʻi, DC, and Louisiana, and his slide collection co-mingled images of leprosy patients taken at Kalihi Hospital and Carville. GMC.

127. Parascandola, "Miracle at Carville."

128. Binford and Connor, *Pathology of Tropical and Extraordinary Diseases,* 207.

129. Nailima Lishman's record is case 368, Box 25 (Medical Examination Records 1907); MER, HSA. She was eventually sent to Molokai on September 27, 1911, and died there on July 1, 1916, at the age of eighteen. HD-3, HSA; 331 Vol. 115, HSA. Her mother, Nellie Nailima Koli, was Kanaka ʻŌiwi; her father, Thomas Lishman, was a white Australian.

130. Entry on page 72, April 23, 1906; 331 Vol. 115, HSA. Elizabeth Napoleon died in Kalaupapa in 1911 at the age of nineteen. Her mother, Elizabeth Kaehukai

(Baker) Napoleon, was also sentenced to Kalaupapa, arriving eight months after her daughter's death. HD-3; HD-4, HSA. Kaʻohulani McGuire's genealogical research about this mother and daughter in the Napoleon family was posted on Kalaupapa National Historical Park's official Facebook page on September 30, 2016, and October 4, 2016. These posts were part of a commemorative series about one hundred years of patients at Kalaupapa.

131. Today hospitals discuss patients without kin as "unbefriended"—people who have no family members or surrogates to make decisions. For example, the letterbook from Kalihi Station reveals multiple visitor permits.

132. Edwards, "Photographic 'Types,'" 245.

133. Sekula, "Body and the Archive," 360.

134. "Report of Insane Asylum Affairs," *Hawaiian Gazette,* January 15, 1901. Davis, *Na Paʻi Kiʻi,* 35.

135. Barbara Brookes, in her readings of nineteenth-century asylum patient photographs, argues that the individuality of patients can be "released" years after their original institutional uses. "Pictures of People," 31. A growing body of scholarship analyzes Indigenous peoples looking back at the camera or subverting imperial optics, even as they were imaged under conditions of duress. See, for instance, Lydon, *Eye Contact;* Mimura, "Dying West?"; Medak-Saltzman, "Transnational Indigenous Exchange"; and Imada, *Aloha America.*

136. Guglyk and Bloombaum, *Maʻi Hoʻokaʻawale,* 80. This seventy-year-old anonymous interviewee, a "part-Hawaiian" man, was thirteen when he was sentenced. By my estimate, he was photographed by the board around 1920.

137. Brown and Phu, *Feeling Photography,* 19–20. This collection amplifies an "affective turn" in photography studies.

138. Within the contemporary setting of a Botswana cancer ward, Julie Livingston has considered how and why Batswana cancer patients readily agreed to pose for clinical photographs. "Figuring the Tumor," 20, 24.

139. Herman Kuhilani's record was no. 320; he was Hawaiian, aged twenty, and unmarried, from Kapahulu, Oʻahu. Kauluhinano, whose record no. was 321, was thirty-eight years old, "½ Hawaiian, ½ Chinese," and single, from Waimanalo, Oʻahu. Hattie Kekai was twenty-four years old, single, and "½ Hawaiian, ½ Portuguese," from Liliha, Honolulu. Kealaaea, or Nalau, record no. 323, was Hawaiian, eighteen years old, and single, from Hotel Street, Honolulu. Kalema Kaaukai, record no. 331, was Hawaiian, thirty years old, and widowed, from Hilo, Hawaiʻi. Cases 320, 321, 322, 323, and 331, Box 18 (Medical Examination Records 1903); MER, HSA. Herman Kuhilani, Kalili Naea, and Kalema Kaaukai were sent to Molokai on September 16, 1903. HD-3, HSA.

140. The "flowering plants" on the hospital grounds are described in *Biennial Report . . . 1890,* 9.

141. Pukui, *ʻŌlelo Noʻeau,* 41.

142. "Profound mourning and expressions of grief were (and still are) a mark of Kanaka life and death," historian David A. Chang emphasizes. *World and All the Things,* 59.

143. Clark, *Kalaupapa Place Names,* 345. I wish to acknowledge Clark's work for selecting and bringing together several moving kanikau in his book. This kanikau originally was published as "Kuu Opuu Rose Ua Mae," *Ke Aloha Aina,* August 19, 1899, p. 3.

144. See references to physicians Fitch, "Appendix E," and Goodhue, above.

145. Inglis has referred to these individual and collective efforts by Kānaka Maoli as struggles to remain "socially alive" in the face of civil death. They submitted petitions to the board asking for treatment, improvements at the settlements, the right to marry and serve as mea kōkua; and teachers and supplies to better nurture their children. Inglis, *Maʻi Lepera,* 61. For more on Hawaiian resistance to leprosy policies and community formation, see Law, *Kalaupapa: A Collective Memory.*

146. Barthes, *Camera Lucida,* 43, 47.

147. McDonald, *Ka Lei,* 125.

148. Cecelia Kalili Naea, known as Kalili Naea, was sent to Molokai on September 16, 1903. She met another inmate, Pepenui Ali, who arrived in Molokai in July 1909. In October 1910, Kalili gave birth to a baby named Rebecca Pepenui Ali, but the baby died three weeks later. In December 1910, Kalili died at age twenty, and Pepenui Ali died in February 1915 at age twenty-four. Kalili Naea's record is case 327, Box 18 (Medical Examination Records 1903); MER, HSA. Pepenui Ali's record is case 772, Box 27 (Medical Examination Records 1909–1910); MER, HSA. Their deaths are recorded in HD-3, HSA.

CHAPTER 3. DRESSING THE BODY: LAUNDRY AND THE
INTIMACY OF CARE

1. Alice Kaelemakule was from Waialua, Oʻahu. She entered leprosy detention in late 1904 at the age of twenty. After exile, she married John Taylor Unea at the Molokai settlement and gave birth to a daughter in August 1911. Unea was about thirty years older than Alice. The baby died at the age of two months. Alice Unea died in the settlement on January 12, 1914, and John Unea in 1920. Alice Kaelemakule and Hattie Piipiilani Kalua's records are cases 471 and 467, Box 21 (Medical Examination Records 1904–1905); MER, HSA, respectively. Kalua entered leprosy detention on December 9, 1904, from Iwilei, Oʻahu. The length of her residence in the settlement is unknown, but she likely arrived in 1905 and was residing there in 1918, when she made a donation to a Red Cross campaign.

2. Several hundred wet glass plate negatives were discovered in a former monastery of the Sacred Hearts Brothers in Kāneʻohe, Hawaiʻi, before the building was demolished in the 1970s. Many were cracked or water damaged. The extant portraits may be the work of Father Paul-Marie (Joseph) Julliotte, who resided in the Molokai settlement as a medical missionary from 1901 to 1907. Ching, "Portraits of Kalaupapa Residents." The photographs may have been taken by more than one priest or lay brother, however. The dates of these images (1901–1925) are my estimates based on BOH patient records and the residencies of Julliotte and other Catholic

fathers and brothers who may have taken photographs in the settlement until ca. 1925.

3. These muʻumuʻu (Mother Hubbard gowns) were missionary-influenced attire worn even in the hot climate of Hawaiʻi.

4. In Hawaiian the actual term for helper is the gender-neutral "mea kōkua," but it became truncated to kōkua or kokua in its use by the state.

5. Catholic missionaries joining the Molokai mission from North America and Western Europe in the late nineteenth and early twentieth centuries were inspired by the "martyr" priest Damien de Veuster from Belgium. Damien established a mission in Kalawao, Molokai, in 1873 and contracted leprosy there in 1884. Although Damien was not the first medical missionary to Kalawao, he was the most prominent, influential, and longest serving of the era. Damien was believed to have developed leprosy while caring for patients in Molokai, but he may have been infected earlier while working in Hilo, Hawaiʻi. Damien and Marianne, two missionaries sainted by the Catholic Church in 2009 and 2012, respectively, have received much attention in Western historiography and popular media for their spiritual and physical sacrifice. Damien, in particular, who died of leprosy at Kalawao in 1889, became a celebrity in Catholic and secular print media at the turn of the century.

6. McClintock, *Imperial Leather,* 71, 211.

7. Quoted in Mouritz, *Path of the Destroyer,* 206. From Hāna, Maui, Ambrose Hutchison later became resident superintendent of the settlement; he died in 1932. Moblo, "Ethnic Intersession," 58–61; HD-7; HSA.

8. Mouritz, *Path of the Destroyer,* 207, 227. Damien learned to dress these sores, but he was only one caregiver among approximately seven hundred patients.

9. Meyer, "Appendix N," cxxvii.

10. Greene, *Exile in Paradise,* 132.

11. "Report of the Special Sanitary Committee." The three men who were signatories to the petition were A. W. B. Nahakualii, John Kaahaihanu, and B. Kaahaihanu.

12. Hōjō Tamio, a writer confined to a Japanese leprosarium, offered vivid descriptions of bodily deterioration and pain in the pre-sulfone antibiotic era: "The bandages wrapping their heads and arms looked as if they were oozing with blackened yellow pus." Tanaka, "Life's First Night," 19.

13. "Letter from a Leper," *Pacific Commercial Advertiser,* October 5, 1878. Settlement agent Rudolf Meyer noted similarly in his 1886 BOH report, "And many really could not work, their hands and feet being too sore." Meyer, "Appendix N," cxxvi. John W. Nakuino may have been J. W. Nakuina from Honolulu, who died in April 1883 at age forty-five. HD-2, HSA.

14. There are no clear statistics on how many mea kōkua lived in the settlement during the formal period of leprosy segregation, from 1866 to 1969. Historian Kerri Inglis estimates that by 1900 there may have been approximately four to five hundred kōkua who had settled on the peninsula. A BOH register listed 203 people as

kōkua between 1868 and 1889, but this number likely did not reflect many others who accompanied patients. Inglis, *Maʻi Lepera,* 86, and "Nā Hoa," 291.

15. "Report of the Special Sanitary Committee." The committee called Luka an "illustration of fidelity and devotion in Hawaiian character," but it is notable that this is one of the very few instances in which health officials or their proxies offered public praise, rather than denigration, for service proffered by kōkua.

16. Emerson, "Report," 122. Emerson was appointed BOH president in 1887.

17. In the United States, custodial institutions for people with intellectual disabilities were supported by "institutional peonage"—the unpaid labor of attendants and resident workers. Beckwith, *Disability Servitude,* 1–3, 44–45. K. Tsianina Lomawaima discusses the vocational labor performed by American Indian students at off-reservation boarding schools that kept these institutions running. *Prairie Light,* 84. On the porousness of boundaries in precolonial Vietnam prisons that allowed mingling between prisoners and family members, see Zinoman, *Colonial Bastille,* 21.

18. The prohibition against children as caregivers seems to have relaxed after the settlement's founding, but adult caregivers were far more common. Molokai superintendent Rudolf Meyer wrote, "All the first shipments of lepers were allowed to take their wives and husbands with them, or a son, and in some instances a daughter, but children were not permitted to accompany them." Meyer, "Appendix N," cxxvi. Children who came as kōkua sometimes remained in the settlement for their entire lives, married, and had children.

19. Nathaniel Bright Emerson, "Leprosy: essay beginning, From one point of view the study of leprosy [bear] to that of other diseases . . . [c. 1880]"; EMR 169; Box 5, NBE.

20. Mouritz, *Path of the Destroyer,* 140.

21. Some of these petitions were discussed in Vols. 15 and 16 Minutes, HSA.

22. The language of "clean" and "unclean" was used by BOH agents and physicians from the 1870s through the Progressive era. Clean was a colloquial description that held medical and juridical weight in its parsing of leprous and non-leprous bodies. Resident physician Fitch, for example, relied on "clean" and "unclean" to distinguish between those infected with leprosy and those who were not. Fitch, "Appendix A," vii. In a later period, physicians George W. McCoy and William J. Goodhue described "kokuas as clean persons who have lived with lepers, usually in conjugal relationship"; in U.S. Treasury, Public Health Service, "Danger of Association," 7. They were the director of the Leprosy Investigation Station and the settlement's medical superintendent, respectively. Goodhue later developed leprosy and left the settlement.

23. The BOH published these settlement rules in 1893, six months after the U.S.-backed overthrow of the Hawaiian Kingdom. They were printed in *Hawaiian Gazette,* July 18, 1893. Kōkua rules were detailed in section 18.

24. Siblings were also allowed to serve as kōkua, but did so with far less frequency.

25. Emerson, "Report," 122.

26. Nathaniel Bright Emerson essay, "Leprosy"; EMR 169; Box 5, NBE.

27. Western medical missionaries, particularly Catholics, were exceptions and given latitude and spiritual dispensation for ministering to leprous people.

28. Issued roughly every year, these official BOH reports included statistics related to public health and mortality in the Hawaiian Kingdom (later the U.S. territory and state of Hawai'i), as well as narrative summaries by government physicians and resident physicians in the leprosy settlement.

29. Fitch's reports were published in 1885 and 1886. Fitch, "Leprosy," and "Appendix E," xxix. Fitch was known as Kauka Pika to his Hawaiian patients.

30. Fitch, "Leprosy," 529; and Fitch, "Appendix E," xxxv.

31. Fitch, "Appendix E," xxxv. He wrote, "The blood and pus saturated garments of lepers laundried by non-lepers, eating, sleeping, drinking with lepers for years fails to reproduce it."

32. Mouritz, "Appendix K," xciii.

33. *Letter from the Surgeon-General;* McGrew, "Leprosy in the Hawaiian Islands"; Morrow, *System of Genito-Urinary Diseases.*

34. Hoolemakani was one of six kōkua who came to Kalawao with twenty patients on August 12, 1868. From Lahaina, Maui, she was the wife of a man named Kalana. By 1900, Hoolemakani had been widowed again. She died in the settlement on May 15, 1915, at the age of seventy-eight. Hoolemakani is discussed in U.S. Treasury, Public Health and Marine-Hospital Service, *Transactions,* 89. Hoolemakani's complex marital and sexual history was detailed alongside that of the kōkua Kalehua in Fitch, "Appendix E," xxix, and *Biennial Report . . . 1892,* 10.

35. Douglas, *Purity and Danger,* 157. Douglas referred to India in this passage.

36. Shah, *Contagious Divides,* 68–69.

37. Douglas, *Purity and Danger,* 156.

38. McClintock, *Imperial Leather,* 48.

39. The theory that leprosy passed down through families invited scrutiny of sexual reproduction, lineal descent, and consanguinity.

40. Kunzel, *Criminal Intimacy,* 1.

41. Morrow, "Personal Observations," 87.

42. As Morrow explained, his quotation was drawn from an earlier 1889 article of his, though I have not been able to locate the original. He quotes from it in *Leprosy,* 632–33.

43. Fitch, "Report of Dr. G. L. Fitch," 120.

44. Fitch, "Appendix E," xxiv–xxix. He also describes white foreign men going native in "Etiology of Leprosy," 296.

45. Emerson quoted Norwegian leprosy researchers Danielsen and Boeck in *Supplement,* 128.

46. Mouritz, *Path of the Destroyer,* 141.

47. Ibid., 148.

48. It is quite possible that patient Q, the laundress Kalehua, and the washerwoman Mouritz discussed in 1886 were the same woman.

49. Mouritz, *Path of the Destroyer,* 150–51.

50. Ibid., 141.

51. In the 1880s, Lombroso studied sexual behavior and crania of incarcerated women to identify "born" female criminal types. His co-authored study with Guglielmo Ferrero, *La donna delinquente (Criminal Woman)* was first published in Italian in 1893, with an English translation issued, in part, as *The Female Offender* in 1895. See also Lombroso and Ferrero, *Criminal Woman,* 4–5, 23–29, on the dissemination of Lombroso's theories of female criminality.

52. Nicholas Turse provides insightful discussion of Mouritz's ethically unsound experiments on kōkua within Western biomedical experimentation in the late nineteenth-century "neocolony" of Hawai'i, but does not analyze the significant gendered and sexualized attention to Indigenous female bodies. "Experimental Dreams."

53. Briggs, "Race of Hysteria," 249–50. See also Owens, *Medical Bondage.*

54. Miller, "Lepers of Hawaii."

55. Priscilla Wald asserts Typhoid Mary as the first healthy carrier. *Contagious,* 98.

56. In addition to "Hawaiian Type" on p. 105 of *Path of the Destroyer,* Mouritz included colored plates of two Hawaiian women with leprosy at the end of his book.

57. See Imada, *Aloha America,* for a detailed discussion of this iconography.

58. Robert Schoofs suggests Father Julliotte's leprosy research was encouraged, if not underwritten, by the U.S. federal government in the form of photographic and laboratory equipment at Molokai. Julliotte may have published his findings in medical journals, although the latter referenced by Schoofs is not currently known. *Pioneers of the Faith,* 339. Julliotte took both clinical photographs of people in medical settings at Molokai and studio portraits. My research indicates that the former, while unattributed to Julliotte, are in Jack London's album of Molokai photographs. Album 55 (Molokai); JL. At least three images bear Julliotte's characteristic handwritten etching. London shot and collected photographs during his visit to Molokai in mid-1907. The men did not meet on that occasion, as Julliotte had recently left the settlement for a Honolulu post.

59. As suggested by CSH photographs, Brother Louis Leissen and Father Philip Blom may have taken photos at Kalaupapa. German-born Leissen served in the Molokai settlement from 1898 to 1925. Dutch-born Blom arrived in Kalaupapa in 1912 and remained there for about three years. Archivist Stuart W. H. Ching provided valuable insights into this collection; more research is required in this area of Catholic-produced photography, which is beyond the immediate scope of this study. See also Ching, "Portraits of Kalaupapa Residents"; Schoofs, *Pioneers of the Faith,* 341, 343.

60. Benjamin, "Work of Art."

61. Photograph Album 1019 includes prints of people in figures 50, 51, and 53, for instance. Photographs collected and compiled in missionary albums were not necessarily contemporaneous with the production of the original negatives, which suggests Catholic fathers and brothers had access to images of patients they did not know personally. At least one album appears to have been assembled as late as the 1930s, while patients were photographed by different fathers or brothers between ca.

1901 and 1915. Photographs of Catholic-run dormitories appear to have been generated by male missionaries, not sisters. I am not aware of photographs taken by sisters of the Order of Saint Francis who resided in the settlement. PA 1019 (Molokai); Box 5; Special Collection I: Photographic Forms: Albums; RG IX.A-2; CSH.

62. Maison de la Bonne Presse, a Paris publisher of Catholic journals and newspapers, printed lantern slides of Father Damien's missionary labors in Molokai, ca. 1900. Typical of an illustrated lecture format, the slides included natural wonders, churches, individual priests, chiefly monarchs of Hawai'i, and groups of patients with Catholic sisters. George Eastman Museum collection, Rochester, New York. CSH is also in possession of lantern slide collections produced commercially for Catholic organizations; these were printed in places like Hawai'i and Washington, DC.

63. Daughton, *Empire Divided,* 39. *Annales de la Propagation de la Foi,* the bimonthly version, reached an estimated 1.5 million French mission supporters. The majority of its readers were French, but the journals were also published in German, English, Spanish, Italian, and seven other languages. My discussion of Catholic media distribution draws on Daughton's book.

64. Daughton, *Empire Divided,* 40.

65. At least one of the photographs published within was taken by Father Julliotte. Alazard, "Un Incendie à Molokaï." The weekly edition was subsequently compiled in an annual format. *Les Missions Catholiques.*

66. Schoofs, *Pioneers of the Faith,* 340. *Les Missions Catholiques* listed financial contributions and donors from many quarters of Western Europe in each issue.

67. Hawaiian girl patients were referenced as such in Catholic missionary slides produced in Paris. George Eastman Museum Collection, Rochester, New York.

68. The Baldwin Home for Leprous Boys and Men opened in Kalawao on the eastern side of the settlement in 1894. The home was run by Catholic brothers from the Congregation of the Sacred Hearts. Catholic supervision and care also extended into gender-segregated institutional homes for non-leprous children of exiled patients: the Kalihi Boys' Home and Kapi'olani Home for Girls, both on O'ahu.

69. Female residents of Bishop Home were described as "inmates" by physicians during this period, including by William J. Goodhue. *Report... Ending December 31st, 1906,* 104.

70. Bashford, *Imperial Hygiene,* 5.

71. *Report... Ending December 31st, 1906,* 104.

72. Lomawaima, "Domesticity in the Federal Indian Schools."

73. "Sing, Jack; Sing, Mary—Kalaupapa." Oral History Interview by Ishmael Stagner and Kenneth Baldridge; February 24, 1979. BYU-Hawaii Oral History Program; BYU-Hawaii Archives and Special Collections, Joseph F. Smith Library, Brigham Young University–Hawaii. Quotation courtesy of Brigham Young University–Hawaii Archives.

74. Hanley and Bushnell, *Pilgrimage and Exile,* 297, 298, 301.

75. Sister Leopoldina Burns is pictured in figure 47. On the sisters, see Hanley and Bushnell, *Pilgrimage and Exile,* n.p.

76. Fitch, "Appendix A," ii, v.

77. Kamokila would later become a fierce opponent of U.S. statehood. For more on her Hawaiian nationalism and anti-statehood advocacy, see Saranillio, *Unsustainable Empire*, 99–129.

78. "Appendix B. Report of Special Committee on Leprosy Investigations," in *Report . . . Ended June 30, 1919*, 61.

79. "Appendix B," 58.

80. Guglyk and Bloombaum, *Maʻi Hoʻokaʻawale*, 38–41.

81. For example, Burke, *Lifebuoy Men, Lux Women*.

82. Quoted in Hanley and Bushnell, *Pilgrimage and Exile*, 297. A letter from a woman named Emma Holi reported that in her youth, she and other girlfriends snuck out to the homes of Dr. William J. Goodhue and Superintendent John D. McVeigh in the settlement. Letters from Emma and Moses Holi, February 19, 1909; 335-12, HSA.

83. In 1909, two boys climbed Kalihi Hospital's high board fence and ventured into the city several times, causing consternation for BOH officials. The board adopted a resolution that rule breakers at Kalihi would be sent to Molokai. "Patients Must Obey the Rules," *Hawaiian Gazette*, July 30, 1909; 334-37, HSA. Adolescent boy inmates later discussed slipping the compound's fence in the 1930s and 1940s, but girls at Kalihi Hospital did not, perhaps because girls faced steeper social consequences. Henry Nalaielua, who entered Kalihi Hospital in 1936 at age ten, made jaunts with other boys to the outside town, as did Edwin Lelepali, who entered Kalihi in 1937 at age ten. Nalaielua, *No Footprints*, 28. Lelepali's oral history is in Langlas, McGuire, and Juvik, "Voices of Kalaupapa."

84. 334-35 Kalihi, HSA. Kahawaii's and Mary Akakao's records are cases 479 and 497, Box 21 (Medical Examination Records 1904–1905); MER, HSA respectively. From Kekaha, Kauaʻi, Mary Akakao was admitted to detention on February 25, 1905, at age twenty; she was recorded as half-Samoan, half-Hawaiian. Akakao died in the settlement at age twenty-two on September 10, 1908. HD-3, HSA. Kahawaii was one of over one hundred patients that signed up for re-examination by the Board of Health in 1909. Nahauowaileia, "Nanaia Na Maʻi o Molokai."

85. This portrait of Kahawaii may have been taken by Father Julliotte; however, it was also included in at least two albums compiled by later Catholic brothers or fathers serving at Kalaupapa settlement. PA 1017 (Molokai), Box 3 and PA 1019 (Molokai), Box 5; Special Collection I: Photographic Forms: Albums; RG IX.A-2; CSH.

86. Mouritz, *Path of the Destroyer*, 140.

87. *Hawaiian Gazette*, July 18, 1893.

88. Meyer, "Appendix N," cxxxvii.

89. *Hawaiian Gazette*, July 18, 1893; *Ka Makaainana*, February 5, 1894; "Na Maʻi Lepera i Hookuu ia Mai," *Kuokoa Home Rula*, December 17, 1909.

90. *Hawaii Holomua* 3, no. 286, August 17, 1893.

91. "Ua Makemake e Noho i Kalaupapa," *Ka Nupepa Kuokoa*, August 7, 1903. McVeigh, who was haole, functioned as judge and jury in the settlement.

92. "E Kaiehuia aku ana," *Ka Makaainana*, February 5, 1894.

93. Perhaps the most famous case of a family refusing to separate was Pi'ilani and Kaluaiko'olau. Pi'ilani wanted to be a kōkua for her husband Kaluaiko'olau, who had been ordered to surrender as a leprosy patient. When they were not allowed to go to Molokai together, they escaped with their young son Kaleimanu to the valley of Kalalau, Kaua'i, in 1893. When haole sheriffs from the pro-U.S. provisional government attempted to capture them, Kaluaiko'olau shot and killed one deputy and wounded two others. Kaluaiko'olau and Kaleimanu died of leprosy, and Pi'ilani emerged from Kalalau valley in 1897. "True Story of Kaluaiko'olau."

94. Lahela Kanewa's record is case 737, Box 16 (Medical Examination Records 1907–1908); MER, HSA. Kanewa's kōkua petition is referenced in Vol. 15 Minutes, HSA. The Kanewa family's numerous visitation permits are recorded in 331 Vol. 115, HSA. Two years later, in May 1910, one of their children, George, was sentenced to Molokai. Joseph Kanewa predeceased his wife Lahela in the settlement in 1911, and Lahela Kanewa died in the settlement on March 18, 1916, at the age of forty-eight. George died in May 1918 at age twenty-two. HD-3 and HD-4, HSA.

95. The BOH denied some of these kōkua petitions from family members without explanation. Petitions approved by the BOH seem to have required favorable character assessments of the inmate and kōkua by powerful settlement superintendent John "Jack" McVeigh. The board followed McVeigh's recommendations uniformly. Vol. 16 Minutes, HSA. However, patients wrote to the BOH, accusing McVeigh of stealing pigs, bribery, and socializing with unmarried women patients from Bishop Home. Handwritten patient letters from Emma and Moses Holi are in 335-12 (1909), HSA.

96. *Hawaiian Gazette,* June 25, 1909; 334-37, HSA. After nineteen of these legislative resolutions passed in 1909, eleven people held in leprosy institutions were released from custody with clearance certificates. The nine people released from Molokai were Charles Wainui, O. Kaimu, J. W. Puiehaka, J. K. Alapai, John Kaapuni, Kahele Kana, Kealiiahonui, Naiwi, and Augusta Freitas. Two boys were released from Kalihi Boys' Home. The territorial resolutions are in 335-11, HSA.

97. "Wehe i Kapili Hookoo ia Loko," *Ka Leo o Ka Lahui,* April 17, 1896. I am grateful to Noelani Arista, who alerted me to this article. Arista's translation used with permission.

98. "Hoomanao Ana i Ka Mea i Hala," *Ka Nupepa Kuokoa,* October 18, 1912.

99. Feet and hands were particularly favored visual subjects, since they were inspected for ulcers that indicated nerve damage from leprosy.

100. In late nineteenth-century photographs, kāhili bearers stand above ali'i. Kāhili, the feather standard, was the sacred symbol of ali'i; attendants held these above the chief's head.

101. Thirty-year-old Jessie Kaena was admitted to Kalihi Hospital on February 12, 1903, and exiled to Molokai on March 24, 1903. Kaena's record is case 251, Box 17 (Medical Examination Records 1903); MER, HSA. Between 1904 and 1910, Jessie

and Kalani had at least four children in the settlement: Lilia Kilikina, born 1904; Helen, born 1906; Joe, born 1908; and Jessie, born 1910. Jessie Kaena died on July 27, 1913, at age forty. Malaea (also spelled Maraea or Maria) Hakalau was from Puʻuhale, Oʻahu, and a widow. She and her fourteen-year-old daughter Imaikalani Hakalau were admitted as suspects to Kalihi Hospital on June 28, 1904. Malaea was sent to Kalaupapa on July 19, 1904. Their records are cases 420 and 421, Box 20 (Medical Examination Records 1904); MER, HSA. HD-3 and HD-5; HSA. Malaea married Pilipo (Philip) Puaalau at Kalaupapa in December 1904. She died in 1915 at age fifty-one. Imaikalani Hakalau gave birth to three children in the settlement between 1910 and 1913. HD-A and HD-C; HSA.

102. The women performers' discrepant pursuit of modern fashion in the form of gowns, hats, and jewelry allowed them to assert themselves as cosmopolitan Native subjects in ways that countered Hawaiian nationalist politics and U.S. empire-building. See Imada, *Aloha America,* especially 83–88.

103. In other extant portraits in CSH, at least two people posed with photographs of loved ones from whom they were separated. One woman named Halekunihi, who was born in Maui and exiled in 1899, held a large framed portrait in her lap that was refracted back to her kin in the newly shot portrait. Another boy whose name is unknown wore a photograph pin on his lapel. In a contemporary U.S. context, Nicole R. Fleetwood has analyzed how vernacular photography strengthens "carceral intimacy" between incarcerated people and their loved ones. "Posing in Prison."

104. L-8 (Letter from John to Mr. Damien, Pauoa, Oahu, February 18, 1889) and L-80 (Letter from D. Waiola to Fr. Damien, Kukuihaele, Hawaii, June 23, 1880); Folder #D-31 (Letters translated by Hawaiian to English by Thomas K. Maunupau); Box VIII-D.1.; Damien Archives, Series D; Diocese Special Collection, Record Group VIII; CSH. In the latter letter, Waiola asked about ten dollars he had sent to Father Damien for clothes for Julia, Andrews, and Moepili of Kohala.

105. *Report . . . Ending June 30, 1907,* 140. Although some unmarried women patients lived in the Bishop Home, where laundry facilities were available, the home would not have been able to launder the majority of clothing for patients in the settlement.

106. Nalaielua, *No Footprints,* 57.

CHAPTER 4. DREAMING IN PICTURES: QUEER KINSHIP
AND SUBALTERN FAMILY ALBUMS

1. Edmond, *Leprosy and Empire;* Bashford, *Imperial Hygiene.* Historian Janine Richardson has written, "[F]or while leprosy meant a life sentence on Molokaʻi, it did not mean the end of reproductive life." Richardson, "None of Them Came for Me," 3.

2. There are no aggregate statistics on how many babies were born in the Molokai settlement during its hundred-year history, but the number was likely in the thou-

sands. In a single twelve-month period in 1907–1908, there were seventy-one births, which increased the settlement population by nearly 10 percent. *Report . . . Ended June 30, 1908*, 115. Non-leprous children of patients were removed from Molokai and placed in gender-segregated group homes: Kapiʻolani Home for Girls (1885–1938) and the Kalihi Boys' Home (1908–1937), both on the island of Oʻahu. Richardson, "None of Them Came for Me," 1.

3. Halberstam, *Queer Time and Place*, 1.

4. Expanding on Halberstam's theorizing of queer time, Alison Kafer argues that disability is already at work in formulations of queer temporality, as people experiencing disability are out of step, "out of time," or "obstacles to the arc of progress." Kafer, *Feminist Queer Crip*, 28, 35. In a related vein, Ellen Samuels describes herself being in "crip time," with its unpredictable loss, incapacity, and liberation. "Six Ways of Looking at Crip Time."

5. I do not disclose the name of this female patient exiled in the mid-1900s. Kaʻohulani McGuire, personal communication, April 16, 2019.

6. Cvetkovitch, *Archive of Feelings;* Brown and Phu, *Feeling Photography*, 19.

7. di Leonardo, "Female World of Cards and Holidays" 442; Holland, "History, Memory, and the Family Album," 9.

8. The practices and uses of photographic portraiture in subordinated and subaltern communities have been analyzed by many scholars. See Wexler, "More Perfect Likeness"; Pegler-Gordon, *In Sight of America;* Smith, "Baby's Picture Is Always Treasured"; Imada, *Aloha America;* Pinney, *Camera Indica.* However, to my knowledge there are few extant collections of vernacular photographs produced over a period of time by institutionalized people, disabled people, and incarcerated people. These include photographs taken by a child from the Heiltsuk Nation institutionalized at St. Michael's Indian Residential School in British Columbia, Canada, in the 1930s and 1940s; vernacular family photographs taken by Japanese American photographer Bill Manbo incarcerated at Heart Mountain, Wyoming, internment camp during World War II; and photographs taken by mostly white American patients confined to the U.S. national leprosarium in Carville, Louisiana, in the twentieth century. Muller, *Colors of Confinement.*

9. Chung-Hoon and Hedgcock, "Racial Aspects of Leprosy," 127.

10. For patient admission demographics, see *Care and Treatment of Leprous Persons*, 5. The 1921 BOH report more precisely records that out of 481 settlement patients, 388 were Hawaiian and part-Hawaiian, 32 Portuguese, 17 Chinese, 14 Filipino, 11 Japanese, and 11 Korean. However, only one American, one Belgian, and three Germans were patients. *Report . . . Ending June 30, 1921*, 37. With interracial relationships, marriage, and sexual encounters in territorial Hawaiʻi, people of various Hawaiian-haole (white), Hawaiian-Asian, and Asian-haole backgrounds received intense social scientific study. See for instance the work of sociologist Romanzo Adams and his social science laboratory based at the University of Hawaiʻi, including *Interracial Marriage in Hawaii.* Beyond sociological studies, however, people who lived at the Molokai settlement retained diverse Indigenous and racial genealogies and identifications far more than formal, state-oriented

classifications. For example, a woman recorded as "Oriental" at birth had a much more complex racial and ethnic background—her father was Japanese and her mother Portuguese and Native Hawaiian. This woman later married a man whose father was Native Hawaiian and whose mother was Chinese-Hawaiian.

11. Chapter XVI, An Act Relating to Divorce, in *Laws of His Majesty Kamehameha V . . . 1870*, 18.

12. Patients interviewed for Gugelyk and Bloombaum's *Ma'i Ho'oka'awale* describe how the BOH incentivized sterilization as leverage when patients sought permission to leave the settlement.

13. The Hawai'i State Department of Health (DOH) administers all medical and social services for former Hansen's disease patient-residents at Kalaupapa. It also regulates visitor traffic into the park. Situated within Kalawao County, Kalaupapa settlement is governed by the state DOH director, who is Kalawao County's mayor. This anomalous legal and administrative jurisdiction is a legacy of Hansen's disease management that began in Hawai'i in 1865. The settlement's relationship with the National Park Service since 1980 is discussed in the epilogue.

14. On Jack Sing Kong, see Bell, "Servant of God," 1. By 1903, Goodhue was recording a complete history of every patient-inmate using photographs "illustrative of the more interesting cases," with some in large folios. Their location is unknown. *Report . . . Ending June 30, 1903*, 163.

15. My broader accounting and assessment of photography at KNHP leads me to a provisional claim that Native Hawaiian and Native Pacific Islander patients had access to equipment and interests in photography, although their collections were not yet fully processed or accessible for research at the time of this study.

16. Seki's camera was a Compco Miraflex with a plastic body manufactured in the 1950s.

17. Kato's civic leadership roles at Kalaupapa include Lions Club chapter treasurer and officer of the Japanese Society of Kalaupapa (later renamed Americans of Japanese Ancestry, or AJA Benevolent Society). He kept careful records for these organizations that are in EK, KNHP, but it is unknown whether he kept records of his own artistic pursuits.

18. HD-7, HSA. Frank Mark may have retained this Protestant affiliation after exile.

19. Langlas, McGuire, and Juvik, "Voices of Kalaupapa."

20. Ibid.

21. The practice of separating infants began after 1908 when a nursery was built in Kalaupapa. *Report . . . to the Legislative Assembly of 1884*, vii. See also Richardson, "None of Them Came for Me"; *Report . . . Ended June 30, 1909*, 197; Ikenaga, "Study of the Care of Children." In response, parents pleaded with the board to allow their infants to remain in the new nursery "near us" until they were of an "age to be sent away" to institutional homes on O'ahu. Vol. 15 Minutes, HSA.

22. Clara Kelehiwa was in all likelihood another Kalaupapa resident-patient. To date, little else is known about her. Frank Mark identifies a woman in a group snapshot who may be Clara. The occasion of their marriage is not featured in this album.

Clara may have died a few years into their marriage, as the 1940 U.S. census indicates Mark was widowed. He was then thirty-four years old.

23. Benjamin Apiki, captioned as "Ben Apiki" in the album, had married in Honolulu in 1925. His part-Japanese wife, Mamie Kaneta, who was non-leprous, was not allowed to join him at the settlement, but later appears to have entered as Benjamin's kōkua (caregiver). The 1940 U.S census listed them as living together as husband and wife in Kalaupapa.

24. Jay Prosser has proposed photography as an "awakening to loss." *Light in the Dark Room,* 8.

25. An infant whom Frank Mark captioned as "Sugihara, Jr.," may be Lydia Sugihara, who was born in October 1929 and died in the settlement in March 1931. She was the namesake of her mother. Her parents were Shigeru Richard Sugihara, a Japanese immigrant exiled in 1924 from Honolulu at age eighteen, and Lydia Kaleikini, a Kanaka 'Ōiwi woman born in Honolulu. Lydia Sugihara was listed in the 1930 U.S. census as an infant ward, meaning she was held in the settlement nursery. The Sugiharas had previously lost children because of the BOH's policy separating non-leprous children from leprous parents. Rachael, born in Kalaupapa in June 1927, was removed to Kapi'olani Girls' Home in May 1928, and Richard Sugihara Jr., born in August 1928, was removed to Kalihi Boys' Home in June 1929. Shigeru Richard Sugihara died in November 1932 and is buried next to one of his children, perhaps Lydia, in the Japanese section of Papaloa Cemetery. HD-7; Vol. 7 Folio; HD-B; and HD-C, HSA.

26. Brown and Davidmann, "Queering the Trans* Family Album," 190.

27. For further description of these islets, see Clark, *Kalaupapa Place Names,* 60, 63,

28. Prosser, *Light in the Dark Room,* 1. Prosser has discussed photographs as unconscious encounters with the dead, but Mark's encounters with death are more self-conscious than unconscious.

29. Mary Ann Apana, also known as Maliana Apana, died in 1933, while Mark likely was still making this album. She was eighteen years old. Lookie, whom Mark captioned "A True Friend," died in 1935. A tombstone in Papaloa Cemetery reads, "In memory of My pal Lookie, 1904–1935, Rest in Peace," and I speculate that this inscription may have been composed by Frank Mark himself. Apana's death is recorded in HD-7, HSA.

30. The woman Costa married in 1925 had been born in the settlement to patients. By 1920, she was living at Bishop Home, the institution for leprous girls and women operated by Catholic Franciscan sisters. She married a patient in 1921 and had divorced this man before marrying Costa.

31. Alfred Costa Photograph Album, KNHP. Alfred Costa is the pseudonym of a late patient.

32. Hof, "Something You Can Actually Pick Up," 381–82.

33. Mikhail Bakhtin defined the chronotope in literature; Martha Langford adapts the chronotope concept to the photographic album. Bakhtin, "Forms of Time"; Langford, *Suspended Conversations,* 44.

34. Swift, "Case of Keanu," 175; U.S. Treasury, Public Health Service, "Danger of Association." The latter used marital and sexual histories to assess the infection rate of "healthy" kōkua living in close proximity to settlement patients.

35. Ikenaga discusses this methodology of compiling and studying patients' complete life histories. "Study of the Care of Children," 24.

36. Langford, *Suspended Conversations,* 102.

37. Ibid., 97.

38. Halberstam, *Queer Art of Failure,* 73; Stockton, *Queer Child;* Edelman, *No Future.*

39. Kafer, *Feminist Queer Crip,* 35.

40. Ka'ohulani McGuire, personal communication, April 16, 2019.

41. Kato was a prolific painter as well as a photographer, and his handwritten signs are still visible in the settlement today.

42. Sloan et al., "Sulfone Therapy," 5.

43. William Malo and Makia Malo, "Coping Strategies for Making the Transition from Isolation Back into the Community," n.d., Speech to XIII International Leprosy Congress held in the Hague, Netherlands, SSC.

44. Saranillio, "Colliding Histories," 285.

45. Fujikane, "Introduction: Asian Settler Colonialism," 7–8.

46. Teaiwa, "Reading Paul Gauguin's Noa Noa," 590.

47. McVeigh Home was named after resident superintendent John "Jack" McVeigh, who had spearheaded the separate facility for white patients in 1908 with private donations. *Report . . . Ended June 30, 1909,* 190. The home opened in 1910. Because of dwindling numbers of white patients, McVeigh was housing some non-white patients by 1921. *Report . . . Ending June 30, 1921,* 39. Elizabeth Kuulei Bell recalled the life of her beloved Mormon elder and fellow Kalaupapa patient Jack Sing Kong. Sing wanted to transfer to McVeigh Home, which Bell knew as the home for "the important white people to live." Sing was Chinese, but he managed to be placed into the nicer home for whites administered by the Board of Health, rather than the Baldwin Home, run by Catholic brothers. Bell, "Servant of God," 1.

48. The Aloha Gang and Haleiwa Gang, respectively, are on Page 1-1; Album 11; Europe 1972 (Aloha Album 1) and Kodak Folder; Box 11; EK.

49. Page 46-1, Album 3; EK.

50. *Report . . . Ended June 30, 1919,* 58.

51. Spence, "Soap, Family Album Work"; Smith, "Baby's Picture Is Always Treasured."

52. Hirsch, *Family Frames,* 107.

53. di Leonardo, "Female World of Cards and Holidays," 442.

54. Ibid., 443.

55. Adamski, "Edward Kato."

56. Page 3-B1 (ca. 1973); Album 17; EK.

57. I am taking a cue from recent turns in queer studies that resist recovering subjects from a range of "negative affects." See Love, *Feeling Backward,* 31.

58. Donna Haraway analyzes intense relationships between human and non-human "companion species." *Companion Species Manifesto.*

59. Naihe Pukai's name also was recorded occasionally as Pukai Naihe. He was from Hanamāʻulu, Kauaʻi, and arrived in the settlement February 1889 at age fourteen. His first wife, Lilia Makaila, died in 1905. Their children were Lui Naihe, born in 1900; Robert Holt, born in 1903; and Victoria Naihe, born in 1905. Lui died in 1901; Robert was removed to Kalihi Boys' Home, and Victoria to Kapiʻolani Girls' Home. Robert was eventually discharged in 1919; Victoria died in 1908 after her discharge from the Girls' Home. Naihe Pukai and his second wife Kamai (or Kamae) Naihe were in a group of at least 133 inmates that signed up for BOH re-examination in 1909. He was not discharged, and he died in the settlement in March 1915 at age forty. 260 Box 30; HD-A; HD-C; HD-3; and HD-5, HSA; Nahauowaileia, "Nanaia Na Maʻi o Molokai."

60. The song "Baby Pakalana" was composed by Kalaupapa patient Helen Freitas Keao about her beloved cat. It was recorded by Molokai-born musician Melveen Leed on her album *Hawaiian Country* in 1975.

61. Gaddis, *Birdman of Alcatraz*, 64.

62. Kaʻohulani McGuire, personal communication, July 19, 2015. One of Gertrude Kaauwai's steak knives is in the KNHP collection.

63. Gertrude Roselani "Spitfire" Seabury Kaauwai, also known as "Gertie," was born in Olowalu, Maui, in 1932 and died in 2010. She was exiled in 1944. Her sister, Elizabeth Kahihikolo, joined her at Kalaupapa in 1956. Kaauwai's quotation about her stepmother is from her interview in *The Soul of Kalaupapa*, while her interview about her cats and separation from her children is in *Kalaupapa Heaven*.

64. Langlas, McGuire, and Juvik, *Voices of Kalaupapa*. Job and Cupcake Akamai were the names of two of Lelepali's dogs.

65. Ibid., 63–64.

66. KALA 21589 (cat painting) and KALA 21592 (dog painting); ER. Elaine Kim Remigio was born in Hāna, Maui, in 1922, arrived in Kalaupapa in 1943, and died in 2008. Her parents were immigrants from Korea to Hawaiʻi. Married in 1940, she was detained at Kalihi Hospital about a year later. She was separated from her young children after exile to Kalaupapa. She married a fellow patient, Justo Remigio, who died in 1989. Elaine bought the community bar from another patient, Mariano Rea, in the early 1990s and renamed it "Elaine's Place." The bar was a gathering space for people to get snacks, have a beer or soda, talk story, and socialize. She retired in 2003 and sold the bar to former patient Gloria Marks.

67. Erving Goffman discusses stigma as the ascription of a "spoiled identity" to a person. *Stigma.*

68. KNHP collection.

69. Nalaielua, *No Footprints*, 38.

70. Bell, "Servant of God."

71. Langlas, McGuire, and Juvik, eds., "Voices of Kalaupapa."

72. Garland-Thomson, *Staring*, 15.

73. *Oral Histories of the Native Hawaiian Elderly*, 276.

74. Foucault, *Birth of the Clinic*; Nalaielua, *No Footprints*, 18–19.

75. Zuromskis, *Snapshot Photography*, 39.

76. Ibid., 38.

77. Law, *Kalaupapa: A Portrait*.

78. Garland Thomson, *Extraordinary Bodies*.

79. Hevey, *Creatures Time Forgot*, 82.

80. The Aloha Gang were friends and family members from Maui and Kalaupapa. Album 11; Europe 1972 (Aloha Album 1); EK.

81. Zuromskis, *Snapshot Photography*, 38.

82. In consultation with one of Pete's close surrogates, who conveyed the late Pete's wishes, I am not publishing his surname.

83. Langford, *Suspended Conversations*, 5, 156.

84. Zuromskis, *Snapshot Photography*, 8, 10, 39.

EPILOGUE: HEALING ENCOUNTERS AT THE SETTLEMENT

1. Newly diagnosed patients in the United States and its territories are treated on an outpatient basis. Between 1949 and the abolition of Hawai'i's leprosy segregation policy in 1969, only thirty-two people were removed to Kalaupapa.

2. Since KNHP was established in 1980, the National Park Service (NPS) and the state of Hawai'i have negotiated a complicated set of land arrangements and responsibilities on the peninsula. NPS generally is responsible for infrastructure— providing non-medical maintenance of roads, utilities, and historical structures. It also has a curatorial facility (Hale Mālama) in the settlement for historical preservation and storage of archival materials. Concurrently the state Department of Health (DOH) manages patient-residents. It is an administrative inheritor of the Hawaiian Kingdom's Board of Health, which first established the settlement in 1865, and the territorial BOH. DOH is responsible for all medical and social services for patients, including food, housing, health care, visitor permits, and waste management. Whereas the rest of Molokai is part of Maui County, the park is administratively placed within Kalawao County and governed by the state DOH. After the last patient dies, the DOH will leave the peninsula and NPS will become the sole management authority. Langlas, McGuire, and Juvik, *Kalaupapa*, 108.

The patchwork of land jurisdictions in the peninsula is a legacy of colonization. The kingdom's BOH acquired land for the settlement on the Makanalua peninsula through purchase or exchange in 1865. The existing residents, or kama'aina, were themselves removed to make way for incarcerated patients. Inglis, *Ma'i Lepera*, 52. Today most of the actual KNHP lands are owned by the state of Hawai'i. KNHP either holds a lease or has a cooperative agreement for use of its lands. For instance, the land on which the settlement is located belongs to the Department of Hawaiian Home Lands, a state agency which manages state lands for the benefit of Native Hawaiians. The lands are leased to NPS until 2041. The eastern portion of the park is under the jurisdiction of the state Department of Land and Natural Resources (DLNR) and is used by the NPS under cooperative agreement. The Kalaupapa airport is under the jurisdiction of the state Department of Transportation (DOT).

3. In mid-2015, there were sixteen former Hansen's disease patients, with approximately nine living full-time in Kalaupapa. The resident staff consists of Hawaiʻi state DOH and federal NPS workers. Some of these workers are local people and Kānaka ʻŌiwi with ties to the peninsula. As of 2018, there were fourteen former Hansen's disease patients, but some live part-time in Kalaupapa.

4. As analyzed in chapter 3, "kōkua" was a social, labor, and administrative category of people who accompanied and cared for patients on an unpaid basis in the nineteenth and early twentieth century. By the 1940s, family members were no longer allowed to come to the settlement as kōkua. However, "kokua" (or "kokuas") is now the local English-language derivative used for non-patient workers at Kalaupapa, including state and federal workers. There are historical continuities between the two categories, as some kokuas today are kin of patients and have an additional incentive to work at Kalaupapa because of familial relationships at the settlement. However, kokuas do not live with the patients, and they are paid for their labor by either the state or the federal government. Kokuas must leave the settlement after their employment ends. Langlas, McGuire, and Juvik, *Kalaupapa,* 25, 40–41.

5. U.S. Department of the Interior, *Draft General Management Plan;* Lincoln, "Planning for Kalaupapa's Future."

6. Wong, "When the Last Patient Dies."

7. Chun, *No Nā Mamo,* 127.

8. The population of Oʻahu is nearly one million, while there are about 7,300 Molokai residents. Molokai and Oʻahu are separated by the rough Kaiwi Channel, which is known for its strong, unpredictable currents, swells, and winds. The hiking trail down from Kalaʻe, Molokai, is unreliable, while air travel is limited and expensive. Tourists have been able to ride mules down the trail, but riders have sustained serious falls. A landslide in December 2018 also damaged a bridge between trail switchbacks, shutting down the trail indefinitely. This has left residents and workers to rely on limited flights in and out of Kalaupapa airport.

9. Langlas, McGuire, and Juvik, "Voices of Kalaupapa."

10. Edwin K. Chung-Hoon, another Native Hawaiian physician, treated patients at Kalaupapa in the 1950s. Young, "Early Physicians," 28–29.

11. Dr. Brady's position at Kalaupapa was funded via an institutional commitment and contractual partnership between 1) the University of Hawaiʻi–Mānoa John A. Burns School of Medicine (JABSOM)'s Department of Native Hawaiian Health (DNHH) and 2) the State Department of Health. Brady already had been working for DNHH as a primary care physician, but divided his clinical appointment between the two units. Two other Hawaiian physicians from DNHH—Martina Kamaka and Peter Donnelly, both in family medicine—also joined the hui (group) treating HD patients at Kalaupapa settlement and Hale Mōhalu. S. Kalani Brady, personal communication, October 12, 2015.

12. When Lau Ola Clinic in Honolulu was closed by the University of Hawaiʻi JABSOM in 2017, Kalani Brady ceased treating patients there. However, he continues to tend to people at Kalaupapa. Brady, personal communication, July 9, 2018.

13. "Local" is a colloquial term referring to people born and raised in Hawaiʻi, usually Chinese, Japanese, Filipino, Portuguese, Hawaiian, or "hapa" ("part," therefore mixed-race) people. The category of local usually excludes whites or "haole." On huakaʻi, see Ledward, "ʻĀina-Based Learning," 35, 37. This field-based pedagogy often is a small-scale Hawaiian decolonizing project, such as farming and cooking internships that teach agricultural skills, food preparation, and healthy eating.

14. All names of huakaʻi participants, Kalaupapa residents, and visitors that are pseudonyms are marked with an asterisk or indicated as such in text. Hawaiian homesteads were created by a 1921 federal law known as the Hawaiian Homes Commission Act. This act aimed to rehabilitate Hawaiians by bringing them back to the land, but its beneficiaries were limited to "native Hawaiians" who could document at least 50 percent blood quantum. See Kauanui, *Hawaiian Blood*.

15. A few days after our trip, Dr. Brady would return with another group of summer interns with Hawaiʻi Pacific Health (HPH), the largest health-care system in Hawaiʻi. Like those on our huakaʻi, these HPH interns were college students who wished to pursue careers in health care. HPH owns four large hospitals on four islands: Wilcox, Pali Momi, Straub, and Kapiʻolani, as well as numerous outpatient clinics.

16. This day, the barge off-loaded used trucks, plastic Adirondack chairs, mattresses, and refrigerators for settlement residents.

17. Wong, "Lost Child of Kalaupapa." Michael Maruyama, the DOH's Hansen's disease branch chief, said, "There's no way of knowing how many children were taken away."

18. Contemporary patient rationales for excluding children from the settlement include their own forced separation from their children; not wishing workers to enjoy access to children when patients were forcibly separated from theirs; not wanting children to stare or make rude remarks at disabled or disfigured patients; and not wanting children to risk being injured by patients with low vision who still drive in the settlement. This policy means patients may not have their moʻopuna (grandchildren) visit. At the same time, NPS and State of Hawaiʻi DOH staff who have children must live separately from them.

19. In the summer of 2018, the bar closed for business and it is unclear if it will open again. With more cellular hotspots set up in the community, residents now have improved internet access in the main village. More people can be seen walking around with their mobile devices.

20. Kaʻohulani McGuire, personal communication, April 16, 2019.

21. Aunty Ellen* had one of her lower limbs amputated and used a wheelchair. She has since passed away.

22. A Hawaiʻi territorial law first passed in 1923 prohibited the taking and exhibition of photographs of leprosy patients confined at institutions without a written permit issued by the Board of Health. L 1923, c 78, §§1, 2 (April 21, 1923). In 1969 this

language was revised to prohibit photography of patients, excepting by professional staff, without the written permission of patients. Haw. Rev. Stat. §326–30; am L 1969, c 152, §7.

23. After Catholic Church services on Sunday, the student group would have been able to linger and chat with patients, but one student had to return to Honolulu and the group left before this brief opportunity.

24. During Brady's historical tour, the group had short, but warm, interactions with Uncle Daniel*, the patient who worked part-time at the KNHP bookstore. The bookstore is in the Americans of Japanese Ancestry (AJA) Buddhist Hall and sells Kalaupapa shirts, books, and park souvenirs.

25. Moku Puakala, a grassy field adjacent to St. Philomena Church in Kalawao, appears empty, but probably contains thousands of iwi (bones). Because thousands of people died on the peninsula from the late nineteenth century on, and individual graves could not be dug fast enough, patients may have been buried in the same ground. Wood, stone, and other materials were in short supply in the settlements, and even if individual markers and crosses had been erected, they would have deteriorated quickly.

26. In summer 2015, the graves of Richard Marks and Gertrude "Gertie" Kaauwai were adorned at Papaloa Cemetery.

27. The settlement celebrated its one-hundredth seal pup birth in January 2017, twenty years after the first recorded modern birth. "Kalaupapa National Historic Park Welcomes 100th Baby Monk Seal," Hawaii News Now, May 12, 2017. KNHP and most of the main Hawaiian Islands are a designated critical habitat for monk seals. U.S. Department of the Interior, National Park Service, *State of the Park Report,* 14.

28. At least eight monk seals have been killed by humans in topside Molokai since 2009, including three in 2018. It is a felony to harass or harm monk seals. "Molokai Leaders Chide Those Killing Monk Seals," *Maui News,* August 3, 2018. Kittinger et al., "Sociocultural Significance," 148. The writers assess heterogeneous Native Hawaiian approaches to monk seals that range from respect to hostility.

29. Brown et al., "Important Hawaiian Monk Seal," 323. Eric Brown is a marine ecologist at Kalaupapa National Historical Park.

30. Wu, "Malnourished Monk Seal Pup."

31. U.S. Department of Commerce, National Oceanic and Atmospheric Administration, National Marine Fisheries Service, "R006."

32. Kelleher, "Remote Home." Kahilihiwa died at Hale Mōhalu, Lēʻahi Hospital, at age seventy-nine in March 2021.

33. Staff and patients at the settlement were also rigidly separated. Fences were erected around staff quarters and a railing around the superintendent's office kept patients at a remove.

34. After the Kalaupapa nursery was built in 1908, patients were not allowed to touch their babies. However, they also did their best to circumvent these restrictions. One anonymous father said parents tried to keep their babies quiet after a home delivery. They held onto them as long as possible after delivery, but usually had

to send them to administrators the morning after. Oral history of Hawaiian male patient, age eight-one, who had spent sixty-seven years in Kalaupapa, in Gugelyk and Bloombaum, *Maʻi Hoʻokaʻawale,* 36–37.

35. Mele has been a sustaining part of the settlement experience and its people since its establishment. Exiled patients were haku mele (composers) of oli (chants) and Hawaiian-language and English songs such as "Bayview Home" and "Sunset of Kalaupapa, Song of the Sunset." The latter was composed around the 1940s by Samson Kuahine, who became blind. He played piano and upright bass; his Baldwin piano remains in Kalaupapa's McVeigh Hall. Inspired by Kalaupapa's history, waters, ʻāina, and people, contemporary musicians continue to write, record, and perform new mele, including "Waimaka Helelei" (the late Dennis Kamakahi and Stephen Inglis), "Ka Ua o Kalaupapa" (Manu Boyd and Hoʻokena), and "Waihānau" (Kainani Kahaunaele).

BIBLIOGRAPHY

MANUSCRIPT AND MEDIA COLLECTIONS

Arnsteiner Patres, Werne, Germany
    Eduard Arning Albums and Research Material
Congregation of the Sacred Hearts of Jesus and Mary U.S.A. Province, Honolulu,
    Hawai'i (CSH)
Hawaiian Historical Society, Honolulu, Hawai'i (HHS)
    Eduard Arning Collection
Hawai'i State Archives, Honolulu, Hawai'i (HSA)
    C. B. Cooper Collection
    Photograph Collection
        Series 259, Minutes of the Board of Health, 1858–1983
        Series 260, Records Related to Hansen's Disease, 1866–1981
        Series 331, Outgoing Letters of the Board of Health, 1865–1981
        Series 334, Incoming Letters of the Board of Health, 1850–1904
        Series 335, Correspondence of the Board of Health, 1905–1917
The Huntington Library, San Marino, California
    Papers of Jack London, Photograph Albums and Large Albums
    Nathaniel Bright Emerson Papers, 1766–1944 (NBE)
Kalaupapa National Historical Park, Kalaupapa, Hawai'i (KNHP)
    Caroline M. Reader Collection, 1978–1998, KALA 12364
    Edward Kato Papers, KALA 17804
    Franklin Mark Album, KALA-00366
    Elaine Remigio Collection
National Hansen's Disease Museum, Carville, Louisiana
    Stanley Stein Collection
National Library of Medicine, Bethesda, Maryland
    Public Health Service Hospitals Historical Collection, 1895–1982 (PHSH)
National Museum of Health and Medicine, Silver Spring, Maryland
    George McCoy Collection, OHA 225. Otis Historical Archives

Queen's Hospital Historical Room, Honolulu, Hawai'i
  Charles Bryant Cooper, M.D., Collection.

SELECTED NEWSPAPERS AND PERIODICALS

Daily Bulletin, Honolulu
Evening Bulletin, Honolulu
The Friend, Honolulu
Hawaiian Gazette
Hawaiian Star
Hawaii Holomua
Ka Hae Hawaii
Ka Leo o Ka Lahui
Ka Nupepa Kuokoa
Ka Oiaio
Ke Aloha Aina
Ke Ola o Hawaii
Ko Hawaii Paeaina
Kuokoa Home Rula
Les Missions Catholiques
Maui News
Pacific Commercial Advertiser
San Francisco Call

BOOKS, ARTICLES, LAWS, AND DIGITAL SOURCES

Abad, Kēhaunani. "The Long Journey Home." *Ka Wai Ola* 30, no. 10 (October 2013): 18–19.

Adams, Romanzo. *Interracial Marriage in Hawaii: A Study of the Mutually Conditional Process of Acculturation and Amalgamation.* New York: Macmillan, 1937.

Adamski, Mary. "Edward Kato, Outstanding Citizen from Kalaupapa." *Honolulu Star-Bulletin,* February 20, 1998.

Agamben, Giorgio. *Homo Sacer: Sovereign Power and Bare Life.* Stanford: Stanford University Press, 1998.

Ahuja, Neel. *Bioinsecurities: Disease Interventions, Empire, and the Government of Species.* Durham: Duke University Press, 2016.

Alazard, Ildephonse. "Un Incendie à Molokaï." *Les Missions Catholiques* 1961 (January 4, 1907): 9–12.

Allen, Harrison. "A Study of Hawaiian Skulls." *Transactions of the Wagner Free Institute of Science of Philadelphia* 4 (January 1896): 7–55.

Amirault, Chris. "Posing the Subject of Early Medical Photography." *Discourse* 16, no. 2 (Winter 1993–1994): 51–76.

An Act to Provide for the Investigation of Leprosy, with Special Reference to the Care and Treatment of Lepers in Hawaii, March 3, 1905, Public Law 176, U.S. Statutes at Large 33 (1905): 1009.

"The Alleged Communication of Leprosy by Inoculation." *British Medical Journal* 1, no. 1535 (May 31, 1890): 1262.

Anderson, Warwick. "The Case of the Archive." *Critical Inquiry* 39, no. 3 (Spring 2013): 532–47.

———. *Colonial Pathologies: American Tropical Medicine, Race, and Hygiene in the Philippines*. Durham: Duke University Press, 2006.

———. "Leprosy and Citizenship." *Positions* 6, no. 3 (August 1998): 707–30.

Andrews, Lew. "'Fine Island Views': The Photography of Alonzo Gartley." *History of Photography* 25, no. 3 (Autumn 2001): 219–39.

"Appendix B. Report of Special Committee on Leprosy Investigations." In *Report of the President of the Board of Health of the Territory of Hawaii for the Twelve Months Ended June 30, 1919*. Honolulu: Advertiser Publishing Co., 1920.

"Appendix O. Copy of Correspondence between the Board of Health and Dr. Edward Arning." In *Appendix to the Report on Leprosy of the President of the Board of Health to the Legislative Assembly of 1886*, lv–lix. Honolulu: P. C. Advertiser Steam Print, 1886.

"Appendix U. Copy of Correspondence between Hon. C. R. Bishop, and others, and the President of the Board of Health, in regard to Dr. Edward Arning." In *Appendix to the Report on Leprosy of the President of the Board of Health to the Legislative Assembly of 1886*, lx–lxviii. Honolulu: P. C. Advertiser Steam Print, 1886.

Armitage, Kimo. *The Healers*. Honolulu: University of Hawai'i Press, 2016.

Arning, Eduard. "Appendix E. Dr. Arning's Report." In *Report of the President of the Board of Health to the Legislative Assembly of 1884*, liii–lxi. Honolulu: P. C. Advertiser Steam Print, 1884.

———. "'Eine Lepra-Impfung beim Menschen' und Demonstration einer Sammlung von Lepraabgüssen." In *Verhandlungen der Deutschen Dermatologischen Gesellschaft: Erster Congress gehalten zu Prag 10–12 Juni 1889*, edited by Filipp von Pick and Albert Neisser, 9–25. Vienna: Wilhelm Braumüller, 1889.

———. "A Lecture by Eduard Arning to the Berlin Anthropological Society in 1887." In *Old Hawaii: An Ethnography of Hawai'i in the 1880s Based on the Research and Collections of Eduard Arning in the Ethnologisches Museum, Berlin*, edited by Adrienne L. Kaeppler, Markus Schindlbeck, and Gisela E. Speidel, translated by Gisela E. Speidel, 49–60. Berlin: Ethnologisches Museum, 2008.

———. "Old Hawai'i: The 1931 Monograph by Eduard Arning." In *Old Hawaii: An Ethnography of Hawai'i in the 1880s Based on the Research and Collections of Eduard Arning in the Ethnologisches Museum, Berlin*, edited by Adrienne L. Kaeppler, Markus Schindlbeck, and Gisela E. Speidel, translated by Gisela E. Speidel, 61–261. Berlin: Ethnologisches Museum, 2008.

Arning, Edward. "Appendix E. Dr. Arning's Report." In *Report of the President of the Board of Health to the Legislative Assembly of 1884*, liii–lxi. Honolulu: P. C. Advertiser Steam Print, 1884.

———. "Appendix I. Report by Dr. Edward Arning." In *Appendix to the Report on Leprosy of the President of the Board of Health to the Legislative Assembly of 1886*, xxxvii–liv. Honolulu: P. C. Advertiser Steam Print, 1886.

Arnold, David. "Leprosy: From 'Imperial Danger' to Postcolonial History—An Afterword." *Journal of Pacific History* 52, no. 3 (2017), 407–19.

Ayau, Edward Halealoha. "Hui Mālama i Nā Kūpuna o Hawai'i Nei Part 1: Empowerment through Education." April 30, 2020. https://kawaiola.news/i-mana-i-ka-'oiwi/hui-malama-i-na-kupuna-o-hawaii-nei-part-1-empowerment-through-education/.

Azoulay, Ariella. "Archive." *Political Concepts: A Critical Lexicon* 1 (Winter 2011). www.politicalconcepts.org/issue1/archive/.

Bakhtin, Mikhail. "Forms of Time and of the Chronotope in the Novel." In *The Dialogic Imagination: Four Essays,* edited by Michael Holquist, translated by Caryl Emerson and Michael Holquist, 84–258. Austin: University of Texas Press, 1981.

Barthes, Roland. *Camera Lucida: Reflections on Photography.* New York: Hill and Wang, 1980.

Bashford, Alison. *Imperial Hygiene: A Critical History of Colonialism, Nationalism and Public Health.* New York: Palgrave MacMillan, 2004.

Baynton, Douglas C. "Disability and the Justification of Inequality in American History." In *The New Disability History: American Perspectives,* edited by Paul K. Longmore and Lauri Umansky, 33–57. New York: New York University Press, 2001.

Beckwith, Ruthie-Marie. *Disability Servitude: From Peonage to Poverty.* New York: Palgrave McMillan, 2016.

Bell, Kuulei. "A Servant of God: Jack Sing Kong." *Mormon Pacific Historical Society,* 13, no. 1 (1992): 1–4.

Benjamin, Walter. "A Short History of Photography." *Screen* 13, no. 1 (Spring 1972): 5–26.

———. "The Work of Art in the Age of Mechanical Reproduction." In *Illuminations,* edited by Hannah Arendt, translated by Harry Zohn, 217–52. New York: Schocken, 1968.

Bergmann, Anna. "Tödliche Menschenexperimente in Kolonialgebieten: Die Lepraforschung des Arztes Eduard Arning auf Hawaii 1883–1886." In *Macht und Anteil an der Weltherrschaft: Berlin und der deutsche Kolonialismus,* edited by Ulrich van der Heyden and Joachim Zeller, 141–48. Münster: Unrast-Verlag, 2005.

Berkowitz, Carin. "Introduction: Beyond Illustrations." *Bulletin of the History of Medicine* 89, no. 2 (2015): 165–70.

Biennial Report of the President of the Board of Health to the Legislature of the Hawaiian Kingdom, Session of 1888. Honolulu: Hawaiian Gazette Co., 1888.

Biennial Report of the President of the Board of Health to the Legislature of the Hawaiian Kingdom, Session of 1890. Honolulu: Hawaiian Gazette Co., 1890.

Biennial Report of the President of the Board of Health to the Legislature of the Hawaiian Kingdom, Session of 1892. Honolulu: Hawaiian Gazette Co., 1892.

Binford, C. H. "The History and Study of Leprosy in Hawaii." *Public Health Reports, 1896–1970* 51, no. 15 (April 10, 1936): 415–23.

Binford, Chapman H., and Daniel H. Connor, eds. *Pathology of Tropical and Extraordinary Diseases.* Vol 1. Washington, DC: Armed Forces Institute of Pathology, 1976.

Bishop, S. E. *Why Are the Hawaiians Dying Out? Or, Elements of Disability for the Survival among the Hawaiian People.* S.n., 1888.

Blaisdell, Kekuni. "Historical and Cultural Aspects of Native Hawaiian Health." *Social Process in Hawaii* 32 (1989): 1–22.

Bloombaum, Milton, and Ted Gugelyk. "Attitudes towards Leprosy." *Social Process in Hawaii* 27 (1979): 68–75.

Bottomley, A. Keith. "Parole in Transition: A Comparative Study of Origins, Developments, and Prospects for the 1990s." *Crime and Justice* 12 (1990): 319–74.

Brenner, Elma. "Recent Perspectives on Leprosy in Medieval Western Europe." *History Compass* 8, no. 5 (May 2010): 386–406. DOI: https://doi.org/10.1111/j.1478-0542.2009.00674.x.

Briggs, Laura. "The Race of Hysteria: 'Overcivilization' and the 'Savage' Woman in Late Nineteenth-Century Obstetrics and Gynecology." *American Quarterly* 52, no. 2 (June 2000): 246–73.

Brilliant, Richard. *Portraiture.* Cambridge: Harvard University Press, 1991.

Brockway, Zebulon Reed. *Fifty Years of Prison Service: An Autobiography.* New York: Country Life Press, 1912.

Brookes, Barbara. "Pictures of People, Pictures of Places: Photography and the Asylum." In *Exhibiting Madness in Museums: Remembering Psychiatry through Collections and Display,* edited by Catherine Coleborne and Dolly MacKinnon, 30–47. New York: Routledge, 2011.

Brown, Elspeth H., and Sara Davidmann. "Queering the Trans* Family Album: Elspeth H. Brown and Sara Davidmann, in Conversation." *Radical History Review* 122 (May 2015): 188–200.

Brown, Elspeth H., and Thy Phu, eds. *Feeling Photography.* Durham: Duke University Press, 2014.

Brown, Eric, Guy Hughes, Randall Watanuki, Thea C. Johanos, and Tracy Wurth. "The Emergence of an Important Hawaiian Monk Seal (Monachus schauinslandi) Pupping Area at Kalaupapa, Moloka'i, in the Main Hawaiian Islands." *Aquatic Mammals* 37, no. 3 (2011): 319–25. DOI 10.1578/AM.37.3.2011.319.

Browne, G. Waldo. *The Paradise of the Pacific: The Hawaiian Islands.* Boston: Dana Estes and Co., 1900.

Buerger, Janet E. "Art Photography in Dresden, 1899–1900: An Eye on the German Avant-Garde at the Turn of the Century." *Image* 27, no. 2 (June 1984): 1–24.

Burch, Susan. "'Dislocated Histories': The Canton Asylum for Insane Indians." *Women, Gender, and Families of Color* 2, no. 2 (Fall 2014), 141–62.

Burke, Timothy. *Lifebuoy Men, Lux Women: Commodification, Consumption, and Cleanliness in Modern Zimbabwe.* Durham: Duke University Press, 1996.

Burns, Stanley. *Early Medical Photography in America, 1839–1883.* New York: Burns Archive, 1983.

Bushnell, O. A. "Dr. Edward Arning: The First Microbiologist in Hawaii." *Hawaiian Journal of History* 1 (1967): 3–30.

———. "Hawaii's First Medical School." In *Hawaii Historical Review: Selected Readings,* edited by Richard A. Greer, 107–21. Honolulu: Hawaiian Historical Society, 1969.

———. "The United States Leprosy Investigation Station at Kalawao." *Hawaiian Journal of History* 2 (1968): 76–94.

Campt, Tina M. *Listening to Images.* Durham: Duke University Press, 2017.

Care and Treatment of Leprous Persons in the Territory of Hawaii. S. Doc. No. 72–570 (1933).

Care and Treatment of Persons Afflicted with Leprosy, S. Rep. 64–306 (1916).

Cartsen, Janet. *Cultures of Relatedness: New Approaches to the Study of Kinship.* Cambridge: Cambridge University Press, 2000.

Caswell, Michelle. *Archiving the Unspeakable: Silence, Memory, and the Photographic Record in Cambodia.* Madison: University of Wisconsin Press, 2014.

Chang, David A. *The World and All the Things upon It: Native Hawaiian Geographies of Exploration.* Minneapolis: University of Minnesota Press, 2016.

Ching, Stuart W. H. "Portraits of Kalaupapa Residents by Father Joseph Julliotte, SS.CC." *Hawaiian Journal of History* 50 (2016): 145–49.

Chun, Malcolm Nāea. *Kāhuna: Traditions of Hawaiian Medicinal Priests and Healing Practitioners.* Honolulu: First People's Productions, 2016.

———. *No Nā Mamo: Traditional and Contemporary Hawaiian Beliefs and Practices.* Honolulu: University of Hawai'i Press, 2011.

Chung-Hoon, Edwin K., and Grace Hedgcock. "Racial Aspects of Leprosy and Recent Therapeutic Advances." *Hawaii Medical Journal* 16, no. 2 (November–December 1956): 125–30.

Clark, John R. K. *Kalaupapa Place Names: Waikolu to Nihoa.* Honolulu: University of Hawai'i Press, 2018.

Cole, Simon A. *Suspect Identities: A History of Fingerprinting and Criminal Identification.* Cambridge: Harvard University Press, 2001.

Compiled Laws of the Hawaiian Kingdom, Published by Authority. Honolulu, 1884.

"The Contagious Nature of Leprosy." *British Medical Journal* 2, no. 1456 (November 24, 1888): 1171–72.

Cottle, G. F. "Photographs of Lepers." *United States Naval Medical Bulletin* 6, no. 2 (July 1912): 342–44.

Cox, Paul, dir. *Kalaupapa Heaven,* 2011.

Cvetkovitch, Ann. *An Archive of Feelings: Trauma, Sexuality, and Lesbian Public Cultures.* Durham: Duke University Press, 2003.

Daland, Judson. "Leprosy in the Hawaiian Islands." *Journal of the American Medical Association* 41 (November 7, 1903): 1125–29.

Danielssen, Daniel Cornelius, and C. W. Boeck. *Om spedalskhed*. Bergen: Christiania, 1847.

Daughton, J. P. *An Empire Divided: Religion, Republicanism, and the Making of French Colonialism, 1880–1914*. New York: Oxford University Press, 2006.

Davis, Lynn. *Na Pa'i Ki'i: The Photographers in the Hawaiian Islands, 1845–1900*. Honolulu: Bishop Museum Press, 1980.

———. *A Photographer in the Kingdom: Christian J. Hedemann's Early Images of Hawai'i*. Honolulu: Bishop Museum Press, 1988.

Daws, Gavan. *Holy Man: Father Damien of Molokai*. Honolulu: University of Hawai'i Press, 1989.

Didi-Huberman, Georges. *Invention of Hysteria: Charcot and the Photographic Iconography of the Salpêtrière*. Cambridge: MIT Press, 2003.

Dolmage, Jay. *Disabled upon Arrival: Eugenics, Immigration, and the Construction of Race and Disability*. Columbus: Ohio State University Press, 2018.

Douglas, Mary. *Purity and Danger*. New York: Routledge, 1966.

Edelman, Lee. *No Future: Queer Theory and the Death Drive*. Durham: Duke University Press, 2004.

Edmond, Rod. *Leprosy and Empire: A Medical and Cultural History*. Cambridge: Cambridge University Press, 2006.

Edwards, Elizabeth. "Photographic 'Types': The Pursuit of Method." *Visual Anthropology* 3, no. 2–3 (1990): 235–58.

Ehring, Franz. "Leprosy Illustration in Medical Literature." *International Journal of Dermatology* 33, no. 12 (December 1994): 872–83.

Elks, Martin A. "Believing Is Seeing: Visual Conventions in Barr's Classification of the "Feeble-Minded." *Mental Retardation* 42, no. 5 (October 2004): 371–82.

Emerson, N. B. "Report of Dr. N. B. Emerson on a Visit Made to the Leper Settlement, March 1882." In *Supplement, Leprosy in Hawaii, Extracts from Reports of Presidents of the Board of Health, Government Physicians and Others, and from Official Records: In Regard to Leprosy before and after the Passage of the Act to Prevent the Spread of Leprosy, Approved January 3rd, 1865*, 122–29. Honolulu: Daily Bulletin Steam Print, 1886.

Erevelles, Nirmalla. *Disability and Difference in Global Contexts: Towards a Transformative Body Politic*. New York: Macmillan, 2011.

"The Etiology of Leprosy." *British Medical Journal* 1, no. 1523 (March 8, 1890): 555–57.

"Expenses of Special Sanitary Committee in Visiting Kalawao." *Pacific Commercial Advertiser Supplement,* June 8, 1878.

Fanon, Frantz. *A Dying Colonialism*. New York: Grove Press, 1965.

Fitch, George L. "Appendix A. General Report by Dr. Fitch." In *Report of the President of the Board of Health to the Legislative Assembly of 1884*, i–ix. Honolulu: P. C. Advertiser Steam Print, 1884.

———. "Appendix E. Report of Dr. G. L. Fitch." In *Appendix to the Report on Leprosy of the President of the Board of Health to the Legislative Assembly of 1886*, xviii–xxxvi. Honolulu: P. C. Advertiser Steam Print, 1886.

———. "The Etiology of Leprosy." *Medical Record: A Weekly Journal of Medicine and Surgery* 42, no. 11 (September 10, 1892): 293–303.

———. "General Report by Dr. Fitch, 1884, to the Honorable Board of Health." In *Supplement, Leprosy in Hawaii, Extracts from Reports of Presidents of the Board of Health, Government Physicians and Others, and from Official Records: In Regard to Leprosy before and after the Passage of the Act to Prevent the Spread of Leprosy, Approved January 3rd, 1865*, 140–45. Honolulu: Daily Bulletin Steam Print, 1886.

———. "Leprosy." *Pacific Medical and Surgical Journal and Western Lancet* 28, no. 10 (October 1885): 526–44.

———. "Report of Dr. G. L. Fitch, Medical Superintendent of the Branch Hospital at Kakaako, and Resident Physician of Honolulu, March 1882." In *Supplement, Leprosy in Hawaii, Extracts from Reports of Presidents of the Board of Health, Government Physicians and Others, and from Official Records: In Regard to Leprosy before and after the Passage of the Act to Prevent the Spread of Leprosy, Approved January 3rd, 1865*, 117–22. Honolulu: Daily Bulletin Steam Print, 1886.

Fleetwood, Nicole R. "Posing in Prison, Family Photographs, Emotional Labor, and Carceral Intimacy." *Public Culture* 27, no. 3 (2015): 487–511.

Forrester, Izola. "The Strange Case of John Early: The True Story of the Closed Door in the Brick Wall between the Outcast Husband and the Faithful Wife." *Munsey's Magazine* 41, no. 6 (September 1909): 773–81.

Foucault, Michel. *The Birth of the Clinic: An Archaeology of Medical Perception*. New York: Vintage, 1973.

———. *The History of Sexuality. Volume I. An Introduction*. Translated by Robert Hurley. New York: Vintage, 1990 [1978].

———. *Society Must Be Defended: Lectures at the Collège de France, 1975–1976*. Edited by Mauro Bertani and Alessandro Fontana. New York: Picador, 2003.

Fujikane, Candace. "Introduction: Asian Settler Colonialism in the U.S. Colony of Hawai'i." In *Asian Settler Colonialism: From Local Governance to the Habits of Everyday Life*, edited by Candace Fujikane and Jonathan Okamura, 1–42. Honolulu: University of Hawai'i Press, 2008.

Gaddis, Thomas E. *Birdman of Alcatraz: The Story of Robert Stroud*. New York: Aeonian Press, 1955.

Garland Thomson, Rosemarie. *Extraordinary Bodies: Figuring Disability in American Culture and Literature*. New York: Columbia University Press, 1997.

———. "Seeing the Disabled: Visual Rhetorics of Disability in Popular Photography." In *The New Disability History: American Perspectives*, edited by Paul K. Longmore and Lauri Umansky, 335–74. New York: New York University Press, 2001.

Garland-Thomson, Rosemarie. *Staring: How We Look*. New York. Oxford University Press, 2009.

Gibson, Mary. *Born to Crime: Cesare Lombroso and the Origins of Biological Criminology.* Westport, CT: Praeger, 2002.

Gilman, Sander A. *Disease and Representation: Images of Illness from Madness to AIDS.* Ithaca: Cornell University Press, 1988.

Goffman, Erving. *Asylums: Essays on the Condition of the Social Situation of Mental Patients and Other Inmates.* New York: Anchor Books, 1961.

———. *Stigma: Notes on the Management of Spoiled Identity.* New York: Simon and Schuster, 1963.

Goodhue, E. S. "The Cure of Leprosy an Established Fact." *American Medicine* 8, no. 3 (March 1913): 187–90.

———. "The Physician in Hawaii." *Journal of the American Medical Association* 34, no. 3 (January 20, 1900): 138–44.

———. "The Surgical Cure of Leprosy Based on a New Theory of Infection." *New York Medical Journal* 98, no. 6 (August 9, 1913): 266–68.

Goodyear-Ka'ōpua, Noelani. "Reproducing the Ropes of Resistance: Hawaiian Studies Methodologies." In *Kanaka 'Ōiwi Methodologies: Mo'olelo and Metaphor,* edited by Katrina-Ann R. Kapā'anaokalāokeola Nākoa Oliviera and Erin Kahunawaika'ala Wright, 1–29. Honolulu: University of Hawai'i Press, 2016.

Gould, Stephen Jay. *The Mismeasure of Man.* New York: Norton, 1996.

Greene, Linda W. *Exile in Paradise: The Isolation of Hawaii's Leprosy Victims and Development of Kalaupapa Settlement, 1865 to the Present.* U.S. Department of the Interior. National Park Service. Alaska/Pacific/Northwest/Western Team. Kalaupapa National Historic Park: 1985.

Greenwell, Jean. "Doctor Georges Phillipe Trousseau, Royal Physician." *Hawaiian Journal of History* 25 (1991): 121–45.

Guglyk, Ted, and Milton Bloombaum. *Ma'i Ho'oka'awale: The Separating Sickness.* Honolulu: Social Science Research Institute, University of Hawai'i, 1979.

Gussow, Zachary. *Leprosy, Racism, and Public Health: Social Policy in Chronic Disease Control.* Boulder: Westview Press, 1989.

Gussow, Zachary, and George S. Tracy. "Stigma and the Leprosy Phenomenon: The Social History of the Disease in the Nineteenth and Twentieth Centuries." *Bulletin of the History of Medicine* 44, no. 5 (September–October 1970): 425–29.

Hagan, M. "Leprosy on the Hawaiian Islands." *Southern California Practitioner* 1, no. 3 (March 1886): 85–91.

Halberstam, J. Jack. *In a Queer Time and Place: Transgender Bodies, Subcultural Lives.* New York: New York University Press, 2005.

———. *The Queer Art of Failure.* Durham: Duke University Press, 2011.

Hale Mohalu: Land of Joy, Land of Pain. Honolulu: Hale Mohalu 'Ohana, 2013.

Haley, Sarah. *No Mercy Here: Gender, Punishment, and the Making of Jim Crow Modernity.* Chapel Hill: University of North Carolina Press, 2016.

Halperin, David M., and Valerie Traub. "Beyond Gay Pride." In *Gay Shame,* edited by David M. Halperin and Valerie Traub, 3–40. Chicago: University of Chicago Press, 2009.

Hanley, Mary Laurence, and O. A. Bushnell. *Pilgrimage and Exile: Mother Marianne of Molokai*. Honolulu: University of Hawai'i Press, 1991.

Haraway, Donna. *The Companion Species Manifesto: Dogs, People, and Significant Otherness*. Chicago: Prickly Paradigm Press, 2003.

Hattori, Anne Perez. "Re-membering the Past: Photography, Leprosy and the Chamorros of Guam, 1898–1924." *Journal of Pacific History* 46, no. 3 (December 2011): 293–318.

Heinrich, Ari (Larissa) N. *The Afterlife of Images: Translating the Pathological Body between China and the West*. Durham: Duke University Press, 2008.

Herman, R. D. K. "Out of Sight, Out of Mind, Out of Power: Leprosy, Race, and Colonization in Hawai'i." *Hūlili: Multidisciplinary Research on Hawaiian Well-Being* 6 (2010): 271–301.

Hevey, David. *The Creatures Time Forgot: Photography and Disability Imagery*. London: Routledge, 1992.

Hirsch, Marianne. *Family Frames: Photography Narrative and Postmemory*. Cambridge: Harvard University Press, 1997.

Hof, Katrina. "Something You Can Actually Pick Up: Scrapbooking as a Form of Forum of Cultural Citizenship." *European Journal of Cultural Studies* 9, no. 3 (2006): 363–84.

Holland, Patricia. "Introduction: History, Memory, and the Family Album." In *Family Snaps: The Meanings of Domestic Photography*, edited by Jo Spence and Patricia Holland, 1–14. London: Virago, 1991.

Hoppe, Trevor. *Punishing Disease: HIV and the Criminalization of Sickness*. Berkeley: University of California Press, 2018.

Ikenaga, Hazel. "A Study of the Care of Children under the Jurisdiction of the Territorial Board of Hospitals and Settlement, 1933–1949." MSW thesis, University of Hawai'i, 1950.

Imada, Adria L. *Aloha America: Hula Circuits through the U.S. Empire*. Durham: Duke University Press, 2012.

———. "Aloha 'Oe: Settler Colonial Nostalgia and the Genealogy of a Love Song." *American Indian Culture and Research Journal* 37, no. 2 (2013): 35–52.

———. "A Decolonial Disability Studies?" *Disability Studies Quarterly* 37, no. 3 (Summer 2017). DOI: http://dx.doi.org/10.18061/dsq.v37i3.

In the Matter of Kaipu, 2 D. Haw. 215 (1904).

Inglis, Kerri A. *Ma'i Lepera: Disease and Displacement in Nineteenth-Century Hawai'i*. Honolulu: University of Hawai'i Press, 2013.

———. "Nā Hoa o Ka Pilikia (Friends of Affliction): A Sense of Community in the Molokai Leprosy Settlement of 19th Century Hawai'i." *Journal of Pacific History* 52, no. 3 (November 2017): 287–301.

Johnson, Walter. "On Agency." *Journal of Social History* 37, no. 1 (Autumn 2003): 113–24.

Jones, David S., Scott H. Podolsky, and Jeremy A. Greene. "The Burden of Disease and the Changing Task of Medicine." *New England Journal of Medicine* 366, no. 25 (June 21, 2012): 2333–38.

Jourdan, Vital. *Le Père Damien de Veuster de la Congrégation des Sacrés-Coeurs, Picpus, Apôtre des Lépreux, 1840–1889.* Paris: Maison-Mère, 1931.

Kaeppler, Adrienne L. "Eduard Arning: Ethnographic Photographer of Hawai'i." In *A Glimpse into Paradise/Blick ins Paradies Historical Photographs of Polynesia,* edited by Marisol Fuchs, Gesa Grimme, and Jeanette Kokott, 86–99. Hamburg, Museum für Völkerkunde, 2014.

———. "Eduard Arning's Hawaiian Collections." *Hawaiian Journal of History* 29 (1995): 179–83.

Kaeppler, Adrienne L., Markus Schindlbeck, and Gisela E. Speidel, eds. *Old Hawaii: An Ethnography of Hawai'i in the 1880s Based on the Research and Collections of Eduard Arning in the Ethnologisches Museum, Berlin.* Translated by Gisela E. Speidel. Berlin: Ethnologisches Museum, 2008.

Kafer, Alison. *Feminist Queer Crip.* Bloomington: Indiana University Press, 2013.

Kaipu v. Pinkham, 51 U.S. 1191 (1907).

Kalisch, Philip A. "The Strange Case of John Early: A Study of the Stigma of Leprosy." *International Journal of Leprosy* 40, no. 5 (1972): 291–305.

Kauanui, J. Kēhaulani. *Hawaiian Blood: Colonialism and the Politics of Sovereignty and Indigeneity.* Durham: Duke University Press, 2008.

———. *Paradoxes of Hawaiian Sovereignty: Land, Sex, and the Colonial Politics of State Nationalism.* Durham: Duke University Press, 2018.

Kealakai, M. A. "He Hoomanao Kanikau no Mrs. Akiu M. Kealakai i Hala." *Ka Oiaio,* August 31, 1894.

Kelleher, Jennifer Sinco. "Remote Home of Leprosy Patients Could Open Door Wider." *Honolulu Star-Advertiser,* May 4, 2015.

Kim, Eleana. *Adopted Territory: Transnational Korean Adoptees and the Politics of Belonging.* Durham: Duke University Press, 2000.

Kim, Eunjung. *Curative Violence: Rehabilitating Disability, Gender, and Sexuality in Modern Korea.* Durham: Duke University Press, 2017.

Kittinger, John N., Trisann Māhealani Bambico, Trisha Kehaulani Watson, and Edward W. Glazier. "Sociocultural Significance of the Endangered Hawaiian Monk Seal and the Human Dimensions of Conservation Planning." *Endangered Species Research* 17 (2012): 139–56. DOI: 10.3354/esr00423.

Kunstphotographie um 1900: Die Sammlung Ernst Juhl. Hamburg: Museum für Kunst und Gewerbe, 1989.

Kunzel, Regina. *Criminal Intimacy: Prison and the Uneven History of Modern American Sexuality.* University of Chicago Press, 2008.

———. "Queer History, Mad History, and the Politics of Health." *American Quarterly* 69, no. 2 (June 2017): 315–19.

Lange, Raeburn. "Leprosy in the Cook Islands, 1890–1925." *Journal of Pacific History* 52, no. 3 (November 2017): 302–24. DOI: 10.1080/00223344.2017 .1379117.

Langford, Martha. *Suspended Conversations: The Afterlife of Memory in Photographic Albums.* Montreal: McGill-Queen's University Press, 2001.

Langlas, Charles, Kaʻohulani McGuire, and Sonia Juvik. *Kalaupapa, 2002–2005: A Summary Report of the Kalaupapa Ethnographic Project*. National Park Service, 2008.

———, eds. "Voices of Kalaupapa: Oral Histories of Six Kalaupapa Hansen's Disease Patients." National Park Service manuscript, May 2007.

Latour, Bruno. *Science in Action: How to Follow Scientists and Engineers through Society*. Philadelphia: Open University Press, 1987.

Law, Anwei Skinses. *Kalaupapa: A Collective History*. Honolulu: University of Hawaiʻi Press, 2012.

———. *Kalaupapa: A Portrait*. Honolulu: Bishop Museum Press, 1989.

Lawrence, Susan C. *Privacy and the Past: Research, Law, Archives, Ethics*. New Brunswick: Rutgers University Press, 2016.

Laws of His Majesty Kamehameha V, King of the Hawaiian Islands. Passed by the Legislative Assembly at Its Session, 1864–65. Honolulu, 1865.

Laws of His Majesty Kamehameha V, Passed by the Legislative Assembly at Its Session, 1870. Honolulu, 1870.

Lederer, Susan. *Subjected to Science: Human Experimentation in America before the Second World War*. Baltimore: Johns Hopkins University Press, 1995.

Ledward, Brandon C. "ʻĀina-Based Learning Is New Old Wisdom at Work." *Hūlili: Multidisciplinary Research on Hawaiian Well-Being* 9 (2013): 35–48.

Leonardo, Micaela di. "The Female World of Cards and Holidays: Women, Families, and the Work of Kinship." *Signs: Journal of Women in Culture and Society* 12, no. 3 (Spring 1987): 440–53.

"Leprosy in the Hawaiian Islands. Its Humanitarian and Financial Burden: An Unparalleled Instance of Public Philanthropy." In *Report of the President of the Board of Health for the Territory of Hawaii for the Year Ending June 30, 1904*, 11–19. Honolulu: Bulletin Publishing Co., 1904.

Les Missions Catholiques. Vol 39. Lyon: Bureaux des Missions Catholiques.

Letter from the Surgeon-General of the Marine-Hospital Service Presenting a Report Relating to the Origin and Prevalence of Leprosy in the United States. S. Doc. No. 57–269 (1902).

Lincoln, Mileka. "Planning for Kalaupapa's Future Means Remembering Its Past." May 7, 2015. www.hawaiinewsnow.com/story/29011284/planning-for-kalaupapas-future-means-remembering-its-past/.

Lindsey, Edward. "Historical Sketch of the Indeterminate Sentence and the Parole System." *Journal of the American Institute of Criminal Law and Criminology* 16, no. 1 (1925): 9–69.

Livingston, Julie. "Figuring the Tumor in Botswana." *Raritan: A Quarterly Review* 34, no. 1 (Summer 2014): 10–24.

———. *Improvising Medicine: An African Oncology Ward in an Emerging Cancer Epidemic*. Durham: Duke University Press, 2012.

Lomawaima, K. Tsianina. "Domesticity in the Federal Indian Schools: The Power of Authority over Mind and Body." In *Deviant Bodies: Critical Perspectives on*

Difference in Science and Popular Culture, edited by Jennifer Terry and Jacqueline Urla, 197–218. Bloomington: Indiana University Press, 1995.

———. *They Called It Prairie Light: The Story of the Chilocco Indian School.* Lincoln: University of Nebraska Press, 1994.

Lombroso, Cesare. *Criminal Man.* Translated by Mary Gibson and Nicole Hahn Rafter. Durham: Duke University Press, 2004.

Lombroso, Cesare, and Guglielmo Ferrero. *Criminal Woman, the Prostitute, and the Normal Woman.* Translated by Nicole Hahn Rafter and Mary Gibson. Durham: Duke University Press, 2004.

Love, Heather. *Feeling Backward: Loss and the Politics of Queer History.* Cambridge: Harvard University Press, 2007.

Luker, Vicki, and Jane Buckingham. "Histories of Leprosy: Subjectivities, Community and Pacific Worlds." *Journal of Pacific History* 52, no. 3 (2017): 265–86.

Lydon, Jane. *Eye Contact: Photographing Indigenous Australians.* Durham: Duke University Press, 2005.

Maehle, Andreas-Holger. "The Search for Objective Communication: Medical Photography in the Nineteenth Century." In *Non-Verbal Communication in Science Prior to 1900*, edited by Renata G. Mazzolini, 563–86. Firenze: Leo S. Olschki, 1993.

Maialoha, S. K. "Na Mea Hou o ke Kahua Maʻi." *Ke Aloha Aina,* September 4, 1909.

McClintock, Anne. *Imperial Leather: Race, Gender, and Sexuality in the Colonial Contest.* New York: Routledge, 1995.

McCurry, Justin. "'Like Entering a Prison': Japan's Leprosy Sufferers Reflect on Decades of Pain." *Guardian,* April 13, 2016.

McDonald, J. T. "A Diagnostic Examination of One Hundred and Fifty Cases of Leprosy." *Journal of the American Medical Association* 40, no. 23 (June 6, 1903): 1567–69.

McDonald, J. T., and A. L. Dean. "The Constituents of Chaulmoogra Oil Effective in Leprosy." *Journal of the American Medical Association* 76, no. 22 (May 28, 1921): 1470–74.

McDonald, Marie A. *Ka Lei: The Lei of Hawaii.* Honolulu: Ku Paʻa, 1989.

McGrew, Henry Goulden. "Leprosy in the Hawaiian Islands." *American Lancet* 12, no. 5 (May 1888): 161–62.

Medak-Saltzman, Danika. "Transnational Indigenous Exchange: Rethinking Global Interactions of Indigenous Peoples at the 1904 St. Louis Exposition." *American Quarterly* 62, no. 3 (2010): 591–615.

Medical Century: The National Journal of Homoeopathic Medicine and Surgery 20, no. 11 (November 1913).

Merry, Sally Engle. *Colonizing Hawaii: The Cultural Power of the Law.* Princeton: Princeton University Press, 2000.

Meyer, R. W. "Appendix N, Report of R. W. Meyer, April 1886." In *Appendix to the Report on Leprosy of the President of the Board of Health to the Legislative Assembly of 1886*, cxxiv–cxli. Honolulu: P. C. Advertiser Steam Print, 1886.

Michael, Jerrold M. "The Public Health Service Leprosy Investigation Station on Molokai, Hawaii, 1909–1913—an Opportunity Lost." *Public Health Reports* 95, no. 3 (May–June 1980): 203–9.

Miller, Joaquin. "Lepers of Hawaii." *San Francisco Call* 78, no. 107, September 15, 1895, 13.

Mimura, Glen M. "A Dying West? Reimagining the Frontier in Frank Matsura's Photography, 1903–1913." *American Quarterly* 62, no. 3 (2010): 687–716.

Mittheilungen und Verhandlungen der Internationalen Wissenschaftlichen Lepra-conferenz zu Berlin im October 1897. Vol. 2. Berlin: August Hirschwald, 1898.

Mobley, Izetta Autumn. "Troublesome Properties: Millie and Christine McKoy, Disability, Photography, and the Enslaved Body." Paper presented at the 89th Annual Meeting of the American Association for the History of Medicine, Minneapolis, April 9, 2016.

Moblo, Pennie. "Blessed Damien of Moloka'i: The Critical Analysis of Contemporary Myth." *Ethnohistory* 44, no. 4 (Autumn 1997): 691–726.

———. "Ethnic Intersession: Leadership at Kalaupapa Leprosy Colony, 1871–1887." *Pacific Studies* 22, no. 2 (June 1999): 27–69.

———. "Institutionalising the Leper: Partisan Politics and the Evolution of Stigma in Post-Monarchy Hawai'i." *Journal of the Polynesian Society* 107, no. 3 (September 1998): 229–62.

The Molokai Settlement (Illustrated), Territory of Hawaii. Honolulu: Board of Health of the Territory of Hawaii, Hawaiian Gazette Co., 1907.

Montgomery, D. W. "Report of the Histological Examination of a Piece of Skin from Keanu's Forearm." *Occidental Medical Times* 4, no. 5 (June 1890): 302–3.

Moran, Michele T. *Colonizing Leprosy: Imperialism and the Politics of Public Health in the United States.* Chapel Hill: University of North Carolina Press, 2007.

Morrow, Prince A. ed. *Leprosy.* New York: William Wood & Co, 1899.

———. "Leprosy." In *A System of Genito-Urinary Diseases, Syphilology and Dermatology.* Vol. 3, edited by Prince A. Morrow, 562–610. New York: D. Appleton and Co., 1894.

———. "Leprosy and Annexation." *North American Review* 165, no. 492 (November 1897): 582–90.

———. "Personal Observations of Leprosy in Mexico and the Sandwich Islands." *New York Medical Journal* 50 (July 27, 1889): 84–89. Reprinted in *New York Medical Journal: A Weekly Review of Medicine,* edited by Frank P. Foster. New York: D. Appleton and Co., 1889.

———. *A System of Genito-Urinary Diseases, Syphilology and Dermatology,* Vol. 3. New York: D. Appleton and Co., 1894.

Mouritz, Arthur. *The Path of the Destroyer: A History of Leprosy in the Hawaiian Islands and Thirty Years Research into the Means by Which It Is Spread.* Honolulu: Honolulu Star Bulletin Co., 1916.

———. "Appendix K. Report of Arthur Mouritz, Resident Physician and Medical Superintendent at the Leper Settlement." In *Appendix to the Report on Leprosy of the President of the Board of Health to the Legislative Assembly of 1886*, lxxii–xcviii. Honolulu: P. C. Advertiser Steam Print, 1886.

Muir, Ernest. *Manual of Leprosy*. Baltimore: Williams and Wilkins Co., 1948.

Muller, Eric L., ed. *Colors of Confinement: Rare Kodachrome Photographs of Japanese American Incarceration in World War II*. Chapel Hill: University of North Carolina Press, 2012.

Mulvey, Laura. "Visual Pleasure and Narrative Cinema." *Screen* 16, no. 3 (Autumn 1975): 6–18.

Musick, John R. *Hawaii, Our New Possessions*. New York: Funk and Wagnalls Co., 1898.

Nahauowaileia, S. K. M. "Na Mea Hou o Kalaupapa." *Kuokoa Home Rula,* September 3, 1909.

———. "Nanaia Na Maʻi o Molokai." *Ka Nupepa Kuokoa,* October 29, 1909.

———. "Papa Inoa o Na Mai Lepera." *Ka Nupepa Kuokoa,* September 3, 1909.

Nakamura, Karen. "The Spectacle of Disability (Studies) in the Age of Trump." Keynote address at UCLA Disability as Spectacle Conference, Los Angeles, April 14, 2017.

Na Kanawai o Ka Moi Kamehameha Ke Alii o Ko Hawaii Pae Aina i Kauia e ka Hale Ahaolelo, Iloko o ka Ahaolelo o Na Makahiki. 1864–65. Honolulu, 1865.

Nalaielua, Henry Kalalahilimoku. *No Footprints in the Sand: A Memoir of Kalaupapa*. Honolulu: Watermark Publishing, 2006.

Ne, Harriet. *Tales of Molokai: The Voice of Harriet Ne*. Lāʻie: Institute for Polynesian Studies, 1992.

Neuse, Wilfried H. G., Norbert J. Neumann, Percy Lehmann, Thomas Jansen, and Gerd Plewig. "The History of Photography in Dermatology: Milestones from the Roots to the 20th Century." *Archives of Dermatology* 132 (December 1996): 1492–98.

Novak Gustainis, Emily R., and Phoebe Evans Letocha. "The Practice of Privacy." In *Innovation, Collaboration and Models: Proceedings of the CLIR Cataloging Hidden Special Collections and Archives Symposium*, March 2015 (CLIR pub. 169), 163–76. Washington, DC: Council on Library and Information Resource.

Ober, William B. "Can the Leper Change His Spots? The Iconography of Leprosy, Part I." *American Journal of Dermapathology* 5, no. 1 (February 1983): 43–58.

O'Day, J. Christopher. "Hawaii and Her Leprosy." *Medical Sentinel* 19, no. 8 (August 1911): 478–85.

———. "A Visit to the Leper Colony of Molokai, Hawaii." *The Urologic and Cutaneous Review* 19, no. 5 (May 1915): 247–52.

Oral Histories of the Native Hawaiian Elderly on the Islands of Hawaii, Kauai, Lanai, Maui and Molokai. Honolulu: Alu Like, Native Hawaiian Resource Center, 1989.

Osorio, Jonathan Kay Kamakawiwoʻole. *Dismembering Lāhui: A History of the Hawaiian Nation to 1887*. Honolulu: University of Hawaiʻi Press, 2002.

Ott, Katherine. "Contagion, Public Health, and the Visual Culture of Nineteenth-Century Skin." In *Imagining Illness: Public Health and Visual Culture,* edited by David Serlin, 85–107. Minneapolis: University of Minnesota Press, 2010.

"Out of the Darkness into the Light." *Paradise of the Pacific* 34, no. 12 (December 1921): 35–37.

Owens, Deirdre Cooper. *Medical Bondage: Race, Gender, and the Origins of American Gynecology.* Athens: University of Georgia Press, 2017.

Paniani, H. P. "Hoomanao Ana i Ka Mea i Hala." *Ka Nupepa Kuokoa,* October 18, 1912.

Parascandola, John. "Miracle at Carville: The Introduction of the Sulfones for the Treatment of Leprosy." *Pharmacy in History* 40, no. 2/3 (1998): 59–66.

Pegler-Gordon, Anna. *In Sight of America: Photography and the Development of U.S. Immigration Policy.* Berkeley: University of California Press, 2009.

Penny, H. Glenn. *Objects of Culture: Ethnology and Ethnographic Museums in Imperial Germany.* Chapel Hill: University of North Carolina Press, 2003.

Phu, Thy, Elspeth H. Brown, and Deepali Dewan. "The Family Camera Network." *Photography and Culture* 10, no. 2 (July 2017): 147–63.

Pinney, Christopher. *Camera Indica: The Social Life of Indian Photographs.* Chicago: University of Chicago Press, 1997.

———. "The Parallel Histories of Anthropology and Photography." In *Anthropology and Photography, 1860–1920,* edited by Elizabeth Edwards, 74–96. New Haven: Yale University Press, 1992.

Povinelli, Elizabeth. "Notes on Gridlock: Genealogy, Intimacy, Sexuality." *Public Culture* 14, no. 1 (2002): 215–38.

Prosser, Jay. *Light in the Dark Room: Photography and Loss.* Minneapolis: University of Minnesota Press, 2005.

Puar, Jasbir. *The Right to Maim: Debility, Capacity, Disability.* Durham: Duke University Press, 2017.

Pukui, Mary Kawena. *ʻŌlelo Noʻeau: Hawaiian Proverbs and Poetical Sayings.* Honolulu: Bishop Museum Press, 1983.

Pukui, Mary Kawena, and Samuel H. Elbert. *Hawaiian Dictionary: Revised and Enlarged Edition.* Honolulu: University of Hawaii Press, 1986.

Pukui, Mary Kawena, Samuel H. Elbert, and Esther T. Mookini. *Place Names of Hawaii.* Honolulu: University of Hawaii Press, 1966.

Pukui, Mary Kawena, E. W. Haertig, and Catherine A. Lee. *Nānā i Ke Kumu (Look to the Source).* Vols. 1 and 2. Honolulu: Hui Hānai, 2001.

Reed, Boardman. "Why Physicians Should Cultivate Photography." *Medical Record: A Weekly Journal of Medicine and Surgery* 36, no. 19 (November 9, 1889): 514–15.

Report of the Board of Health for the Biennial Period Ending December 31, 1897. Honolulu: Hawaiian Gazette Co., 1898.

Report of the President of the Board of Health of the Territory of Hawaii for the Eighteen Months Ending December 31, 1902. Honolulu: Bulletin Publishing Co., 1903.

Report of the President of the Board of Health of the Territory of Hawaii for the Fiscal Year Ended June 30, 1922. Honolulu: Honolulu Star-Bulletin, 1923.

Report of the President of the Board of Health of the Territory of Hawaii for the Six Months Ending June 30, 1903. Honolulu: Bulletin Publishing Co., 1903.

Report of the President of the Board of Health of the Territory of Hawaii for the Six Months Ending December 31st, 1906. Honolulu: Hawaiian Gazette Co., 1907.

Report of the President of the Board of Health of the Territory of Hawaii for the Twelve Months Ending June 30, 1907. Honolulu: Bulletin Publishing Co., 1907.

Report of the President of the Board of Health of the Territory of Hawaii for the Twelve Months Ended June 30, 1908. Honolulu: Bulletin Publishing Co., 1908.

Report of the President of the Board of Health of the Territory of Hawaii for the Twelve Months Ended June 30, 1909. Honolulu: Bulletin Publishing Co., 1909.

Report of the President of the Board of Health of the Territory of Hawaii for the Twelve Months Ended June 30, 1915. Honolulu: Hawaiian Gazette Co., 1915.

Report of the President of the Board of Health of the Territory of Hawaii for the Twelve Months Ended June 30, 1919. Honolulu: Advertiser Publishing Co., 1920.

Report of the President of the Board of Health of the Territory of Hawaii for the Twelve Months Ending June 30, 1921. Honolulu: Honolulu Star-Bulletin, 1921.

Report of the President of the Board of Health of the Territory of Hawaii for the Twelve Months Ended June 30, 1923. Honolulu: Honolulu Star-Bulletin, 1924.

Report of the President of the Board of Health of the Territory of Hawaii for the Year Ending June 30, 1904. Honolulu: Bulletin Publishing Co., 1904.

Report of the President of the Board of Health to the Legislative Assembly of 1884. Honolulu: P. C. Advertiser Steam Print, 1884.

"Report of the Special Sanitary Committee on the State of the Leper Settlement at Kalawao." *Pacific Commercial Advertiser Supplement,* June 8, 1878.

Reverby, Susan M. *Examining Tuskegee: The Infamous Syphilis Study and Its Legacy.* Chapel Hill: University of North Carolina Press, 2009.

Richardson, Janine M. "'None of Them Came for Me:' The Kapiʻolani Home for Girls, 1885–1938." *Hawaiian Journal of History* 42 (2008): 1–26.

Rifkin, Mark. "Debt and the Transnationalization of Hawaiʻi." *American Quarterly* 60, no. 1 (2008): 43–66.

Rodriguez, Dylan. *Forced Passages: Imprisoned Radical Intellectuals and the U.S. Prison System.* Minneapolis: University of Minnesota Press, 2006.

Rony, Fatima Tobing. *The Third Eye: Race, Cinema, and Ethnographic Spectacle.* Durham: Duke University Press, 1996.

Rothman, David J. *The Discovery of the Asylum: Social Order and Disorder in the New Republic.* New York: Routledge, 2002.

Samuels, Ellen. "Examining Millie and Christine McKoy: Where Enslavement and Enfreakment Meet." *Signs* 37, no. 1 (September 2011): 53–81.

———. "Six Ways of Looking at Crip Time." *Disability Studies Quarterly* 37, no. 3 (Summer 2017). DOI: http://dx.doi.org/10.18061/dsq.v37i3.

Saranillio, Dean Itsuji. "Colliding Histories: Hawaiʻi Statehood at the Intersection of Asians 'Ineligible to Citizenship' and Hawaiians 'Unfit for Self-Government.'" *Journal of Asian American Studies* 13, no. 3 (October 2010): 283–309.

————. *Unsustainable Empire: Alternative Histories of Hawai'i Statehood.* Durham: Duke University Press, 2018.

Schoofs, Robert. *Pioneers of the Faith: History of the Catholic Mission in Hawaii, 1827–1940.* Honolulu: Sturgis, 1978.

Schuessler, Jennifer. "Your Ancestors Were Slaves. Who Owns the Photos of Them?" *New York Times,* March 22, 2019.

Schweik, Susan. "Kicked to the Curb: Ugly Law Then and Now." *Harvard Civil Rights–Civil Liberties Law Review* 46, no. 1 (Winter 2011): 1–16.

————. *Ugly Laws: Disability in Public.* New York: New York University Press, 2009.

Segregation of Lepers, 5 Haw. 162 (1884).

Sekula, Allan. "The Body and the Archive." *October* 39 (Winter 1986): 3–64.

Shah, Nayan. *Contagious Divides: Epidemics and Race in San Francisco's Chinatown.* Berkeley: University of California Press, 2001.

Sharpe, Christina. *In the Wake: On Blackness and Being.* Durham: Duke University Press, 2016.

Silva, Noenoe K., and Pualeilani Fernandez. "Mai Ka 'Āina O Ka 'Eha'eha Mai: Testimonies of Hansen's Disease Patients in Hawai'i, 1866–1897." *Hawaiian Journal of History* 40 (2006): 75–97.

Simpson, Audra. "On Ethnographic Refusal: Indigeneity, 'Voice' and Colonial Citizenship." *Junctures* 9 (2007): 67–80.

Sloan, N. R., E. K. Chung-Hoon, M. E. Godfrey-Horan, and G. H. Hedgcock. "Sulfone Therapy in Leprosy: A Three Year Study." *International Journal of Leprosy* 18, no. 1 (January–March 1950): 1–9.

Smith, Linda Tuhiwai. *Decolonizing Methodologies: Research and Indigenous Peoples* London: Zed Books, 1999.

Smith, Shawn Michelle. "'Baby's Picture Is Always Treasured': Eugenics and the Reproduction of Whiteness in the Family Photograph Album." *Yale Journal of Criticism* 11, no. 1 (Spring 1998): 197–220.

Snyder, Sharon L., and David T. Mitchell. *Cultural Locations of Disability.* Chicago: University of Chicago Press, 2006.

Sontag, Susan. *Illness as Metaphor and AIDs and Its Metaphors.* New York: Doubleday, 1989.

————. *On Photography.* New York: Farrar, Straus and Giroux, 1977.

Spence, Jo. "Soap, Family Album Work . . . and Hope." In *Family Snaps: The Meanings of Domestic Photography,* edited by Jo Spence and Patricia Holland, 200–207. London: Virago, 1991.

"State Medical Society of Pennsylvania." *Boston Medical and Surgical Journal* 130, no. 24 (June 14, 1894): 600–601.

Steeno, Omar P. "Eduard Arning: 1855–1936." Unpublished manuscript, 2001.

Stepan, Nancy Leys. *Picturing Tropical Nature.* Ithaca: Cornell University Press, 2001.

Stevenson, Lisa. *Life Beside Itself: Imagining Care in the Canadian Arctic.* Berkeley: University of California Press, 2014.

Stockton, Kathryn Bond. *The Queer Child, or Growing Sideways in the Twentieth Century.* Durham: Duke University Press, 2009.

Stoler, Ann Laura. *Along the Archival Grain: Epistemic Anxieties and Colonial Common Sense.* Princeton: Princeton University Press, 2009.

———. *Carnal Knowledge and Imperial Power: Race and the Intimate in Colonial Rule.* Berkeley: University of California Press, 2010.

Strathern, Marilyn. "Displacing Knowledge: Technology and the Consequences for Kinship." In *Conceiving the New World Order: The Global Politics of Reproduction,* edited by Faye D. Ginsburg and Rayna Rapp, 346–64. Berkeley: University of California Press, 1995.

Supplement, Leprosy in Hawaii, Extracts from Reports of Presidents of the Board of Health, Government Physicians and Others, and from Official Records: In Regard to Leprosy before and after the Passage of the Act to Prevent the Spread of Leprosy, Approved January 3rd, 1865. Honolulu: Daily Bulletin Steam Print, 1886.

Swift, Sidney Bourne. "The Case of Keanu." *Occidental Medical Times* 4, no. 4 (April 1890): 171–75.

Tanaka, Kathyrn M. "'Life's First Night' and the Treatment of Hansen's Disease in Japan: A Translation and Introduction to Hōjō Tamio's Novella." *Asia-Pacific Journal* 13, no. 4 (January 19, 2015): 1–34.

Tayman, John. *The Colony: The Harrowing Story of the Exiles of Molokai.* New York: Scribner, 2006.

Teaiwa, Teresia. "Reading Paul Gauguin's Noa Noa with Epeli Hau'ofa's Kisses in the Nederends: Militourism, Feminism, and the 'Polynesian Body.'" In *Inside Out: Literature, Cultural Politics, and Identity in the New Pacific,* edited by Vilsoni Hereniko and Rob Wilson, 249–63. Oxford: Rowman and Littlefield, 1999.

Tebb, William. *The Recrudescence of Leprosy and Its Causation: A Popular Treatise.* London: Swan Sonnenschein and Co., 1893.

Thompson, J. Ashburton. "Leprosy in Hawaii: A Critical Enquiry." In *Mittheilungen und Verhandlungen der Internationalen Wissenschaftlichen Lepra-Conferenz zu Berlin im October 1897.* Vol. 2, 270–91. Berlin: August Hirschwald, 1898.

"The True Story of Kaluaiko'olau, or Ko'olau the Leper." [Original by Kahihina Kelekona]. Translated by Francis N. Frazier. *Hawaiian Journal of History* 21 (1987): 1–41.

Trask, Haunani-Kay. "The Birth of the Modern Hawaiian Movement: Kalama Valley, O'ahu." *Hawaiian Journal of History* 21 (1987): 126–53.

Tuck, Eve, and K. Wayne Yang. "R Words: Refusing Research." In *Humanizing Research: Decolonizing Qualitative Inquiry with Youth and Communities,* edited by Django Paris and Maisha T. Winn, 223–47. Los Angeles: Sage, 2014.

Turse, Nicholas. "Experimental Dreams, Ethical Nightmares: Leprosy, Isolation, and Human Experimentation in Nineteenth-Century Hawaii." In *Imagining Our Americas: Toward a Transnational Frame,* edited by Sandhya Shukla and Heidi Tinsman, 138–67. Durham: Duke University Press, 2007.

U.S. Department of Commerce. National Oceanic and Atmospheric Administration. National Marine Fisheries Service. Pacific Islands Regional Office. "R006:

The Legacy of Mama Eve." June 23, 2017. www.fisheries.noaa.gov/feature-story/
r006-legacy-mama-eve.

U.S. Department of the Interior. National Park Service. Pacific West Region. Kalaupapa National Historic Park. *Draft General Management Plan and Environmen-
tal Impact Statement*. Kalawao, Hawai'i, April 2015.

U.S. Department of the Interior. National Park Service. *State of the Park Report for
Kalaupapa National Historical Park*. State of the Park Series no. 21. Washington,
DC, 2015.

U.S. Department of the Interior. *Report of the Governor of Hawaii to the Secretary of
the Interior, 1920*. Washington, DC: GPO, 1920.

U.S. Treasury Department. Public Health and Marine-Hospital Service. *Transactions of the Second Annual Conference of State and Territorial Health Officers with
the United States Public Health and Marine-Hospital Service*. Washington, DC:
GPO, 1904.

U.S. Treasury Department. Public Health and Marine-Hospital Service. "V. A
Report upon the Treatment of Six Cases of Leprosy with Nastine (Deycke)." In
Studies upon Leprosy, by Walter R. Brinckerhoff and James T. Wayson, 3–11 and
plates I–X. Washington, DC: GPO, 1909.

U.S. Treasury Department. Public Health Service. "XX. The Danger of Association
with Lepers at the Molokai Settlement." In *Studies upon Leprosy, Public Health
Bulletin* 61 (July 1913), by George W. McCoy and William J. Goodhue, 7–10.
Washington, DC: GPO, 1913.

U.S. Treasury Department. Public Health Service. "The Treatment of Leprosy, with
Especial Reference to Some New Chaulmoogra Oil Derivatives." In *Public
Health Reports* 35, no. 4 (August 20, 1920), by J. T. McDonald, 1959–1974. Wash-
ington, DC: GPO, 1921.

U.S. Treasury Department. Public Health Service. "XXXV. Statistical Report on
Cases of Leprosy Which Have Left Segregation on Parole." In *Studies Upon Lep-
rosy, Public Health Bulletin* no. 130 (December 1922), by H. E. Hasseltine, 12–24.
Washington, DC: GPO, 1923.

U.S. Treasury Department. Public Health Service. "XXXVI. The Treatment of Leprosy with Derivatives of Chaulmoogra Oil." In *Studies upon Leprosy, Public Health
Bulletin* no. 141 (July 1924), by H. E. Hasseltine. 1–11. Washington, DC: GPO, 1924.

Vincent, Ethan, dir. *The Soul of Kalaupapa: Voices of Exile*. 2012. www.ethanvincent
.com/soul-of-kalaupapa.

Wald, Priscilla. *Contagious: Cultures, Carriers, and the Outbreak Narrative*. Durham: Duke University Press, 2008.

Wayson, James T. "Notes on Kalahi [*sic*] Hospital." *Archives of Dermatology and
Syphilology* 3, no. 1 (January 1921): 45–46.

Wayson, N. E. "Leprosy in Hawaii." *Leprosy Review* 3 no. 1 (1932): 9–17.

Weston, Kath. *Families We Choose: Lesbians, Gays, Kinship*. New York: Columbia
University Press, 1997.

Wexler, Alice. *The Woman Who Walked into the Sea: Huntington's and the Making
of a Genetic Disease*. New Haven: Yale University Press, 2008.

Wexler, Laura. "'A More Perfect Likeness': Frederick Douglass and the Image of the Nation." *Yale Review* 99, no. 4 (October 2011): 145–69.

———. "The State of the Album." *Photography and Culture* 10, no. 2 (July 2017): 99–103.

Wong, Alia. "A Lost Child of Kalaupapa." *Honolulu Civil Beat,* July 20, 2011. www .civilbeat.org/2011/07/12168-a-lost-child-of-kalaupapa/.

———. "When the Last Patient Dies." *Atlantic,* May 27, 2015.

Wong, Sterling. "Iwi Kūpuna Returning Home from Germany after More than a Century." December 1, 2017. https://kawaiola.news/moolelo/iwi-kupuna-returning-home-germany-century/.

Woods, Fred E. *Kalaupapa: The Mormon Experiences in an Exiled Community.* Salt Lake City: Brigham Young University, 2017.

———. *Reflections of Kalaupapa.* Lāʻie: Y Mountain Press, 2017.

Worboys, Michael. "Tropical Diseases." In *Companion Encyclopedia of the History of Medicine,* edited by W. F. Bynum and Roy Porter, 512–26. New York: Routledge, 1993.

Wu, Nina. "Malnourished Monk Seal Pup Rescued from Molokai." *Honolulu Star-Advertiser,* July 19, 2018.

Yanagisako, Sylvia Junko. *Producing Culture and Capital: Family Firms in Italy.* Princeton: Princeton University Press, 2002.

Young, Ben. "Early Physicians of Hawaiʻi and Reflections on the Emergence of Hawaiian Doctors." *Hūlili: Multidisciplinary Research on Hawaiian Well-Being* 10 (2015): 1–48.

Zimmerman, Andrew. "Adventures in the Skin Trade: German Anthropology and Colonial Corporeality." In *Worldly Provincialism: German Anthropology in the Age of Empire,* edited by H. Glenn Penny and Matti Bunzl, 156–78. Ann Arbor: University of Michigan Press, 2003.

———. *Anthropology and Antihumanism in Imperial Germany.* Chicago: University of Chicago Press, 2001.

Zinoman, Peter. *The Colonial Bastille: A History of Imprisonment in Vietnam, 1862–1940.* Berkeley: University of California Press, 2001.

Zuromskis, Catherine. *Snapshot Photography: The Lives of Images.* Cambridge: MIT Press, 2013.

INDEX

Note: Page references in *italics* refer to illustrative matter.

Act to Prevent the Spread of Leprosy (1865), xiii, 1–2, 8, 22, 75, 242n4, 257n28

Act to Provide for Investigation of Leprosy (1905), 273n111

affective care, 111–114, 126, 158–159, 186. *See also* kōkua (unpaid caregivers)

affective excess, 108–110, 118

African Americans, 21, 30, 136, 246n41, 253n120, 254n127, 257n29, 257n35, 274n126. *See also* slavery

Agamben, Giorgio, 19

Akakao, Mary, 147, 282n84

Akim, Mary (Keawe, Malia), 80–82, 266n36

Alapai, Edward, 147

Alazard, Ildephonse, 141

Alexander, Maria, 76, 266n25

Ali, Pepenui, 276n148

Aloha Gang, 180, 202, 288n48, 290n80

Aloisa, Louis, 273n112

Alvarez, Luis, 261n97

American Indians: 21, 254n127; boarding schools and, 126–127, 144, 278n17, 285n8. *See also* Indigenous people

"Among My Souvenirs" (song), 187

Anderson, Warwick, 72, 246n41, 250n82

animal companionship, 191–196, *197*, 289n60, 289n64

annexation of Hawai'i by United States, xiii, 5, 44, 61, 71, 73, 99, 252n110, 267n47, 272n98. *See also* Territory of Hawai'i

anthropology: British, 110, 259n62; German, 40, 43–46, 110, 257n27, 259n64, 260n78; medicine and, 39–40, 43–44; photography and, 247n47; physical, 54, 67, 78, 110. *See also* Arning, Eduard; salvage ethnography

anthropometry, identification system, 78, 110, 259n62

antibiotics. *See* sulfone antibiotic drugs

Apana, Mary Ann (Maliana), 171, 287n29

Apiki, Benjamin, 287n23

Apolo, Henry K., 100

archive of kin, 15–16, 18–20, 123. *See also* Board of Health (BOH); kinship

archive of skin: as term, 12; circulation of, 11, 14, 72–73, 97, 99, 105–107; disability and race in, 14–15; 102–107; production of, 72–75; as visual spectacle, 15. *See also* Board of Health (BOH); disability; medical photography

Arning, Eduard: as art photographer, 65–66, 262nn100–101; background of, 37–38, 39–40; Board of Health (BOH) and, 45, 47, 57, 261n93; carceral medicine and, 9–10, 45–46, 59; Emerson's support of, 64; as ethnographer, 38–39, 42–45, 57; Keanu and, 47–54, 57–58, 63, 66, 258n47, 258n50, 259nn54–55; on

mele (songs), 114, 210, 294n35. *See also*
names of specific songs
methodologies, research; vii–viii, 27–29,
74; Indigenous communities and, 27,
253n118; speculation and, 30. *See also*
ethics of restraint
Meyer, Rudolf, 277n13, 278n18
microbiology, xi–xii, 7, 40, 47–49, 135,
255n8
microscopic evidence, 81–83, 93
Les Missions Catholiques (publication),
141–142, 281n65, 281n66
Moku Puakala, Kalawao, 293n25
Molokai. *See* Makanalua peninsula; Kalaupapa settlement, Molokai; Kalawao
settlement, Molokai; Molokai settlement; topside Molokai
Molokai settlement: criteria for exile to, 9;
establishment of, 2, 290n2; Hawaiian
terms for, 2; Kānaka ʻŌiwi as largest
group at, 3, 242n8; medical missionaries
at, 10, 276n2, 280n59; medical photography at, 14, 59, 60, 104–105, 264n12,
262n104, 272n105; as natural prison, 2,
10; non-Hawaiian population of, 242n8,
243n11; number of incarcerated people
at, 4; photography at, 10–11, 16, 17, 68,
122, 139, 140–141, 142, 144, 148, 154–155,
157, 161, 163–164, 167, 169–170, 172,
184–185, 187–190, 192–194, 205; physicians at, 7, 14, 19, 35, 209, 255n9, 258n47,
273n116, 278n22; as term, xi. *See also*
archive of kin; archive of skin; Board of
Health (BOH); Kalawao settlement,
Molokai; Kalaupapa settlement,
Molokai; medical tourism
monk seals (Hawaiian), 222, 226–228, 231,
293nn27–28
moral hygiene, 138–149
Moran, Michelle, 107
Morrow, Prince A., 59–61, 99, 133, 261n82,
271n96
Mother's Day, 183–186
Mouritz, Arthur A., 14, 47, 127, 130, 134–
138, 149, 243n9, 257n26
mourning and grief, viii, 97, 151, 172, 188,
254n129, 275n142. *See also* kanikau;
loneliness

Mulvey, Laura, 15
mumps outbreaks, 6. *See also* epidemics
Museum für Völkerkunde. *See* Berlin
Ethnological Museum
muʻumuʻu, 119, 122, 277n3. *See also* clothing
Mycobacterium leprae (leprosy bacilli), xi, 4,
7, 47–48, 81–83, 93. *See also* leprosy
(Hansen's disease)

Naea, Cecelia Kalili, 111, 116, 118, 276n148
Nahauowaileia, S. K. M., 32–33, 254n128.
See also Maialoha, S. K.
Nailima, Joseph Hoaeae, 67–69, 262n105,
262n107, 263n109
Nailima, Kealoha, 54, 55, 57, 67–69,
260n65, 262n105, 262n107
Nailima, Kuheleloa (Kahalewai's brother),
69, 263n109
Nailima, Kuheleloa (Kahalewai's son), 69,
263n110
Nailima, Louis (Lui), 67, 262n105
Nailima, Louis Kahalewai, 67–69,
262n105, 262n107, 263nn109–110
Naiwi, 82, 267n41
Nakamura, Karen, 23
Nakuina, Emma Kaʻilikapuolono Metcalf,
83, 90, 267n46
Nakuina, Emma Kalanikupaulakea, 83, 90,
267n46
Nakuina, Moses, 90, 267n46
Nakuino, John W., 125–126, 277n13
Nalaielua, Henry, 158, 252n109, 282n83
Naluaai, 105, 274n118
Napoleon, Elizabeth Francis, 110, 274n130
National Institute of Health, 10, 106,
247n52
National Leprosarium, Carville, Louisiana,
xiii, 92, 107–108, 179, 181, 183, 215,
254n130, 273n111, 274n126, 285n8
National Park Service (NPS), 206–207,
286n13, 290n2, 291n3, 292n18. *See also*
Kalaupapa National Historical Park
(KNHP)
Native American Graves and Repatriation
Act (NAGPRA, 1990), 58
Native Hawaiians. *See* Kānaka ʻŌiwi
Native Hawaiian self-determination move-
ment, 26, 252n110

statehood, 177, 282n77. *See also* annexation of Hawai'i by United States; State of Hawai'i; Territory of Hawai'i

sterilization, coerced, 17, 147, 164, 195, 216, 286n12. *See also* eugenics

St. Francis Catholic Church, Kalaupapa, 141, 223, 228

stigma: defined by Goffman, 289n67; leprosy and, 4, 26, 131, 206, 216, 244n20, 251n91, 254n130; tuberculosis and, 244n18

Stockton, Kathryn Bond, 175

Stoler, Ann, 56, 67, 72, 90, 248n55

Stroud, Richard, 194–195

Sugihara, Lydia, 287n25

Sugihara, Lydia Kaleikini, 287n25

Sugihara, Shigeru Richard, 287n25

sulfone antibiotic drugs, xiii, 92, 97, 108, 158, 164, 176, 204–205, 241n1. *See also* Promin (sulfone drug); therapeutic treatments for leprosy

"Sunset of Kalaupapa, Song of the Sunset" (song), 294n35

Sunter, Sarah, 88–90, 268nn58–59

surveillance. *See* carceral medicine; criminality; medical incarceration; medical photography

suspect, as category, 9, 75, 95, 241n1 (intro.). *See also* Board of Health (BOH)

syphilis, 35, 40, 47, 58–59, 80, 99, 130, 132, 133, 135, 243n10, 254n127, 257n36, 258n52. *See also* epidemics

temporality: 11, 31, 37, 157, 174, 191, 230; crip and queer, 175–176; 285n4; non-normative, 161–162. *See also* emphemerality

temporary medical release, 161, 177, 205

Territory of Hawai'i: 24; Asian Americans in, 177; census by United States of, 10, 247n50; leprosy policies in, 163; parole (leprosy) in, 90, 95; tourism and, 98; U.S. Public Health Service and, 90–91, 101, 106. *See also* Board of Health (BOH); annexation of Hawai'i by United States

theft of burials, 58, 66, 261n80. *See also* iwi; repatriation

therapeutic treatments for leprosy: 90–95; chaulmoogra oil, 90, 92, 94–95, 97,

269n66, 269n75, 273n112; ethyl hydnocarpate, 94; radium, 97; sulfone antibiotic drugs, xiii, 92, 97, 108, 158, 164, 176, 204–205, 241n1 (intro.); wound care, 123–125, 145, 168. *See also* leprosy (Hansen's disease); medical experimentation

topside Molokai: as term, 253n119; 29, 191, 204, 207, 212, 224

tourism: 23–25, 98, 165, 177; dark, 28, 220–221; by people on medical release, 177, 179, 183, 199–202. *See also* medical tourism

Trousseau, Georges, 84, 267n49

tuberculosis, 4, 6, 40, 100, 244n18, 245nn31–32. *See also* epidemics

typhoid, 132, 136

"Typhoid Mary" (Mary Mallon), 132, 136, 280n55

Uncle Leonard, 228–231

Unea, John Taylor, 276n1

United States: American Indian boarding schools in, 126–127, 144, 278n17, 285n8; annexation of Hawai'i by, 5, 44, 61, 71, 99, 252n110, 267n47, 272n98; census of Hawai'i by, 10, 247n50; epidemics in, 6, 245n32; immigration restriction of Asians in, 243n10; leprosy cases in, 100; leprosy legislation in, 108; overthrow of Hawaiian Kingdom by, 5, 23, 44, 98, 99, 267n49; vaccination ruling in, 8. *See also* Territory of Hawai'i; U.S. Public Health Service

U.S. Committee on Public Health and National Quarantine, 100–101

U.S. Leprosy Investigation Station, Hawai'i, xiii, 91, 101, 106, 247n52, 269n75, 270n76, 273n111–112, 278n22. *See also* Kalihi Hospital and Detention Station, Honolulu

U.S. Public Health Service, 90–91, 99–101, 106

venereal disease, 6, 66, 132, 135. *See also* epidemics; sexuality; syphilis

Vietnam, 127, 278n17

Founded in 1893,
UNIVERSITY OF CALIFORNIA PRESS
publishes bold, progressive books and journals
on topics in the arts, humanities, social sciences,
and natural sciences—with a focus on social
justice issues—that inspire thought and action
among readers worldwide.

The UC PRESS FOUNDATION
raises funds to uphold the press's vital role
as an independent, nonprofit publisher, and
receives philanthropic support from a wide
range of individuals and institutions—and from
committed readers like you. To learn more, visit
ucpress.edu/supportus.

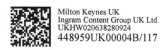